12 Strokes

Ferdinand K. Hui
Alejandro M. Spiotta
Michael J. Alexander • Ricardo A. Hanel
Blaise William Baxter
Editors

12 Strokes

A Case-based Guide to Acute Ischemic Stroke Management

Springer

Editors
Ferdinand K. Hui
Department of Radiology
Johns Hopkins Hospital
Baltimore, MD
USA

Alejandro M. Spiotta
Department of Neurosurgery
Medical University of South Carolina
Charleston, SC
USA

Michael J. Alexander
Department of Neurosurgery
Cedars-Sinai Medical Center
Los Angeles, CA
USA

Ricardo A. Hanel
Baptist Neurological Institute
Jacksonville, FL
USA

Blaise William Baxter
Department of Radiology
Lehigh Valley Health Network
Allentown, PA
USA

ISBN 978-3-030-56856-6 ISBN 978-3-030-56857-3 (eBook)
https://doi.org/10.1007/978-3-030-56857-3

This Springer imprint is published by the registered company Springer Nature Switzerland AG
The registered company address is: Gewerbestrasse 11, 6330 Cham, Switzerland

Foreword

Stroke Intervention is a revolution.

It can be argued that the discovery of penicillin in 1928 revolutionized medicine, providing a method to counter bacterial infections, a lethal condition so commonly encountered during the Great War. Stroke intervention is a highly impactful intervention that can improve the lives of a tremendous number of patients constrained by the high cost of devices, the need for highly experienced operators, and the exquisite coordination of many experts and stakeholders.

This book aims at those constraints, bringing together in one place technical, systemic, and procedural insights that the Stroke Interventionalist needs in preparation and in reflection for our patients.

It is with humility we place our thoughts in the reader's hands, hoping to speed up the delivery of care our patients so desperately need.

Citius, Fortius

Ferdinand K. Hui
Department of Radiology, Johns Hopkins Hospital
Baltimore, MD, USA

Alejandro M. Spiotta
Department of Neurosurgery, Medical University of South Carolina
Charleston, SC, USA

Michael J. Alexander
Department of Neurosurgery, Cedars-Sinai Medical Center
Los Angeles, CA, USA

Ricardo A. Hanel
Baptist Neurological Institute
Jacksonville, FL, USA

Blaise William Baxter
Department of Radiology, Lehigh Valley Health Network
Allentown, PA, USA

Preface

Therapeutic nihilism prevailed when stroke thrombectomies were done even as recently as 10 years ago. The entire thrombectomy process, including interfacility communication, triage, transportation, image acquisition, and the procedure itself, was unnecessarily physically and mentally cumbersome. The observed angiographic improvement was exciting but the actual functional improvement was modest. The delivery of stroke thrombectomy was painstaking. This therapeutic futility magnified the burden of being on call. Expectations were low.

Now, it is both surprising and gratifying to see residents and trainees talk about stroke thrombectomy with a much higher expectation of efficacy. The triage workflow at most busy thrombectomy-capable hospitals largely automates much of these once-cumbersome processes. Effective devices that have been proven with level 1A evidence are now available and familiar. The focus on stroke thrombectomy is now, fortunately, no longer on its effectiveness, but how to meaningfully improve access and optimize delivery.

As such, *Twelve Strokes* aims to provide the critical knowledge that can help readers achieve these aims. Improving access to stroke is of particular importance because patients often misinterpret their symptoms or can't speak for themselves if they have aphasia. More importantly, access needs to be organized because stroke therapies are all extremely time-sensitive. Scalable, choreographed protocols are necessary for our emergency medical systems to "capture" stroke patients and automatically transport and triage to time-sensitive treatments. Many of the chapters in the first part on Fundamentals and Systems provide valuable insight in improving access to stroke care.

As much as the literature may represent stroke thrombectomy as an efficient, effective, reproducible procedure, anyone in practice can attest to the myriad of often challenging technical details that can easily complicate one procedure to the next. C Miller Fisher's famous quote that neurology is learned stroke by stroke speaks of the tremendous variability in stroke syndromes. As such, our treatment approaches should certainly not be comprised of a one-size-fits-all approach.

Twelve Strokes examines the primary technical principles that underlie the current thrombectomy approaches. Instead of continuing the conceptual dichotomy of stent versus aspiration, many of the chapters look at underlying principles and then discuss ways in which the currently available devices and approaches can best exploit them. The variety, creativity, and detail in many of these chapters help the reader develop a deeper understanding that might assist their ability to successfully take care of their next patient that "doesn't follow the textbook."

The anatomic and pathophysiologic classification of the core 12 chapters will help the reader organize their thinking and approach. This knowledge, particularly because it is organized based on common, challenging syndromes, will arm the reader to be able to quickly recognize patterns and deftly adapt their management approaches to the needs of the patient. Oftentimes, it is the recognition of a particularly challenging anatomy or pathology ahead of time that will force a physician to take a few more moments to prepare a variety of possible approaches and mentally prepare for a complex and difficult procedure, which can contribute to a favorable final outcome.

Our expectations have become and should be quite high for patients treated with thrombectomy. The thought, detail, insight, and organization of *Twelve Strokes* will help the reader meet these needs of stroke patients with large vessel occlusions.

Michael Chen, MD
Department of Neurological Surgery
Rush University Medical Center
Chicago, IL, USA

Contents

Contributors

Ramez N. Abdalla, MD Departments of Radiology and Neurological Surgery, Northwestern University, Feinberg School of Medicine, Chicago, IL, USA

Department of Radiology, Ain Shams University, Cairo, Egypt

Todd A. Abruzzo Barrow Neurological Institute at Phoenix Children's Hospital, Phoenix, AZ, USA

University of Arizona College of Medicine, Phoenix, AZ, USA

Phoenix Children's Hospital, Phoenix, AZ, USA

Tarek Abuelem, MD Department of Neurosurgery, St. Vincent Arkansas Neuroscience Institute, Little Rock, AR, USA

Amin Aghaebrahim, MD Baptist Medical Center, Baptist Neurological Institute, Jacksonville, FL, USA

Michael J. Alexander, MD Department of Neurosurgery, Neurovascular Center, Cedars-Sinai Medical Center, Los Angeles, CA, USA

Eyad Almallouhi, MD Medical University of South Carolina, Department of Neurology, and Neurosurgery, Charleston, SC, USA

Tommy Andersson, MD, PhD Department of Clinical Neuroscience, Karolinska Institutet, Stockholm, Sweden

Department of Neuroradiology, Karolinska University Hospital, Stockholm, Sweden

Department of Medical Imaging, AZ Groeninge, Kortrijk, Belgium

Sameer A. Ansari, MD, PhD Departments of Radiology, Neurology, and Neurological Surgery, Northwestern University, Feinberg School of Medicine, Chicago, IL, USA

Rose A. Arslanian, BS Department of Radiology, University of Massachusetts Medical School, Worcester, MA, USA

Adam S. Arthur, MD, MPH Semmes-Murphey Clinic, Department of Neurosurgery, University of Tennessee Health Science Center, Memphis, TN, USA

Mohamad A. Asfour Baptist Medical Center, Lyerly Neurosurgey, Jacksonville, FL, USA

Robin M. Babadjouni, MD Department of Neurosurgery, Cedars-Sinai Medical Center, Los Angeles, CA, USA

Mark Bain, MD Cerebrovascular Center, Neurological Institute, Cleveland Clinic, Cleveland, OH, USA

Zachary R. Barnard, MD Department of Neurosurgery, Neurovascular Center, Cedars-Sinai Medical Center, Los Angeles, CA, USA

Blaise William Baxter, BSc, MD, FRCPC Department of Radiology, Lehigh Valley Health Network, Allentown, PA, USA

Donald R. Cantrell, MD, PhD Departments of Radiology and Neurological Surgery, Northwestern University, Feinberg School of Medicine, Chicago, IL, USA

Russell Cerejo, MD Cerebrovascular Center, Allegheny Health Network, Pittsburgh, PA, USA

Ronil V. Chandra Monash Health and Monash University, NeuroInterventional Radiology, Melbourne, VIC, Australia

Michael Chen, MD Department of Neurological Surgery, Rush University Medical Center, Chicago, IL, USA

Stephanie H. Chen, MD Department of Neurosurgery, University of Miami, Miami, FL, USA

Juyu Chueh, PhD Department of Radiology, University of Massachusetts Medical School, Worcester, MA, USA

Charlotte Y. Chung, MD, PhD Department of Radiology and Imaging Sciences, Emory University School of Medicine, Atlanta, GA, USA

Roberto Crosa, MD Médica Uruguaya, CEN Neuro Endovascular Center, Montevideo, Uruguay

Guilherme Dabus, MD, FAHA Interventional Neuroradiology and Neuroendovascular Surgery, Miami Cardiac & Vascular Institute, Baptist Neuroscience Center, Miami, FL, USA

Angelique Sao Mai S. Do, MD Department of Neurosurgery, Cedars-Sinai Medical Center, Los Angeles, CA, USA

David Dornbos III, MD Department of Neurosurgery, University of Tennessee Health Sciences Center and Semmes-Murphey Clinic, Memphis, TN, USA

John J. Entwistle, DO Department of Neurosurgery, Carilion Clinic, Roanoke, VA, USA

Johanna T. Fifi, MD Department of Neurology and Neurosurgery, Mount Sinai Health System, New York, NY, USA

David J. Fiorella, MD, PhD Department of Neurosurgery, Stony Brook University, Stony Brook, NY, USA

Matthew J. Gounis, PhD Department of Radiology, University of Massachusetts Medical School, Worcester, MA, USA

Manuel F. Granja, MD Baptist Medical Center, Baptist Neurological Institute, Jacksonville, FL, USA

Ricardo A. Hanel, MD Baptist Medical Center, Baptist Neurological Institute, Jacksonville, FL, USA

Julian Hardman, MD Cerebrovascular Center, Neurological Institute, Cleveland Clinic, Cleveland, OH, USA

Ferdinand K. Hui Department of Radiology, Division of Interventional Neuroradiology, The Johns Hopkins Hospital, Baltimore, MD, USA

Muhammad Shazam Hussain, MD Cerebrovascular Center, Neurological Institute, Cleveland Clinic, Cleveland, OH, USA

Ashutosh Jadhav, MD, PhD Barrow Neurological Institute, Phoenix, AZ, USA

Liwei Jiang, MD Department of Radiology, Brigham and Women's Hospital, Boston, MA, USA

Sarah Johnson, BE, PhD Student Department of Biomedical Engineering, National University of Ireland Galway, Galway, Ireland

Tudor G. Jovin, MD Barrow Neurological Institute, Phoenix, AZ, USA

Sami Al Kasab, MD Medical University of South Carolina, Department of Neurology, and Neurosurgery, Charleston, SC, USA

Department of Neurosurgery, Medical University of South Carolina, Charleston, SC, USA

Jaims Lim, MD Department of Neurosurgery, Jacobs School of Medicine and Biomedical Sciences, University at Buffalo, Buffalo, NY, USA

Department of Neurosurgery, Gates Vascular Institute at Kaleida Health, Buffalo, NY, USA

Italo Linfante, MD, FAHA Interventional Neuroradiology and Neuroendovascular Surgery, Miami Cardiac & Vascular Institute, Baptist Neuroscience Center, Miami, FL, USA

Peter E. McHugh, BE, ScM, PhD Department of Biomedical Engineering, National University of Ireland Galway, College of Engineering and Informatics, Galway, Ireland

Philip M. Meyers, MD Department of Neurological Surgery, Columbia University Medical Center, New York, NY, USA

Jacob Morey, BS Icahn School of Medicine at Mount Sinai, New York, NY, USA

Matias Negrotto, MD Hospital Maciel, Montevideo, Uruguay

Eric C. Peterson, MD Department of Neurosurgery, University of Miami, Miami, FL, USA

Matthew B. Potts, MD Departments of Radiology and Neurological Surgery, Northwestern University, Feinberg School of Medicine, Chicago, IL, USA

Ajit S. Puri, MD Department of Radiology, University of Massachusetts Medical School, Worcester, MA, USA

Ansaar T. Rai, MD, MBA Department of Neuroradiology, West Virginia University School of Medicine, Morgantown, WV, USA

Dennys Reyes, MD Interventional Neuroradiology and Neuroendovascular Surgery, Miami Cardiac & Vascular Institute, Baptist Neuroscience Center, Miami, FL, USA

Monica Scarsella, MD Cerebrovascular Center, Neurological Institute, Cleveland Clinic, Cleveland, OH, USA

Belinda Shao, BA Department of Neurological Surgery, Columbia University Medical Center, New York, NY, USA

Adnan H. Siddiqui, MD, PhD Department of Neurosurgery, Gates Vascular Institute at Kaleida Health, Buffalo, NY, USA

Departments of Neurosurgery and Radiology, Jacobs School of Medicine and Biomedical Sciences, University at Buffalo, Buffalo, NY, USA

Jacobs Institute, Buffalo, NY, USA

Eleonora Francesca Spinazzi, MD Department of Neurological Surgery, Columbia University Medical Center, New York, NY, USA

Alejandro M. Spiotta, MD Department of Neurosurgery, Medical University of South Carolina, Charleston, SC, USA

Robert M. Starke, MD Department of Neurosurgery, University of Miami, Miami, FL, USA

Madhav Sukumaran, MD, PhD Departments of Radiology and Neurological Surgery, Northwestern University, Feinberg School of Medicine, Chicago, IL, USA

Gabor Toth, MD Cerebrovascular Center, Cleveland Clinic, Cleveland, OH, USA

Pavan S. Upadhyayula, BA Department of Neurological Surgery, Columbia University Medical Center, New York, NY, USA

Kunal Vakharia, MD Department of Neurosurgery, Jacobs School of Medicine and Biomedical Sciences, University at Buffalo, Buffalo, NY, USA

Department of Neurosurgery, Gates Vascular Institute at Kaleida Health, Buffalo, NY, USA

Muhammad Waqas, MBBS Department of Neurosurgery, Jacobs School of Medicine and Biomedical Sciences, University at Buffalo, Buffalo, NY, USA

Department of Neurosurgery, Gates Vascular Institute at Kaleida Health, Buffalo, NY, USA

Dileep R. Yavagal, MD Department of Neurology, University of Miami, Miami, FL, USA

Leonard Leong Litt Yeo, MBBS, MRCP Department of Clinical Neuroscience, Karolinska Institutet, Stockholm, Sweden

Department of Neuroradiology, Karolinska University Hospital, Stockholm, Sweden

Divison of Neurology, National University Health System, Singapore and Yong Loo Lin School of Medicine, National University of Singapore, Singapore, Singapore

Benjamin Zussman, MD Wellstar Health System, Atlanta, GA, USA

Part I
Fundamentals and Systems

Chapter 1
Evidence on Mechanical Thrombectomy in Acute Ischemic Stroke

Matias Negrotto and Sami Al Kasab

Goals of This Chapter

1. Review the literature that forms the basis of mechanical thrombectomy in acute ischemic stroke for large vessel occlusion.
2. Critically analyze steps to follow on stroke protocol and the decision to make endovascular treatment.
3. Critically analyze the importance of imaging studies in this pathology.

Landmark Papers

Langhorne P1, Williams BO, Gilchrist W, Howie K. Do Stroke Units Save Lives? Lancet. 1993 Aug 14; 342(8868): 395–8

This seminal paper initiated the fertile ground for stroke treatment. This paper clearly demonstrated the newly introduced meta-analysis technique and identified that stroke units improved patient outcomes.

The authors performed a statistical overview of randomized controlled trials reported between 1962 and 1993 in which the management of stroke patients in a specialist unit was compared with that in general wards. They identified ten trials, eight of which used a strict randomization procedure. 1586 stroke patients were

M. Negrotto (✉)
Hospital Maciel, Montevideo, Uruguay

S. Al Kasab
Medical University of South Carolina, Department of Neurology, and Neurosurgery, Charleston, SC, USA

F. K. Hui et al. (eds.), *12 Strokes*, https://doi.org/10.1007/978-3-030-56857-3_1

included: 766 allocated to a stroke unit and 820 to general wards. The odds ratio (stroke unit vs. general wards) for mortality within the first 4 months (median follow-up of 3 months) after the stroke was 0.72 (95% CI 0.56–0.92), consistent with a reduction in mortality of 28% ($2p < 0.01$). This reduction persisted (odds ratio 0.79, 95% CI 0.63–0.99, $2p < 0.05$) when calculated for mortality during the first 12 months. The conclusion was that management of stroke patients in a stroke unit was associated with a sustained reduction in mortality.

The National Institute of Neurological Disorders and Stroke rt-PA Stroke Study Group. Tissue Plasminogen Activator for Acute Ischemic Stroke. N Engl J Med 1995; 333 (24): 1581–7

r-tPA treatment: In 1995 the first study with a positive impact was published, being statistically significant regarding the use of IV r-tPA in ischemic stroke: NINDS2. It showed, at $n = 333$, that patients treated with IV r-tPA compared to placebo within 3 hours of onset of symptoms had at least 30% better outcome in terms of disability at 3 months. The patients with IV r-tPA had a 3-month mortality rate of 17% vs. 21% ($p = 0.30$); however, the percent hemorrhage was 6.4% vs. only 0.6 in control ($p < 0.001$). The findings were statistically significant with a clear benefit of IV r-tPA treatment, with a required number of treatment (NNT) of eight to obtain favorable results.

Hacke W, Kaste M, Bluhmki E, Brozman M, Dávalos A, Guidetti D, et al.; ECASS Investigators. Thrombolysis with Alteplase 3 to 4.5 Hours After Acute Ischemic Stroke. N Engl J Med 2008; 359 (13): 1317–29

In 2008, the second statistically significant study was published that supported treatment with IV r-tPA: ECASS III. This work increased the therapeutic window, extending the use of IV r-tPA within the first 4.5 hours of symptom onset. There was no difference in mortality, but it was favorable in terms of morbidity with an NNT of 14 for "favorable results." Thus, from the results of these two seminal works, we have begun to implement this technique, with a level of evidence class 1A in the guidelines of the American Heart Association/American Stroke Association (AHA/ASA) of 2013/2014. Restoration of blood flow in patients with ischemic stroke is effective in reducing long-term morbidity. For patients meeting national and international eligibility guidelines, IV r-tPA improves functional outcomes at 3 and 6 months when given within the first 4.5 hours. It should be delivered as soon as possible, with better results shown the early it is given. Therefore, its administration must be initiated whenever there is a correct indication. This approach will help minimize start-to-treat times, a key efficacy factor for r-tPA [11, 12].

Acute large vessel ischemic strokes pose a significant challenge to intravenously administered thrombolytic therapy. Large vessel occlusion (LVO) is defined as the presence of occlusion of a large intracranial vessel (including both the anterior and posterior circulations) with a corresponding perfusion deficit on CT perfusion imaging indicative of an acute ischemic stroke that would be technically eligible for IA endovascular intervention. Specific segments (intracranial internal carotid artery (ICA), M1 and M2 segments of the middle cerebral artery, A1 and A2 anterior cerebral segments of the anterior cerebral artery, the basilar artery, V4 segment of the vertebral artery, and P1 and P2 segments of the posterior cerebral artery) are included [13].

Presence of an LVO is a significant predictor of outcome in patients undergoing stroke therapy, and unless recanalized, these patients do poorly [14, 15]. IV r-tPA has not been shown to be effective for recanalization of these proximal vessels [16] due to a large thrombus burden [17]and hence has limited efficacy in impacting outcomes [18].

Large vessel occlusions (LVOs) are responsible for significant proportions of AIS [19]and portend a dismal prognosis [20]. They are a major source of morbidity, mortality, and healthcare cost, and developing a focused treatment strategy for these patients was important. The data presented below strongly support endovascular therapy as a significant independent predictor of outcome compared with IV thrombolysis alone for large vessel occlusions.

Endovascular Treatment

The EVT of AIS has rapidly evolved rapidly over the past 20 years [21–23]. The first three multicenter, prospective, randomized, controlled trials (IMS III, SYNTHESIS, MR RESCUE) using first-generation devices (MERCI system) failed to show benefit of intra-arterial revascularization. In 2015, controlled clinical trials with a level of evidence class 1A (MR CLEAN, ESCAPE, EXTEND-IA, SWIFT PRIME, REVASCAT) forever changed the treatment paradigm for ischemic stroke. These studies demonstrated clear efficacy of endovascular treatment by mechanical thrombectomy in patients with ischemic stroke of less than 6 hours of evolution, with occlusion of large vessels of the anterior circulation. It was not only a crucial point in history of stroke but also in the history of medicine. For those who have lived through the transition from having no proven acute intervention to the introduction of thrombolytic and now endovascular therapy, this was an unforgettable moment. It was the most important event in stroke since the introduction of tPA in 1995.

Broderick JP, Palesch YY, Demchuk AM, Yeatts SD, Khatri P, Hill MD, et al. Endovascular Therapy After Intravenous t-PA versus t-PA Alone for Stroke. N Engl J Med. 2013;368:893–903 (IMS 3)

In March 2013, in a single issue the *New England Journal of Medicine* published three studies that evaluated the efficacy of endovascular treatment for ischemic stroke (IMS III, MR RESCUE, SYNTHESIS). In IMS III, a total of 656 participants underwent randomization (434 participants to endovascular therapy and 222 to intravenous tPA alone) at 58 study centers between August 25, 2006, and April 17, 2012 in the United States, Canada, Australia, and Europe. Eligibility criteria included receipt of intravenous tPA within 3 hours after symptom onset and a moderate-to-severe neurologic deficit (defined as an NIHSS score ≥10 or, after approval of amendment 3, a score of 8 to 9 with CT angiographic evidence of an occlusion of the first segment of the middle cerebral artery [M1], internal carotid artery, or basilar artery at institutions where CT angiographic imaging at baseline was the standard of care for patients with acute stroke). Participants randomly assigned to the endovascular-therapy group underwent angiography as soon as possible, either at the hospital that initiated treatment with intravenous tPA or at another participating hospital. Participants who had no angiographic evidence of a treatable occlusion received no additional treatment, and those with a treatable vascular occlusion received endovascular intervention. The angiographic procedure had to begin within 5 hours and be completed within 7 hours after the onset of stroke.

Reperfusion rates, as measured by a TICI score of 2b (partial reperfusion of half or more of the vascular distribution of the occluded artery) to 3, were 38% for an occlusion in the internal carotid artery, 44% for an occlusion in M1, 44% for a single M2 occlusion, and 23% for multiple M2 occlusions.

The trial was stopped early because of futility, according to the prespecified criteria. There was no significant difference between the endovascular-therapy and intravenous tPA groups in the overall proportion of participants with a modified Rankin score of 2 or less. It failed to show a benefit in functional outcome with the use of additional endovascular therapy, as compared with the standard therapy of intravenous tPA alone. The safety profiles were similar in the two treatment groups.

In MR RESCUE, 127 patients were randomized to embolectomy and studied clinical outcomes in subgroups with and without a "penumbral pattern" on MRI or CT of each treatment arm. They did not observe better revascularization, tissue reperfusion, and clinical outcomes in the embolectomy group compared to the standard care group.

The other trial, SYNTHESIS, compared the efficacy of thrombolytic treatment with respect to endovascular treatment with stent during the first 4.5 h. It included 362 patients (181 in each group). The study did not show significant differences in the rate of good prognosis (30.4% endovascular vs. 34.8% intravenous), in the hemorrhagic complications or mortality.

Numerous concerns regarding various aspects of these trials were raised by the neurointerventional community. First, only one of the three trials, MR RESCUE, routinely identified LVO with either computed tomography or magnetic resonance angiography (CTA or MRA, respectively). In IMS III, CTA was performed in only 47% of patients, and approximately 20% of patients in the interventional arm either did not have an LVO or had an inaccessible, distally located thrombus. In SYNTHESIS Expansion, approximately 10% of patients in the interventional arm did not have a LVO. Moreover, modern devices, such as retrievable stents (stentrievers) and the Penumbra System (Penumbra, Inc., Alameda, California, USA), were used in only a minority of patients. The use of older, less effective endovascular technology resulted in significantly low rates of successful recanalization, defined as thrombolysis in cerebral infarction (TICI) grade 2b or 3. The rates of TICI 2b or 3 recanalization were 40% in IMS III, 27% in MR RESCUE, and not reported in SYNTHESIS Expansion. In the IMS III trial, Solitaire was used in 5 of 434 patients randomized to endovascular treatment. In the SYNTHESIS Expansion trial, Solitaire (ev3/Covidien) and Trevo (Concentric/Stryker) were used in 23 of the 181 patients assigned to endovascular treatment. In MR RESCUE, no patient was treated with Solitaire or Trevo retriever. The low rates of Solitaire or Trevo use in all the abovementioned studies could partially explain the relatively low rates of partial or complete recanalization seen in these studies. Furthermore, patients with minor ischemic deficits were included, so these trials demonstrated that the benefit of endovascular treatment may be seen in patients with major ischemic deficits and not in those with minor ischemic stroke. Last but not least, patients in the interventional arm of SYNTHESIS Expansion were not administered IV-tPA, the use of which is supported by class I evidence, and were treated in a delayed fashion compared to the medical arm.

Despite the negative results, these studies pointed the way for new trials that justified this treatment modality (Table 1.1).

Table 1.1 Characteristics of trials mentioned above

Trial	Trial period	Location	Total no. of patients	No. of centers
MR CLEAN	2010–2014	Europe	500	30
ESCAPE	2013–2014	North America, Europe, South Korea	315	22
EXTEND-IA	2012–2014	Australia and New Zealand	70	14
SWIFT PRIME	2013–2014	North America, Europe	196	39
REVASCAT	2012–2014	Spain	206	4
DAWN	2014–2017	North America, Europe, Australia	206	32
DEFUSE 3	2016–2017	North America	182	38

O. Bekhemer, F. Beumer, V. Berg, H Lingsma, Y. Schonewile, V. Nederkoom: The Randomized Trial of Intraarterial Treatment for Acute Ischemic Stroke (MR CLEAN). The New England Journal of Medicine, January 2015, vol 372

The MR CLEAN was the first positive trial to be published in January 2015. It included 500 patients (233 intervention and 267 control group), aged more than 18 years and whose NIHSS was more than 2, with less than 6 hours of evolution since the onset of symptoms to treatment, confirming proximal vascular occlusion by CT angiography, with ASPECTS score of 7–10. IV r-tPA was performed on 90% of the patients (87% intervention vs. 91% control) with the disadvantage of a wait between the initiation of IV thrombolytic and endovascular therapy. No significant changes were observed in terms of mortality; however, there was a statistically significant decrease in morbidity with an mRS of 0–2: 33% with endovascular treatment vs. 19% control group. It had a relatively low reperfusion rate (59% TICI 2b/3), which was also explained by delayed onset of endovascular therapy.

One concern is that the sample size was rather small (500 patients); however, it allowed to estimate the primary effect parameter with sufficient precision. The use of multiple IAT modalities per patient was not restricted. This is a limitation of the trial design, because it will restrict the possibilities of comparing different treatment modalities and only allowed to give a global judgment whether or not IAT is effective. On the other hand, this pragmatism allows us to follow current practice closely and allows new mechanical devices and treatment strategies into the trial.

Time since onset is a serious concern. The arguments for a 6- or even 8-hour time window from onset of stroke symptoms to treatment are mostly based on tradition (previous studies of IAT also used this window) and the absence of an association of complications and treatment effect with time since onset in previous, mostly neutral trials [5].

M. Goyal, A. Demchuk, B. Menon, M. Eesa, J. Rempel, J. Thornton, D. Roy: Randomized Assay of Rapid Endovascular Treatment of Ischemic Stroke (ESCAPE). The New England Journal of Medicine, February 2015

ESCAPE included a total of 315 patients (165 intervention vs. 150 control), with an NIHSS of more than 12, an ASPECTS of more than 5, and a therapeutic window of 12 hours, with diagnosis of proximal occlusion by CT angiography and perfusion for evaluation of circulation. IV r-tPA was made in 76% of the patients (72.7% intervention vs. 78.6% control group). This study was stopped early because of the clear benefit and efficacy of endovascular treatment in the control group. A TICI 2b/3 reperfusion rate of 72% was observed, with a favorable outcome mRS of 0–2 of 53% with intervention vs. 29% control group (NNT = 4) and a decrease in mortality of 10% vs. 19% in the control group.

The trial was based on the premise that patients with large vessel occlusion of the anterior circulation with small to moderate infarct core and moderate to good collaterals identified on computed tomography (CT)-based imaging would benefit most from endovascular treatment if reperfusion was achieved quickly after imaging. In the ESCAPE trial, achieving a short imaging-to-reperfusion time significantly improved the chance of achieving a functionally independent outcome. Speed of treatment can be achieved in dedicated stroke centers with teamwork, parallel workflow, and a focus on quality improvement. Endovascular-capable hospitals should identify eligible patients by using quick and reliable imaging techniques and focus on achieving reperfusion as quickly and efficiently as possible [24].

B. Campbell, P. Mitchell, T. Kleinig, H. Dewey, L. Churilov, N. Yassi: Endovascular Therapy for Ischemic Stroke with Perfusion-Imaging Selection (EXTEND -IA). The New England Journal of Medicine, February 2015

EXTEND-IA was the smallest trial with $n = 70$ (35 intervention vs. 35 control). The selection criteria were based on perfusion images in patients with LVO, no age limits, no NIHSS limits, and time to treatment of less than 4.5 hours. RAPID software imaging was used for all the patients. IV r-tPA was done in 100% of patients; a TICI 2b/3 reperfusion rate of 86% was observed, with a favorable outcome mRS of 0–2 of 71% with intervention vs. 40% control group and a decrease in mortality of 9% vs. 20% in the control group.

They concluded that early endovascular thrombectomy with Solitaire FR after IV r-tPA resulted in greater reperfusion and early neurologic recovery than r-tPA alone in a population with LVO and salvageable tissue on CT perfusion imaging.

J. Saver, M. Mayank, A. Bonafe, M. Diener, P. Elad, I. Levy: Stent-Retriever Thrombectomy After Intravenous t-PA vs. t-PA Alone in Stroke (SWIFT PRIME). The New England Journal of Medicine, February 2015

In SWIFT PRIME, 196 cases were recruited (98 intervention vs. 98 control), aged 18–80 years, with an NIHSS of between 8 and 29 and ASPECTS of more than 6. 98% received IV r-tPA before 4.5 hours. Large vessel occlusion was diagnosed by CT angiography or MR angiography. RAPID software imaging was used for 80% of patients. A TICI 2b/3 reperfusion rate of 88% was achieved, with a favorable outcome mRS of 0–2 of 60% with intervention vs. 36% control group, with no significant changes in symptomatic intracranial hemorrhage (0% vs. 3%, $P = 0.12$).

There was no significant decrease in mortality.

In the SWIFT PRIME publication, the rate of functional independence, defined as a modified Rankin scale (mRS) score of 0 to 2, in the intervention group was 60%

which was higher than that in MR CLEAN (33%) and similar to that observed in the ESCAPE trial (53%) and the EXTEND-IA trial (71%).

The better outcome results probably reflect "the earlier start of the intervention, the exclusion of patients with large core infarcts on the basis of imaging, and the greater reperfusion rate in this trial."

Jovin, A. Chamorro, E. Cobo, M. Miquel, C. Molina, A. Rovira: Thrombectomy Within 8 Hours After Symptom Onset in Ischemic Stroke (REVASCAT). The New England Journal of Medicine, February 2015

REVASCAT assessed the efficacy of mechanical thrombectomy within 8 hours of symptom onset. 206 patients were included (103 vs. 103), aged between 18 and 80 years, with an NIHSS of more than 6, diagnosis of proximal occlusion by CT angiography, and ASPECTS of greater than 7. 73% received IV r-tPA; TICI 2b/3 was 66%, with clear favorable outcome mRS of 0–2 of 44% with intervention vs. 28% control group, with no significant changes in mortality. This study contributed evidence to support the efficacy of neurovascular thrombectomy in patients with anterior circulation stroke who could be treated within 8 hours after the onset of symptoms.

THE REVASCAT was stopped before formal stopping boundaries were reached, because of ethical considerations.

The magnitude of the observed benefit in the abovementioned trials was dramatic. The findings clearly show a superior outcome following treatment with IV thrombolysis and thrombectomy using modern thrombectomy devices compared with best medical treatment alone. The successes from these RCTs have been mostly attributed to improved thrombectomy devices with faster and higher rates of recanalization and better study protocols with documentation of vessel occlusion before randomization.

Raul G. Nogueira, MD; Ashutosh P. Jadhav, MD, PhD; Diogo C. Haussen, MD; Alain Bonafe, MD; Ronald F. Budzik, MD; Parita Bhuva, MD; et al. Thrombectomy 6 to 24 Hours After Stroke with a Mismatch Between Deficit and Infarct. N Engl J Med. January 4, 2018

The DAWN Trial is the first to evaluate the late-window and wake-up stroke patient population. This was a multicenter, prospective, randomized, open-label trial with a Bayesian adaptive-enrichment design and with blinded assessment of end points.

This study supports the use of the Trevo retriever beyond the 8-hour time limit in wake-up, unclear-onset, and late-presenting ischemic stroke subjects.

The investigators selected patients arriving after 6 hours from symptom onset for inclusion in the trial by using imaging and clinical scores to identify those with "target mismatch" – a small core infarct volume but a large area of brain at risk for ischemia yet still potentially salvageable. RAPID software imaging was used for all the patients.

From September 2014 through February 2017, a total of 206 patients were enrolled in the trial; 107 were randomly assigned to the thrombectomy group and 99 to the control group.

For the DAWN trial, patients with a large vessel occlusion stroke presenting between 6 and 24 hours (average of 13 hours) underwent computed tomographic (CT) perfusion or magnetic resonance diffusion-weighted imaging. Patients were selected for inclusion and randomization to thrombectomy or control if they had a small infarct core in relation to their National Institutes of Health Stroke Scale (NIHSS) score. The exact requirements varied with age.

Patients had to have a mismatch between the severity of the clinical deficit and the infarct volume, which was defined according to the following criteria: Patients aged over 80 had to have an NIHSS score of over 10 and a core volume of less than 21 mL. For patients younger than 80 years, requirements were an NIHSS score of over 10 and a core volume of less than 31 mL or an NIHSS score of over 20 and a core volume of less than 51 mL.

Results showed a 2-point difference in the 90-day weighted modified Rankin scale (mRS) score in favor of the thrombectomy group, which translated into a 73% relative reduction of dependency in activities of daily living. In addition, there was a 35% absolute increase in the number of patients achieving functional independence (mRS score, 0 to 2), with a number needed to treat for this end point of 2.8.

> The results of this trial expanded the population of patients who can benefit from mechanical thrombectomy for stroke, to significantly reduce functional impairment in the mostly severely affected patients.
>
> The DAWN trial also showed that patients treated earlier had better outcomes, so the concept "time is brain" is unchanged, it is just that eligibility for treatment should not be restricted by time windows.

G.W. Albers, M.P. Marks, S. Kemp, S. Christensen, J.P. Tsai, S. Ortega-Gutierrez, et al. Thrombectomy for Stroke at 6 to 16 Hours with Selection by Perfusion Imaging. The New England Journal of Medicine, January 24, 2018

DEFUSE 3 was a multicenter, randomized, open-label trial, with blinded outcome assessment, of thrombectomy in patients 6 to 16 hours after they were last known to be well and who had remaining ischemic brain tissue that was not yet infarcted.

From May 2016 through May 2017, a total of 182 patients underwent randomization (92 to the endovascular-therapy group and 90 to the medical-therapy group) at 38 centers in the United States (Fig. 1.1).

Patients with proximal middle-cerebral-artery or internal-carotid-artery occlusion, an initial infarct size of less than 70 ml, and a ratio of the volume of ischemic tissue on perfusion imaging to infarct volume of 1.8 or more were randomly assigned to endovascular therapy (thrombectomy) plus standard medical therapy (endovascular-therapy group) or standard medical therapy alone (medical-therapy group). RAPID software imaging was used for all the patients.

The primary outcome was the ordinal score on the modified Rankin scale (range, 0 to 6, with higher scores indicating greater disability) at day 90. Endovascular therapy plus standard medical therapy was associated with a more favorable distribution of disability scores on the modified Rankin scale at 90 days than standard medical therapy alone. Mortality at 90 days was 14% in the endovascular-therapy group and 26% in the medical-therapy group ($P = 0.05$). The rate of symptomatic intracranial hemorrhage did not differ significantly between the two groups.

DAWN Clinical – infarct mismatch	DEFUSE 3 Target mismatch
• Age ≥ 80 • NIHSS ≥ 10 • Ischemic core ≤ 21 ml	• Ischemic core < 70 ml
• Age ≤ 80 • NIHSS ≥ 10 • Ischemic core ≤ 31 ml	• Mismatch ratio ≥ 1.8
• Age < 80 • NIHSS ≥ 10 • Ischemic core 31 ml – 51 ml	• Mismatch volume ≥ 15

Fig. 1.1 DAWN and DEFUSE 3 selection criteria

Recommendations and Level of Evidence

- Pre-hospital stroke management: Stroke patients are dispatched at the highest level of care available in the shortest time possible. Travel time is equivalent to trauma or myocardial infarction calls [25].
- Emergency evaluation and diagnosis of acute ischemic stroke: The evaluation and initial treatment of patients with stroke should be performed expeditiously. Because time is critical, a limited number of essential diagnostic tests are recommended [25].
- Early diagnosis and brain and vascular imaging: An emergency brain imaging study is recommended prior to initiating any specific treatment for acute stroke (class I, level of evidence A) [26].
- Noninvasive intracranial vascular study: If endovascular therapy is contemplated, this study is strongly recommended during the initial imaging evaluation of the acute stroke patient but should not delay intravenous r-tPA if indicated (class I, level of evidence A) [26].
- When evaluating patients with AIS within 6 hours of last known normal with LVO and an Alberta Stroke Program Early Computed Tomography Score (ASPECTS) of ≥6, selection for mechanical thrombectomy based on CT and CTA or MRI and MRA is recommended in preference to performance of additional imaging such as perfusion studies (class I, level of evidence B) [26].
- When selecting patients with AIS within 6 to 24 hours of last known normal who have LVO in the anterior circulation, obtaining CTP or DWI-MRI, with or without MRI perfusion, is recommended to aid in patient selection for mechanical thrombectomy, but only when patients meet other eligibility criteria from one of the RCTs that showed benefit from mechanical thrombectomy in this extended time window (class I, level of evidence A) [26].
- Intravenous r-tPA (0.9 mg/kg, maximum dose 90 mg) is recommended for administration to eligible patients who can be treated in the time period of 3 to 4.5 hours after stroke onset (class I, level of evidence B) [26].
- Patients eligible for intravenous r-tPA should receive intravenous r-tPA even if endovascular treatments are being considered (class I, level of evidence A) [27].
- Observing patients after intravenous r-tPA to assess for clinical response before pursuing endovascular therapy is not required to achieve beneficial outcomes and is not recommended (class III, level of evidence B-R) [26].
- Endovascular treatment 0 to 6 hours after onset: Patients should receive this therapy if they meet the following criteria (class I, level of evidence A) [26]:
  (a) Prestroke mRS score 0 to 1.
  (b) Acute ischemic stroke receiving intravenous r-tPA within 4.5 hours of onset according to guidelines from professional medical societies.
  (c) Large vessel occlusion.
  (d) Age ≥ 18 years.
  (e) NIHSS score of ≥6.
  (f) ASPECTS of ≥6.
  (g) Treatment can be initiated (groin puncture) within 6 hours of symptom onset.

- Endovascular treatment 6 to 24 hours after onset: Patients should receive this therapy if they meet the following criteria (class I, level of evidence A) [26]:
  (a) In selected patients with AIS within 6 to 16 hours of last known normal who have LVO in the anterior circulation and meet other DAWN or DEFUSE 3 eligibility criteria, mechanical thrombectomy is recommended (class I, level of evidence A).
  (b) In selected patients with AIS within 16 to 24 hours of last known normal who have LVO in the anterior circulation and meet other DAWN eligibility criteria, mechanical thrombectomy is reasonable (class IIa, level of evidence B-R).
- The technical goal of the thrombectomy procedure should be a TICI 2b/3 angiographic result to maximize the probability of a good functional clinical outcome (class I, level of evidence A) [26].

A finding of intracranial large vessel occlusion(s) during the initial diagnostic evaluation is strongly associated with worse functional outcome and higher mortality rate. Patients with emergent large vessel occlusion (ELVO) are a heterogeneous group requiring rapid and effective revascularization with the likelihood of benefit decreasing over time elapsed from symptom onset [27].

As already mentioned, endovascular treatment in cases not meeting strict criteria is allowable. Each patient should be discussed quickly, analyzing the level of occlusion, NIHSS at presentation, vascular anatomy, established infarct core, Alberta Stroke Program Early CT Score (ASPECTS), age, baseline functional status, and collateral circulation.

The role of mechanical thrombectomy could be significantly expanded if patients are selected based on risk of severe disability and favorable parenchymal/collateral imaging findings, instead of time and occlusion location [28].

- Type of device: The use of retrievable stents is recommended with the highest level of evidence by American Heart Association (AHA), Canadian Stroke Best Practices (CSBP), and European Stroke Organisation (ESO) guidelines, with lower levels of recommendations given to consider other devices based on local protocols. An analysis of the MR CLEAN data showed that choice of device did not influence outcomes in that data set. The majority were treated with the Trevo device at 53%, Solitaire device at 13%, and other devices at 17% [29]. The other devices which can be used for mechanical thrombectomy is the aspiration Penumbra System (Penumbra, Inc., California, USA). Two randomized controlled trials compared the safety and efficacy of aspiration thrombectomy compared to stentriever and showed similar safety and efficacy profiles between the two techniques. The ASTER trial concluded that among patients with ischemic stroke in the anterior circulation undergoing thrombectomy, first-line thrombectomy with contact aspiration compared with stent retriever did not result in an increased successful revascularization rate at the end of the procedure [30]. The second trial is the COMPASS trial which confirmed the findings in ASTER [31, 32].

Interestingly, COMPASS showed that the use of aspiration first-line technique was associated with lower cost of approximately 4551 USD compared to stentriever.

- Type of anesthesia: Conscious sedation is preferred over general anesthesia (unless medically indicated) by both AHA and CSBP recommendations, albeit with reduced levels of evidence (class IIb level C and level B, respectively), whereas the ESO guideline leaves this as an individual patient decision. Several RCTs are underway to address this issue [33].

Time – RAPID Software to Select Patients for Late-Window Endovascular Therapy

The substantial clinical benefits of late-window thrombectomy that were recently documented in the DAWN and DEFUSE 3 studies led to expansion of the treatment window for thrombectomy from 6 to 24 hours in the 2018 American Heart Association stroke guidelines.

DEFUSE and DAWN trials had a great impact on how ischemic stroke patients who present between 6 and 24 hours are assessed and treated. They had profound implications for treatment of stroke due to LVO, because they validate the biological (rather than chronological) approach to patient selection for endovascular therapy. They also allow many more patients with LVO stroke to be treated with mechanical thrombectomy.

The new clinical trial data and guidelines have led a large number of stroke centers to begin using advanced imaging with computed tomography perfusion (CTP) or magnetic resonance imaging (MRI) to evaluate patients who present with a possible large vessel occlusion in an extended time window. These techniques can provide quantitative estimates of ischemic core and penumbra without user input and have excellent interobserver agreement [34].

The new AHA guidelines recommend that DAWN or DEFUSE 3 eligibility should be strictly adhered to in clinical practice; therefore, it is important to understand how these trials selected eligible patients as it is explained in Fig. 1.1. The only imaging modalities that have been shown to be effective for selecting patients for late-window thrombectomy are CTP and MRI. Both trials used the Rapid Processing of Perfusion and Diffusion (RAPID) automated software platform (iSchemaView, Menlo Park, CA) to determine imaging eligibility for all patients. Imaging selection for patients in both DEFUSE 3 and DAWN required either CTP or MRI, with the majority being selected by CTP. As it was mentioned above, RAPID was also used in EXTEND-IA and SWIFT PRIME trials. RAPID software provides automated analysis in less than 2 minutes. In evidence-based trials, RAPID imaging technology has given healthcare professionals the data needed to make more informed treatment decisions, becoming an extremely valuable tool in the treatment of acute stroke.

Summary

1. The understanding of the natural history of ischemic stroke and its treatment relies on multiple landmark papers. Endovascular thrombectomy is of benefit to most patients with acute ischemic stroke caused by occlusion of the proximal anterior circulation, irrespective of patient characteristics. Medical systems of care must be equipped to provide this life-saving treatment in a timely fashion to patients with acute ischemic stroke due to large vessel occlusion.
2. We think that the concept "time is brain" is unchanged but we should have in mind the concept of "penumbra is brain." Eligible patients should still be treated as quickly as possible; it is just that eligibility for treatment should not be restricted by time windows. No matter the time, if we have salvageable tissue in imaging studies, endovascular treatment should be done. We have to validate the biological (rather than chronological) approach to patient selection for endovascular therapy.

Bibliography

1. Fisher M, Aminoff M, Boller F, Swaab D. Handbook of clinical neurology, vol. 92 (3rd series). Stroke. Part I. M Fisher, Editor: Elsevier B.V; 2009.
2. Gomez CR. Editorial: time is brain! J Stroke Cerebrovasc Dis. 1993;3(1):1–2.
3. Bekhemer O, Beumer F, Berg V, Lingsma H, Schonewile Y, Nederkoom V. The randomized trial of intraarterial treatment for acute ischemic stroke (MR CLEAN). N Engl J Med. 2015;372:11.
4. Goyal M, Demchuk A, Menon B, Eesa M, Rempel J, Thornton J, Roy D. Randomized assay of rapid endovascular treatment of ischemic stroke (ESCAPE). N Engl J Med. 2015;372:1019.
5. Campbell B, Mitchell P, Kleinig T, Dewey H, Churilov L, Yassi N. Endovascular therapy for ischemic stroke with perfusion-imaging selection (EXTEND -IA). N Engl J Med. 2015;372:1009.
6. Saver J, Mayank M, Bonafe A, Diener M, Elad P, Levy I. Stent-retriever thrombectomy after intravenous t-PA vs. t-PA alone in stroke (SWIFT PRIME). N Engl J Med. 2015;372:2285.
7. Jovin T, Chamorro A, Cobo E, Miquel M, Molina C, Rovira A. Thrombectomy within 8 hours after symptom onset in ischemic stroke (REVASCAT). N Engl J Med. 2015;372:2296.
8. Kidwell CS, Jahan R, Gornbein J, Alger JR, Nenov V, Ajani Z, et al. A trial of imaging selection and endovascular treatment for ischemic stroke. N Engl J Med. 2013;368:914–23 (MR RESCUE).
9. Ciccone A, Valvassori L, Nichelatti M, Sgoifo A, Ponzio M, Sterzi R, et al. Endovascular treatment for acute ischemic stroke. N Engl J Med. 2013;368:904–13 (SYNTHESIS).
10. Broderick JP, Palesch YY, Demchuk AM, Yeatts SD, Khatri P, Hill MD, et al. Endovascular therapy after intravenous t-pa versus t-pa alone for stroke. N Engl J Med. 2013;368:893–903 (IMS 3).
11. Hacker W, Donney G, Fieschi C, Kaste M, von Kummer R, Broderick JP, Brott T, Frankel M, Grotta JC, Haley EC Jr, Kwiatkowski T, Levine SR, Lewandowski C, Lu M, Lyden P, Marler JR, Patel S, Tilley BC, Albers G, Bluhmki E, Wilhelm M, Hamilton S. Association of outcome with early stroke treatment: pooled analysis of ATLANTIS, ECASS, and NINDS rt-PA stroke trials. Lancet. 2004;363:768–74.

12. Tissue plasminogen activator for acute ischemic stroke. The National Institute of Neurological Disorders and Stroke rt-PA Stroke Study Group. N Engl J Med. 1995;333:1581–7.
13. Maas MB, Furie KL, Lev MH, et al. National Institutes of Health Stroke Scale score is poorly predictive of proximal occlusion in acute cerebral ischemia. Stroke. 2009;40:2988–93. - Nedeltchev K, Schwegler B, Haefeli T, et al. Outcome of stroke with mild or rapidly improving symptoms. Stroke. 2007;38:2531–5.
14. Rai AT, Jhadhav Y, Domico J, et al. Procedural predictors of outcome in patients undergoing endovascular therapy for acute ischemic stroke. Cardiovasc Intervent Radiol Published Online First: 14 December. 2012; https://doi.org/10.1007/s00270-011-0323-7.
15. Nogueira RG, Liebeskind DS, Sung G, et al. Predictors of good clinical outcomes, mortality, and successful revascularization in patients with acute ischemic stroke undergoing thrombectomy: pooled analysis of the Mechanical Embolus Removal in Cerebral Ischemia (MERCI) and multi MERCI trials. Stroke. 2009;40:3777–83.
16. Demchuk AM, Christou I, Wein TH, et al. Specific transcranial Doppler flow findings related to the presence and site of arterial occlusion. Stroke. 2000;31:140–6.
17. Zivin JA, Fisher M, DeGirolami U, et al. Tissue plasminogen activator reduces neurological damage after cerebral embolism. Science. 1985;230:1289–92.
18. Lee JH, Kim YJ, Choi JW, et al. Multimodal CT:. Favorable outcome factors in acute middle cerebral artery stroke with large artery occlusion. Eur Neurol. 2013;69(6):366–74.
19. Smith WS, Lev MH, English JD, et al. Significance of large vessel intracranial occlusion causing acute ischemic stroke and TIA. Stroke. 2009;40:3834–40.
20. Nogueira RG, Smith WS. Emergency treatment of acute ischemic stroke: expanding the time window. Curr Treat Options Neurol. 2009;11:433–43.
21. Penumbra pivotal stroke trial investigators. The Penumbra pivotal stroke trial: safety and effectiveness of a new generation of mechanical devices for clot removal in intracranial large vessel occlusive disease. Stroke. 2009;40:2761–8.
22. Castano C, Dorado L, Guerrero C, et al. Mechanical thrombectomy with the Solitaire AB device in large artery occlusions of the anterior circulation. A pilot study. Stroke. 2010;41:1836–40.
23. Costalat V, Machi P, Lobotesis K, et al. Rescue, combined, and stand-alone thrombectomy in the management of large vessel occlusion stroke using the Solitaire device: a prospective 50-patient single–center study. Stroke. 2011;42:1929–35.
24. Menon BK, Sajobi TT, Zhang Y, Rempel JL, Shuaib A, Thornton J, et al. Analysis of workflow and time to treatment on thrombectomy outcome in the endovascular treatment for small core and proximal occlusion ischemic stroke (ESCAPE) randomized, controlled trial. Circulation. 2016;133:2279.
25. Jauch EC, Saver JL, Adams HP Jr, Bruno A, Connors JJ, Demaerschalk BM, Khatri P, McMullan PW Jr, Qureshi AI, Rosenfield K, Scott PA, Summers DR, Wang DZ, Wintermark M, Yonas H. Guidelines for the early management of patients with acute ischemic stroke: a guideline for healthcare professionals from the American Heart Association/American Stroke Association. Stroke. 2013;44:870–947.
26. Powers WJ, Rabinstein AA. Guidelines for the early management of patients with acute ischemic stroke: 2019 update to the 2018 guidelines for the early management of acute ischemic stroke. A guideline for healthcare professionals from the American Heart Association/American Stroke Association. Stroke. 2019;50:e344.
27. Khatri P, Yeatts SD, Mazighi M, et al. Time to angiographic reperfusion and clinical outcome after acute ischemic stroke: an analysis of data from the Interventional Management of Stroke (IMS iii) phase 3 trial. Lancet Neurol. 2014;13:567–74.
28. Bhole R, Goyal N, Nearing K, Belayev A, Doss VT, Elijovich L. Implications of limiting mechanical thrombectomy to patients with emergent large vessel occlusion meeting top tier evidence criteria. J Neuro Intervent Surg. 2016;0:1–5. https://doi.org/10.1136/neurintsurg-2015-012206.
29. Dippel D, Majoie C, Roos Y, et al. Influence of device choice on the effect of intra-arterial treatment for acute ischemic stroke in MR CLEAN. Stroke. 2016;47:2574–81.

30. Lapergue B, Blanc R, Gory B, Labreuche J, Duhamel A, Marnat G. Effect of endovascular contact aspiration vs stent retriever on revascularization in patients with acute ischemic stroke and large vessel occlusion: the ASTER randomized clinical trial. JAMA. 2017;318(5):443–52.
31. Lapergue, Blanc, Gory, Labreuche, Duhamel, Marnat, et al. Effect of endovascular contact aspiration vs stent retriever on revascularization in patients with acute ischemic stroke and large vessel occlusion: the ASTER randomized clinical trial. JAMA. 2017;318(5):443–52. https://doi.org/10.1001/jama.2017.9644.
32. Turk AS 3rd, et al. Aspiration thrombectomy versus stent retriever thrombectomy as first-line approach for large vessel occlusion (COMPASS): a multicentre, randomised, open label, blinded outcome, non-inferiority trial. Lancet. 2019;393(10175):998–1008.
33. Sedation vs. Intubation for Endovascular Stroke Treatment (SIESTA). ClinicalTrials.gov NCT02126085.
34. Gregory W, Albers MD. Use of imaging to select patients for late window endovascular therapy. Stroke. 2018;49:00. https://doi.org/10.1161/STROKEAHA.118.021011.

Chapter 2
In Vitro Clot Modeling and Clinical Applications

Sarah Johnson, Juyu Chueh, Ajit S. Puri, Peter E. McHugh, Rose A. Arslanian, and Matthew J. Gounis

Introduction

Stroke is a leading cause of death and disability in the USA and poses a significant economic burden to society. According to the heart disease and stroke statistics from 2018, an additional 4% of the adult population will have experienced a stroke by 2030 [1]. Recent randomized controlled trials have demonstrated a convincing benefit from stent retriever-mediated mechanical thrombectomy for selected acute ischemic stroke (AIS) patients with large vessel occlusion in the anterior circulation [2–5]. Early reperfusion of ischemic penumbra is associated with favorable outcomes and reduced mortality. The dependencies of the efficacy and safety of endovascular treatment on clot composition and mechanics were highlighted in prior studies [6, 7]. Understanding the clot composition prior to thrombectomy using imaging modalities such as MR or CT may help determine the most appropriate treatment strategy. Current in vitro clot modeling techniques produce clinically representative clot analogs with different mechanical features for device efficacy testing and with various histological patterns for improving clot imaging quality. In this chapter, we will review several methods of clot preparation and characterization and discuss the clinical applications of the clot analogs.

S. Johnson
Department of Biomedical Engineering, National University of Ireland Galway, Galway, Ireland

J. Chueh (✉) · A. S. Puri · R. A. Arslanian · M. J. Gounis
Department of Radiology, University of Massachusetts Medical School, Worcester, MA, USA
e-mail: juyu.chueh@umassmed.edu

P. E. McHugh
Department of Biomedical Engineering, National University of Ireland Galway, College of Engineering and Informatics, Galway, Ireland

F. K. Hui et al. (eds.), *12 Strokes*, https://doi.org/10.1007/978-3-030-56857-3_2

In Vitro Clot Modeling

Clot Analogs Made with Biological Blood Components

There are many protocols in the literature to produce clot analog material. It is important to make clot models that represent mechanical features of clots that cause stroke in order to predict efficacy of thrombectomy technology. There is large variability of the composition and mechanical features in emboli that cause large vessel occlusions likely related to the source of clot. Common variables to generate clot analogs include donor species, the addition of thrombin, the use of radiopacifying media, and the variation in red blood cell (RBC) and fibrin content. The variation in hematologic values from different donors, as well as varying concentrations of thrombin, contrast agent, fibrinogen, platelets, and calcium, can result in very different clot composition and structure [8].

Bovine, porcine, ovine and human blood are commonly used for the preparation of clot analogs. Thrombin-induced clotting is initiated by mixing whole blood with thrombin [9, 10]. The blood-thrombin mixture is then injected into a silicone tube for clotting and aging prior to use. Barium sulfate is incorporated into the blood to enhance or offer radiopacity and can decrease elasticity leading to being prone to fragmentation. Calcium-mediated clotting can also be achieved without the addition of thrombin. Asakura et al. [11] collected porcine blood without heparin. The blood was added to citric acid to remove calcium. The mixture was centrifuged and the plasma was mixed with lactic acid Ringer's solution to produce a fibrin clot. Fibrin clots were also formed using human blood from healthy volunteers for rheologic analysis [12]. The blood samples were centrifuged at a slow spin of 110 g for 15 minutes to remove the platelet-rich plasma (PRP). The PRP was spun at a high spin at 1000 g for 15 minutes to yield the platelet-poor plasma (PPP). Gel-filtered platelets were prepared from the PRP and were stored in platelet buffer at 37 °C for up to 2 hours. Human fibrinogen was partially purified from the PPP by adding saturated ammonium sulfate and incubating at 4 °C for 1 hour. Thrombin-induced clotting was used in this study. The rheologic results revealed that introducing platelets to human plasma and fibrin during clot preparation increases the clot stiffness and reduces strain hardening. Recently, Fitzgerald et al. have shown that platelet-rich emboli harvested during thrombectomy correspond to or are more frequently encountered in LVO cases with large artery atherosclerosis as the underlying etiology [13].

Ovine blood has been demonstrated to be a suitable substitute for human blood for coagulation studies [14] and the corresponding blood clots have been shown to be histologically similar to human clots [7, 15]. Citrated ovine blood was used to prepare different clot analogs with varying RBC and fibrin content [15]. The whole blood was centrifuged and separated into the plasma, buffy layer, and RBC-rich layer. The plasma and RBCs were harvested separately and then recombined in controlled ratios to give clot analogs with varying compositions – 0%, 5%, 40%, and 80% RBC content. Calcium chloride ($CaCl_2$) was added to the solution to reverse the action of the sodium citrate, and the samples were incubated at 37 °C for 30 minutes to initiate clotting. Murine blood has also been used in the formation of clot analogs. Citrated murine blood was centrifuged at a low spin [16]. The PRP layer was then collected and brought to 37 °C in a water bath. The clot analog was formed by adding $CaCl_2$ and thrombin to the PRP and was left at room temperature for 2 hours until fully coagulated before testing.

Clot Models Formed Under Dynamic Conditions

One experimental approach to in vitro thrombogenesis is Chandler's loop technique, whereby the clot is formed under dynamic flow conditions in a closed loop. This technique has been found to produce a more heterogeneous clot [3, 17]. A modified version of the Chandler's loop technique was developed to make a fibrin-rich clot analog [15]. Silicone tubing was mounted on a multi-rotator device and partially filled with citrated ovine whole blood. Calcium chloride was injected into the tubing and the ends of the tubing were then fixed, thus forming a closed loop. The tubing was rotated at a rate of 25 rpm for 1 hour. The resulting clot analog revealed a predominance of fibrin with several clumps of RBCs. A similar method was adopted by Shao et al. forming clots from swine blood mixed with barium sulfate and bovine thrombin [18]. The mixture was injected into a polyvinyl chloride tube, ensuring there were no air bubbles. The tube was coiled using a connector and set into a plexiglass ring rotation unit, which was mounted on a rotating shaft of an MR-16 blood clot detector and slowly rotated for 15 minutes at 15 rpm. Poole et al. also produced clots using a similar modified Chandler method from citrated human, bovine, rat, and rabbit blood mixed with $CaCl_2$ [19].

Clot Analogs Made of Polymeric Materials

In training environments, it is not always possible to use clot analogs that are derived from blood products due to local regulations. Furthermore, clot analogs derived from blood products are always subject to biological variability associated with normal variations in hematological values as well as a variability associated with techniques deployed to collect blood. Therefore, it is attractive to have synthetic alternatives. Moderately stiff synthetic clots made from polyacrylamide were used to evaluate the clot capture efficiency of various vena cava filters in a physiological venous flow loop [20]. These devices were also tested using clots formed in vitro from both human and ovine blood. This study found that although the polymeric clots were more convenient and easier to use than the clots formed from blood, there were differences in shape, density, and elasticity, and this in turn affected the device performance.

Synthetic clot material formed by combining polyacrylamide and alginate (PAAM-Alg) with a cross-linking agent was tested by Merritt et al. [21]. Rheometry was used to compare the shear and dynamic moduli of the synthetic polymeric clots with clots formed in vitro using human blood. The PAAM-Alg analogs were found to closely mimic the clots formed using human blood and were easily adjustable to mimic various thrombi classifications.

Clot Characterization

Mechanical Characterization

Clot analogs are an attractive option for the preclinical testing and development of treatment devices, as they can be produced from blood proteins and components present in the clotting cascade and have a similar chemical structure to native clots [22]. In addition, they are also a useful tool for the investigation and characterization of clot material properties and their mechanical behavior as a function of their constituents. As discussed earlier, there are many protocols in the literature for the manufacture of clot analogs. The mechanical properties of these analogs, such as strength, permeability, and elasticity, can easily be manipulated by altering the concentrations of fibrinogen, thrombin, platelets, RBCs, and calcium [23]. Many studies have investigated the effect of clot composition on their mechanical properties. It is important to use clot models that have similar bulk mechanical characteristics as the emboli that lead to LVO in stroke patients in order to optimize device technology and techniques on the bench.

Tensile Testing

Krasokha et al. investigated the tensile strength of clot analogs, produced in vitro from porcine blood and combined with thrombin and barium sulfate [24]. They found that the analog material reached high levels of stress and strain, approximately 9k Pa and 240%, respectively, before failure. This indicates that the material is highly elastic. Similar results were obtained by Brown et al. [25] from their extension testing of fibrin clots, formed from purified human fibrinogen. The samples were stretched to three times their relaxed length before failing. Similar failure strains were observed by Saldivar et al. [26] during the tensile testing of their clot analogs formed in vitro from thrombin and human fibrinogen. It was found that mechanical failure was a consequence of fibrinolytic activity due to an increased concentration of plasmin. This finding has clinical relevance in that it shows that fibrinolysis has a profound impact on the mechanical properties of the clot suggesting that pre-thrombectomy administration of recombinant tissue plasminogen activator severely damages the fibrin structure which may produce more clot fragmentation during thrombectomy. Ongoing trials will answer the question if pre-thrombectomy r-tPA versus direct to thrombectomy for LVO patients imparts any difference in clinical outcomes.

Compression Testing

Mechanical testing of soft tissues, such as clot material, can be quite challenging particularly for tensile testing where grasping the clot material is necessary. Therefore, very soft tissues are often tested in compression to determine their mechanical behavior. Krasokha et al. performed unconfined compression testing of clots formed in vitro using porcine and human whole blood and investigated the effect of the addition of barium sulfate. It was found that both the porcine and human clot analogs demonstrated increased stiffness due to the addition of barium sulfate. Similarly these results were validated by Chueh et al. [10], who also determined that the addition of barium sulfate greatly reduced the elasticity of clot analogs formed from bovine, porcine, and human whole blood. However, differences in structure and composition were observed between analog clot material and the specimens retrieved from the AIS patients.

Compression testing was employed to determine the mechanics of fibrin clot under compression [27]. Fibrin clot analogs were prepared by mixing human citrated PPP with calcium chloride and human thrombin. The origin of the nonlinear rheology of the fibrin networks under compression was investigated using confocal microscopy and rheological measurements [22]. Visual observations of the 3D networks displayed buckling of the fibrin fibers along the direction of the compressive force. Fiber bending was also found to increase with compressive force and the deformation of the individual fibers depended greatly on their orientation in the network. Fibrin clots formed in vitro showed plastic deformation under compressive loading as cross-linked clot samples did not recover or spring back [26]. This suggests that fiber integrity is essential for sustaining consistent clot response when samples experience large levels of stress both in vitro and in vivo.

Other Test Methods

Rheology and large-amplitude oscillatory shear (LAOS) deformations were used to study the nonlinear viscoelastic properties of clot analogs, formed from whole porcine blood, PRP, and PPP [28, 29]. The rheology results indicate that clots formed from PRP had the highest stiffness, followed by clots formed with whole blood and PPP, respectively. This behavior can be explained by platelet contraction, which causes the increased stiffness of the network [30]. The high volume of RBCs in the whole blood prevents this contraction. This can be noted between clots formed from PRP and whole blood during the LAOS experiments as the fibrin network is stiffer when there are no RBCs present [28].

Nanoindentation was performed to determine the mechanical properties of murine clot material produced from PRP in vivo [16]. This test method has many advantages over other test methods as it can obtain small-scale measurements. The indenter tips are easily customizable and high-resolution load and displacement measurements can be obtained. The moduli values for the clot material were found to be within the range for soft materials. Indentation testing may be very appropriate for studying the response of clot analogs specific to stent retriever thrombectomy, where the struts impose chronic outward force into the clot as the mechanism of action for thrombectomy [31].

During the thrombectomy procedure, the clot experiences sliding contact along the inside of the vessel and/or the inside of the catheter. The resistance to sliding (friction) of clot material as a function of composition was studied to investigate if clot composition may contribute to friction and the resistance to clot removal [7]. The results from the study found that fibrin-rich clots had a significantly larger coefficient of friction than clots with high RBC content, which may contribute to fibrin-rich clots requiring more retrieval attempts [32]. Moreover, the emboli tend to roll along the surface of the stent retriever, which may help to explain the recent finding that longer stent retrievers have a statistically higher first-pass effect [33]. Essentially, the longer stent provides more real estate for the rolling clot so that the risk of complete disengagement during the first pass is reduced.

Histological Characterization

Clot composition has a definite impact on the performance of mechanical thrombectomy devices and can be assessed using various histological methods [34]. Clots with high RBC content are associated with a high rate of successful intra-arterial thrombectomy [35], whereas fibrin-rich clots are often resistant to mechanical thrombectomy, resulting in an extended procedure time and unfavorable clinical outcome. The most commonly used staining methods are hematoxylin-eosin staining (H&E) and Martius Scarlet Blue (MSB) [10, 15]. H&E highlights nuclei in blue-black, RBCs in orange red, and fibrin in deep pink. MSB stains fresh fibrin red, aged fibrin blue, and RBCs yellow. Immunostaining is conducted to identify platelets using antibodies for platelet glycoprotein IIIa with CD61 [36]. Inflammatory cells such as neutrophils have recently been found to have impacts on clot stability and can be detected with neutrophil elastase staining [37]. Other methods such as Elastica van Gieson staining stain nuclei black-brown [38]. Clinical samples are stained with Gomori methenamine silver for fungus [39]. For quantitative measurements of clot components, the stained slide is imaged at low magnification and the clot image is subjected to segmentation to differentiate each clot constituent (Fig. 2.1).

Thermal and Electrical Characterization

The efficacy of ultrasound-assisted thrombolysis as a treatment of ischemic stroke is being widely investigated. To determine the role of ultrasound hyperthermia in blood clot disruption, the acoustic-mechanical and thermal properties of both human and porcine blood clots formed in vitro were measured [40]. Direct calorimetric measurements using E-type thermocouples were performed to evaluate the specific heat of the clots, and the comparative steady-state method was used for the determination of their thermal conductivity. An insertion loss method was used to measure

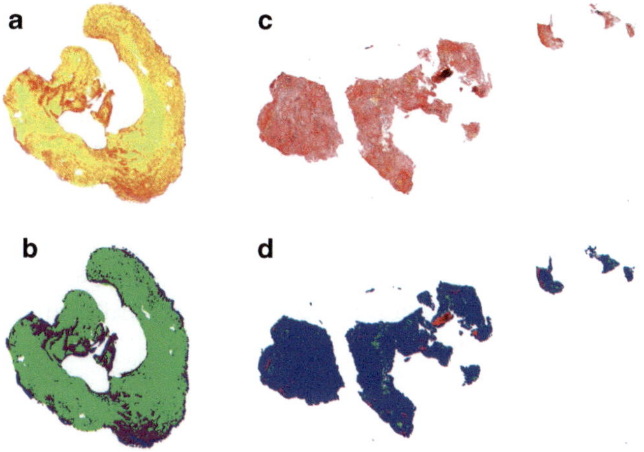

Component	Percentage	Percentage
RBC	76.64	2.05
Fibrin	4.67	95.86
RBC and fibrin	18.69	2.09

Fig. 2.1 Paraffin-embedded sections of human clot (**a**) erythrocyte-rich clot. (**c**) fibrin-rich clot. The corresponding (**b** and **d**, respectively) segmented masks show erythrocytes in green, fibrin in blue, and fibrin/erythrocyte mixed area in purple. (Table) Quantitative analysis of the percentage of erythrocytes, fibrin, and mixed erythrocytes and fibrin by area

the ultrasound attenuation in the clots. The specific heat values of human and porcine clots were found to be $3.5 \pm 0.8 \times 10^3$ J/kg.K and $3.2 \pm 0.5 \times 10^3$ J/kg.K, respectively, and the coefficients of thermal conductivity were 0.55 ± 0.13 W/m/K and 0.59 ± 0.11 W/m.K, respectively. The magnitudes of amplitude attenuation varied between 0.10 and 0.3 Np/cm in the porcine clots and 0.09 and 0.23 Np/cm in the human samples. The measured attenuation coefficients were in the range of published values for other soft biological materials such as liver, kidney, and brain [40]. The results obtained from this study will allow for the numerical estimates of a magnitude of the thermal evaluation during ultrasound sonification of thrombus for enhanced thrombolysis. This knowledge may be useful in the development of high-intensity focused ultrasound and other therapies.

Aging and Storage

It has been found that aged clot material behaves differently to fresh clot material. Previously published experiments have been carried out on clot material with substantial variations in age, from 1 hour to 10 days [17]. Aged human thromboemboli were found to have a reduced elasticity when compared to soft, highly elastic fresh red thromboemboli. These fresh thromboemboli are also less likely to fragment when compared to aged specimens. Similar results have been produced with analog clot material, where increased stiffness was observed as the clot samples aged [24]. This is an important consideration particularly relevant to LVOs in patients with atrial fibrillation, where the clot material may have formed over long periods of time.

Krueger et al. investigated the effect of clot aging and storage temperature on clot samples [17]. Spontaneous and thrombin-induced samples were aged for 1 or 5 days at 4 °C or 37 °C. The results from the study show that thrombus can affect the results of the thrombectomy procedure and clot stability appeared to decrease with age. It was hypothesized that this was due to cell lysis. Storage temperature as a singular factor was not found to affect the results and only had an effect in combination with other parameters tested.

Clinical Applications

Comparison with Human Clots – Microstructure/ Mechanical Behavior

Analog clot material is becoming increasingly prevalent in preclinical testing of devices as a cheaper and more readily available alternative to human clot tissue [22]. However, a limitation of this material is the fundamental difference between the clot analogs formed in vitro and the complex human material [10]. Research into the morphology of AIS thrombi has revealed that no two thrombi are histologically identical, due to ranging fibrin and RBC composition [39, 41, 42], presence of neutrophil extracellular traps [43] and von Willebrand factor [44], and platelet content [45].

Human thrombi have been found to be very heterogeneous, with large variation in structure and composition [10, 21, 39, 41, 46, 47]. Most analog clot materials have a homogeneous composition, though some heterogeneous clots have been formed [21, 48, 49]. A paper by Chandler et al. proposed forming the clot samples in a closed loop in order to simulate the physiological blood flow environment [48]. Clots formed using this method are found to have a fibrin-rich pattern and are more firm and elastic in comparison to clots formed under static conditions, which are generally RBC dominant with increased heterogeneity [15]. Similarly, an experimental approach by Kan et al. [49] prepared the clot analogs by sedimentation to ensure that the clots had a layered structure consisting of a fibrin-rich and a RBC-rich component.

Clot analogs have been developed with ranging compositions that are mechanically relevant and histologically similar to thrombi removed from AIS patients (Fig. 2.2) [10, 15, 39]. Recalcified porcine analogs and thrombin-induced analogs formed from human blood were found to have similar elasticity and stiffness to clots from cerebral thromboemboli [10]. In addition, it was noted that there was no

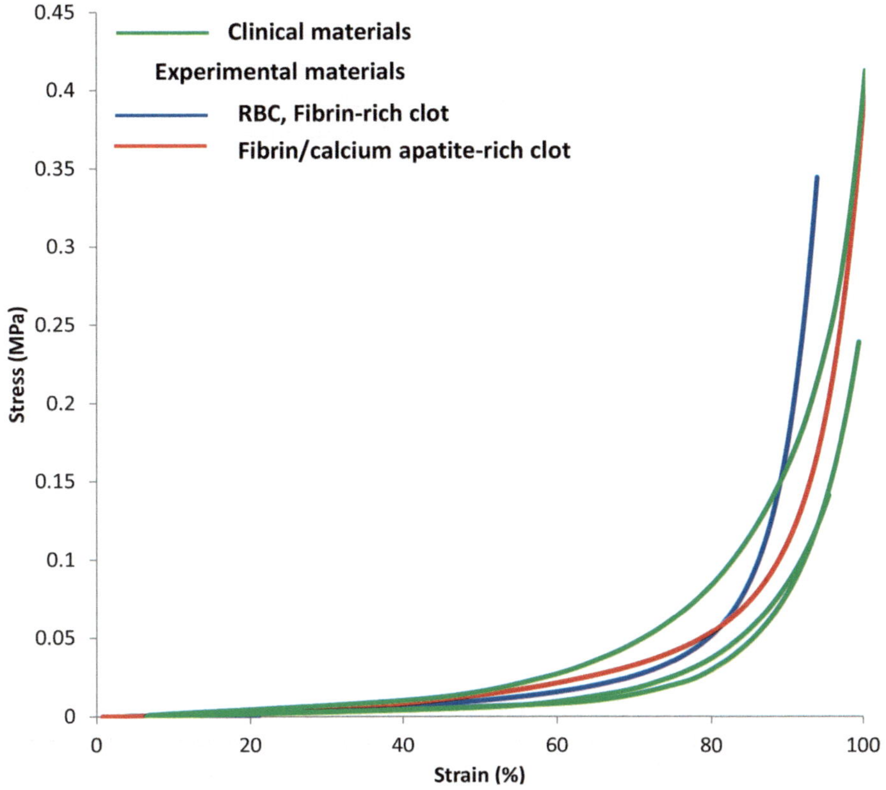

Fig. 2.2 Characterization of clots stiffness is conducted using dynamic mechanical analyzer. The stress-strain curves demonstrate the similarity in stiffness between the clinical and experimental clot specimens

significant difference in stiffness between thrombin-induced bovine or porcine in vitro analogs and clot samples collected by carotid endarterectomy. Calcifications in AIS thrombi are rare but often challenging. Previous SEM results demonstrated that the calcified materials found in the cerebral thromboemboli were mainly composed of calcium phosphate apatite [10]. An innovative method has been developed to facilitate calcium phosphate mineralization in the fibrin gel by diffusion to incorporate calcification into the clot modeling process [50].

Clot Attachment to the Wall

Various animal models of vascular occlusion for thrombectomy device testing are created by injecting the clot analogs into the target vessels [51–53]; however, the extent of clot attachment to the vessel wall is still undetermined in these embolic models. The potential effects of clot-vessel wall interaction on the performance of the thrombectomy devices have been mentioned in previous work [54, 55].

Clot stability in injured arteries has been widely discussed from the viewpoint of molecular and cellular biology [56–61]. In the cases of hemostasis or rupture of atherosclerotic plaque, exposure of the underlying fibrous matrix triggers deposition and activation of platelets which are mediated by von Willebrand factor (vWF)/glycoprotein (GP)Ib-IX-V and/or collagen/GPVI interactions, depending in part on the shear condition [62–67]. The activated GPIIb/IIIa interacts with adhesive proteins in plasma to aggregate the platelets, which accelerates the thrombus formation [68]. The thrombus stability on the vessel wall is associated with platelet myosin contractility [59], fibrin, and GPIIb/IIIa-dependent contraction [62]. Similar platelet reactions initiated by the intact inflamed endothelium are described in the previous work. During the inflammatory state, adhesion molecules like vWF and P-selectin are secreted from the Weibel-Palade bodies (storage granules of endothelial cells) and interact with platelets via GPIb-IX-V. The vWF released from the Weibel-Palade bodies is stickier than that found in the plasma [68]. Dynamic platelet aggregation not only occurs during thrombosis but also at the occlusion site after embolization. Zhang et al. observed cluster of platelets at the site of embolus 1 hour after the embolization; in addition, GPIIb/IIIa and plasminogen activator inhibitor-1 immunoreactivity was present between the embolus and the vessel wall [69].

Several methods have been developed to analyze the force required to detach the adherent cells from the substrates [70]. Cells, including cultured fibroblasts, osteoblastic cells, cancer cells, or leukocytes, are often seeded on the tissue engineering scaffolds such as glass or tissue-culture polystyrene plate coated with endothelial cells, collagen, or fibronectin [71–74]. Cells may then be mechanically separated from the substrate by using centrifuge assay, spinning disk device, flow chambers, or micromanipulation [72, 75, 76]. Although these approaches provide insight into single cell-scaffold interactions, the typical measurement range of force (of the order of piconewtons to nanonewtons) is not sufficient to remove the clot from the vessel wall [70, 74, 76, 77].

Clot-vessel wall adhesion analysis was performed with the use of the rabbit stenosis model that was developed for creation of embolic occlusion. The clot was injected into the common carotid artery and lodged at the stenosis for 6 hours to allow clot attachment to the vessel wall. The occluded vessel segments were explanted and subjected to the debonding test with the use of a customized rig [78]. Investigation of the clot-vessel interactions in terms of adhesion force and histological characteristics can be used as a means of bridging the gap between pathophysiological consequences of endothelial dysfunction and performance of thrombectomy devices. Such information will provide important information to establish physiologically representative models of cerebrovascular occlusion and prevent overestimating the successful rate of the mechanical thrombectomy in preclinical tests.

Mechanical Thrombectomy for Treatment of Acute Ischemic Stroke

Recent randomized clinical trials have shown that mechanical thrombectomy is an effective treatment for patients with large vessel occlusion in the anterior circulation. The US Food and Drug Administration in early 2018 further cleared the extended use of the Trevo clot retrieval device (Stryker Neurovascular) from 6 to 24 hours after stroke onset, based on the results of the DAWN trial [79]. There has been rapid evolution in thrombectomy devices and approaches over the past decade; however, to date, there are no universally accepted standards for device or treatment selection due to little-known scientific information about what combinations of techniques or devices will yield the best outcome [80].

Device Safety: Distal Embolization

While several clinical trials have shown better recanalization rate with the newer thrombectomy devices, improved recanalization rates with the newer thrombectomy devices are not synonymous with better clinical outcomes [2–5]. The leading hypothesis to explain this conundrum is that patients who benefit from thrombectomy need to be correctly identified. Therefore, most comprehensive stroke centers currently deploy advanced imaging to identify patients with viable penumbra. Other plausible contributors to poor patient outcome may be related to creation of distal emboli, arterial wall response to the thrombectomy devices, baseline NIH stroke scale, and time to recanalization [81–83]. Among these parameters, generation of clot fragmentation during treatment with subsequent distal shower of emboli is a procedure-related adverse event which can be technically modified.

Clot debris generated during mechanical thrombectomy or that form in situ due to local vessel damage during thrombectomy can result in distal embolization. According to the previous in vitro studies with the use of the thrombin-induced clot models, thousands of microemboli were formed during the thrombectomy procedure [6, 84]. The impact of these microemboli on the microcirculation remains unknown. This may lead to poor clinical outcomes, even in the setting of good proximal revascularization. Several adjunctive endovascular techniques such as balloon guide catheter-assisted stent retriever thrombectomy as well as stent retriever thrombectomy with aspiration via a distal access catheter are used in acute stroke interventions to reduce the risk of distal embolization [6]. Subsequently, numerous clinical studies have shown that deployment of balloon guide catheters during thrombectomy is significantly associated with improved rates of good clinical outcomes [85–89]. This evidence strongly suggests that reducing distal embolization during thrombectomy improves functional outcomes in patients.

The growing use of the experimental clot models for thrombectomy device testing continues with a goal to provide clinicians with treatment strategies based on laboratory findings; therefore, it is critical to have clot models that are clinically representative in terms of their bulk mechanical behaviors as well as compositional features. The prior in vitro work used the clot models that have similar mechanical characteristics to the clot specimens retrieved from the patients with AIS. The results suggested that applying proximal flow control with the use of a balloon guide catheter during clot removal not only achieved effective and successful mechanical thrombectomy but also significantly reduced the risk of distal embolization.

Particle Characterization

Continuous detection of microembolic signals in a number of clinical conditions has been performed using the technique of transcranial Doppler ultrasonography [90–93], but this technique is associated with the following limitations. Firstly, an acoustic temporal bone window required for the Doppler signal to reach the cerebral vasculature is unsatisfactory in certain patients. Secondly, the operator must be highly trained and experienced with the technique to be successful; otherwise this technique may lead to high levels of variability in signal-to-noise ratio. For particle detection in the in vitro systems, there are a wide range of characterization methods that can be used to measure particles [94]. These methods include but are not limited to dynamic imaging particle analysis [95], light-scattering technique [96–98], the Coulter counter [6, 99], and filtration methods [100, 101].

Dynamic imaging particle analysis uses digital images to measure the size and shape of each particle. Real-time detection of emboli generation during thrombectomy is particularly useful in optimizing techniques, since each action during the procedure can have an associated impact on clot fragmentation. The sample containing the particles streams by the microscope optics in the flow cell, and thousands of particle images are captured per second. The camera triggering frequency is determined based on the sample flow rate and is fixed during the experiment. Consequently, particles may be counted multiple times if flow rate is significantly reduced during the counting operation. Data post-processing is required to remove the particles that are imaged more than once. During the dynamic light-scattering (DLS) measurement, the Brownian motion of particles in suspension scatters the laser light and causes variations in scattering intensity. The fluctuations in the scattered light intensity are used to gain information about the particle size. Only small sample volume is required to obtain the mean particle size. However, this method does not provide detailed information about the particle size distribution. The size and size distribution of the particles can be measured in electrolytes using the Coulter principle (Fig. 2.3). When a particle travels through an orifice, the resulting current fluctuation is converted to a voltage pulse, which is proportional to the volume of the particle. Analysis of a broad size distribution can be achieved by using different apertures/orifices.

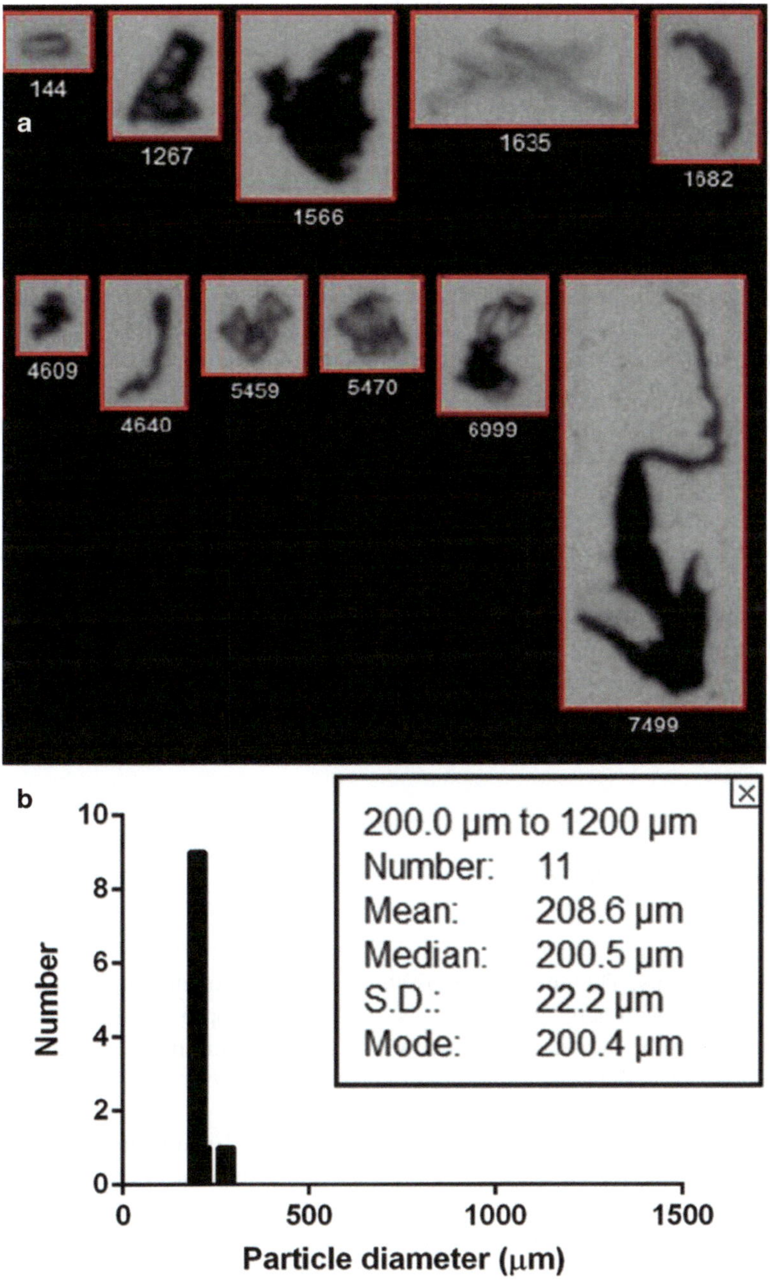

Fig. 2.3 (**a**) Images of the clot fragments acquired using dynamic imaging particle analysis. (**b**) The imaging results are correlated well with the Coulter counter data. Both techniques show that there are 11 emboli with size >200 µm generated during mechanical thrombectomy in an in vitro setup

Device Efficacy: Clot Integration Factor

Successful first-pass recanalization is associated with better clinical outcomes and is a new measure for thrombectomy device testing [102]. During the stent retriever thrombectomy, the ability of the stent retriever to retain the clot in the stent struts during clot retrieval is affected by the device design. Loss of interaction between clot and stent retriever when passing the tortuous cerebral arteries can result in partial or failed thrombectomy. The clot retriever is in a collapsed configuration for deployment across the occlusion and self-expands radially to compress the occlusive clot against the vessel wall prior to clot retrieval [103]. The recommended time for the clot to be fully engaged within the stent retriever prior to withdrawal in the instructions for use varies from 3 to 5 minutes, depending on the thrombectomy device. However, in actual clinical practice, the interaction time between clot and device ranges from 30 seconds to more than 5 minutes [104–107]. The invention of the clot integration factor (CIF) made quantitative assessment of device-clot interaction possible during stent retriever thrombectomy (Fig. 2.4) [108]. By comparing the CIF immediately following device deployment as well as 5 minutes following device deployment, it was found that a better device-clot interaction was achieved by increasing the interaction time. Sufficient image contrast level between the clot analog and the stent strut allowed successful segmentation of the stent retriever during post-image processing during CIF measurements; however, it is not always achievable in daily clinical practice. However, evaluating the angiogram carefully during stent engagement of the clot may inform the time required for optimal device-clot interaction [109].

Thrombolytic Drug Testing

Early reperfusion of ischemic penumbra is associated with favorable outcomes and reduced mortality. The only approved pharmacological treatment, IV recombinant tissue plasminogen activator (r-tPA), is available for approximately 5% of stroke patients due to the narrow time window and several contraindications that limit its use. Moreover, with large clot burdens in proximal vessels, r-tPA is less effective in achieving recanalization.

Marosfoi et al. investigated a novel shear-activated nanotherapeutic (SA-NT) that releases recombinant tissue-type plasminogen activation when exposed to high levels of hemodynamic stress, combined with temporary endovascular bypass (TEB) [55] . The aim of this study was to determine if this approach could be used to concentrate r-tPA at occlusion sites by utilizing the high shear stresses that are created by stent placement. The microscale aggregates remain intact when flowing in blood under physiological conditions and break up into individual nanoscale components when exposed to high shear stress [110]. These nanoparticles adhere to the surface of the clot and concentrate the r-tPA at these sites.

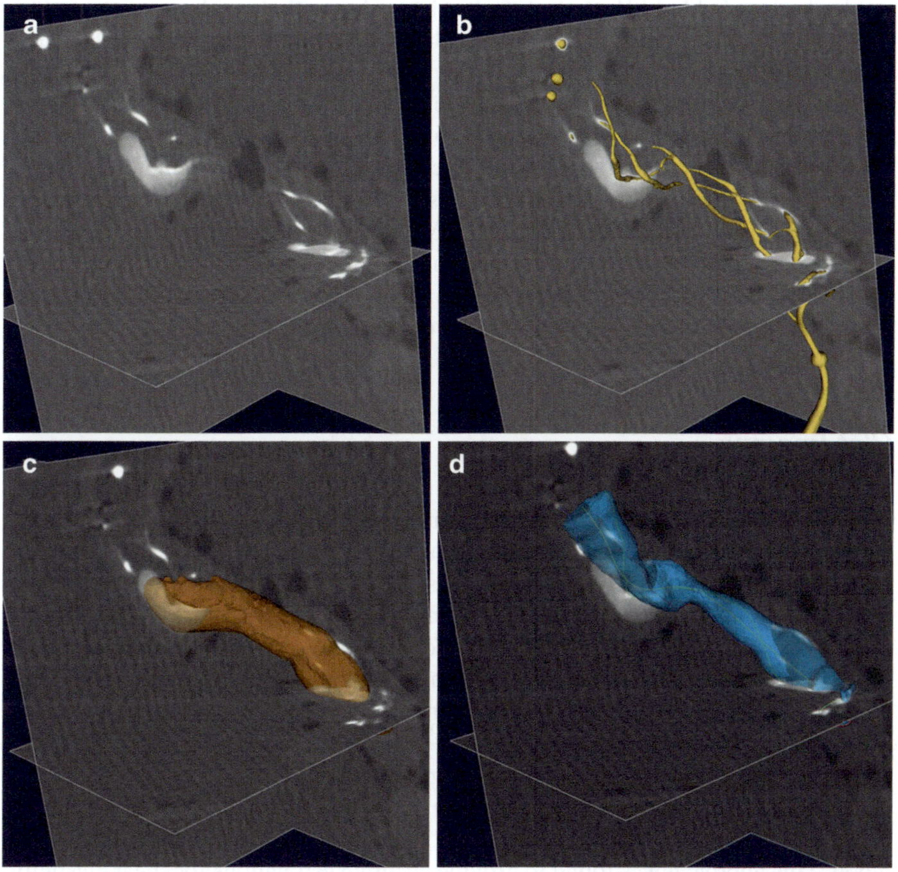

Fig. 2.4 Example views with three orthogonal planes of a reconstructed VasoCT image (**a**), the location of the three marker wires (**b**), the result of the level-set segmentation of the clot (**c**), and the determination of the inner volume of the device bounded by the extracted marker wires (**d**)

A rabbit model of a carotid occlusion was used to test this hypothesis. The angiographic recanalization of three cases, TEB alone, intra-arterial delivery of soluble r-tPA alone, and TEB combined with two doses of intra-arterial infusion of SA-NT or soluble r-tPA, was analyzed. Vascular injury was also compared with thrombectomy using a stent retriever. The results show that the shear-targeted delivery of the r-tPA using the SA-NT resulted in the highest rate of complete recanalization when compared to the controls. SA-NT also had a higher likelihood of achieving complete recanalization when compared with TEB alone, intra-arterial r-tPA alone, or TEB with soluble r-tPA. The histological analysis showed loss of endothelium in the area where the TEB was deployed. However, there was significantly less vascular injury using a TEB compared to the stent retriever procedure.

r-tPA results in early reperfusion in only 13–50% of patients with occlusions of the intracranial internal carotid artery or the first segment of the middle cerebral artery [111–113]. Recent studies have shown that combining intravenous thrombolysis (IVT) using r-tPA with mechanical thrombectomy (MT) is superior to direct MT in terms of clinical outcomes at 90 days [2, 3, 5, 114, 115]. However, most of these studies compared IVT-eligible and IVT-ineligible patients, although both groups are inherently different [115, 116]. In contrast, when analysis was confined to studies with a low risk of selection bias (i.e., comparable IVT-eligible patients in both treatment groups), the results indicate that direct MT may offer comparable safety and efficacy to IVT+MT [117]. On the contrary, it has also been suggested that r-tPA may cause harm as it may promote the blood-brain barrier breakdown, potentiate vessel wall damage by stent retrievers, and induce thrombus fragmentation, leading to more challenging interventions [116].

Clot Imaging

Distinguishing between red and white thrombi and determining clot age could potentially be very useful in evaluating what treatment strategy to pursue [118]. The definition of clot characteristics that are associated with successful recanalization could help to inform treatment decisions and identify patients at risk [119]. From a clinical aspect, imaging of a clot in situ before treatment could assist in establishing the clot type and, in turn, could assist the physician in selecting the most appropriate treatment method to administer or establish what device to use that would ensure a greater success rate in each case [22].

Non-invasive imaging techniques are a promising tool in the characterization of clot material. Huang et al. [120] used shear-wave dispersion ultrasound vibrometry to measure elasticity and viscosity of clot analogs formed from porcine whole blood. This approach was found to provide accurate estimations for shear elasticity; however, it did not measure viscosity accurately. Alternatively, dynamic ultrasound elastography was implemented by Schmitt et al. [121] to evaluate the storage and loss moduli of similar analogs also formed from porcine whole blood. Fang et al. [118] also used ultrasound to distinguish between newly formed and aged clots formed in vitro from porcine whole blood. This study recognized ultrasound as a useful tool to distinguish between clot types that, in turn, may be used to assist in establishing personalized thrombolytic treatment planning.

Computed tomography (CT) imaging has been shown to be a feasible option for differentiating thrombi according to their hematocrit. The study by Kirchhof et al. [47] supported this hypothesis by demonstrating that CT is a suitable technique for distinguishing clots as white, mixed, and red by estimating the number of erythrocytes present based on the attenuation number. Phantom clot samples were prepared in vitro with varying hematocrit levels. The results from the study show that the CT numbers of white, mixed, and red clots vary significantly and suggest that clots with a larger hematocrit level have larger CT numbers than clot samples with a lower hematocrit level. These findings were supported by Riedel et al. [122] who found that erythrocyte-rich clots were shown to have higher attenuation values than platelet-rich clots using non-contrast CT.

Magnetic resonance imaging (MRI) has also been utilized to analyze the histological composition of clots [123]. Erythrocyte-rich and fibrin-rich clots were created in vitro and injected into the common carotid artery in a swine model. Some of the samples were imaged in vivo, while other samples were randomly selected for in vitro imaging. The erythrocyte component of the clots were found to show high fluid-attenuated inversion recovery (FLAIR) signal intensity and iso-intensity in T2-weighted imaging, compared to the fibrin-rich samples which demonstrated low FLAIR and low-intensity T2-weighted signals. Similar results were achieved in both the in vitro and in vivo stroke models.

Liebeskind et al. [41] provided a correlative study of the hyperdense middle cerebral artery sign (HMCAS) and gradient-echo MRI blooming artifact (BA) with the pathology of thrombi retrieved from patients with AIS. This study combined noncontrast CT and gradient-echo MRI to study 50 consecutive cases of acute middle cerebral artery occlusion before mechanical thrombectomy was performed. The occlusions retrieved from the thrombectomy procedure were analyzed using histology. It was found that the CT HMCAS and gradient-echo MRI BA reflected the pathology of the thrombus and that the RBC content determined the appearance of HMCAS and BA. The absence of HMCAS or BA was found to indicate a fibrin-predominant occlusion. Thus, using CT and MRI, characteristics have been found to aid in the differentiation of clot compositions within thrombi [124, 125].

FEA Model Development/In Silico Models

Finite element analysis (FEA) is commonly accepted as a powerful tool used in the medical device industry to analyze the performance of devices during development. While predictive computational models simulating clot behavior in vivo are valuable for vascular research and device design, relatively little has been reported on the computational modeling of clot tissue mechanics in the literature to date. Simple finite element models have been developed to simulate simple experiments to validate the results [16, 126, 127]. However, few complex computational models of clot material and the thrombectomy procedure exist.

Under the current FDA guidance for non-clinical testing of neurothrombectomy devices, devices must be shown to have the capability of capturing clots of variable size, coagulation, and composition in order to determine device effectiveness [128]. Currently the majority of this testing is performed in vitro; however, the use of finite element modeling to simulate these procedures could significantly reduce the number of in vitro experiments required and provide a more time- and cost-effective approach to device testing and development.

A recent study by Gu et al. [129] used FEA as a method to evaluate the mechanical performance of a semi-enclosed tubular mechanical embolus retrieval device. This model was also used to optimize the geometric design of the device. The FE model successfully modeled the shape-setting, crimping, and deployment of the device, followed by the embolus capture. The results showed that the maximum stress value was not exceeded at any point during the procedure and a number of recommendations were obtained to further improve and optimize the structure of the device. Similarly, Romero et al. [130] developed computational models of their "GP" thrombus aspiration device. These models were used to examine the performance of the device under different blood flow conditions. The models were also used to evaluate the device performance with clots of varying size. The minimum pressure necessary to extract the clot was also established through the simulations.

FEA is recommended by the FDA in the guidelines for the non-clinical testing of stents and associated delivery systems, for conducting stress and fatigue analysis on the devices seeking approval [22, 131]. Although this recommendation is not currently included in the guidelines for non-clinical testing of neurothrombectomy devices, as these devices are experiencing increased use for the treatment of stroke, it is possible that the criteria for FDA approval may become more rigorous in the future and this may lead to the requirement of finite element analysis of these devices.

The INSIST project has been recently funded by the European Commission as part of the Horizon 2020 research and innovation program. This is a collaborative project between nine laboratories from all over Europe. The main goal of the project is to perform in silico clinical trials for biomedical products for the treatment of acute ischemic stroke. This involves the generation of populations of virtual stroke patients, in silico models of treatments, and in silico models of the biophysical aspects of the human response to stroke. This project aims to validate these models and to provide proof of concept by running and validation of in silico clinical stroke trials from the perspective of the three participating stakeholders – pharmaceutical, the medical device industry, and health professionals.

Conclusion

Clot analogs are valuable tools to develop and characterize the next generation of thrombectomy technologies. Fully characterized clinically relevant clot material has been developed in vitro with varying compositions and mechanical properties to mimic the large range of stiffness and elasticity of AIS thrombi found in vivo. Development of advanced imaging technologies is desired to visualize clot composition for prediction of device performance. Finally, exciting developments are underway to analyze the clot material extracted during thrombectomy as a diagnostic assay to inform stroke etiology.

References

1. Benjamin EJ, Virani SS, Callaway CW, Chamberlain AM, Chang AR, Cheng S, et al. Heart disease and stroke statistics-2018 update: a report from the american heart association. Circulation. 2018;137:e67–e492.
2. Saver JL, Goyal M, Bonafe A, Diener HC, Levy EI, Pereira VM, et al. Stent-retriever thrombectomy after intravenous t-pa vs. T-pa alone in stroke. N Engl J Med. 2015;372:2285–95.

3. Campbell BC, Mitchell PJ, Kleinig TJ, Dewey HM, Churilov L, Yassi N, et al. Endovascular therapy for ischemic stroke with perfusion-imaging selection. N Engl J Med. 2015;372:1009–18.
4. Goyal M, Demchuk AM, Menon BK, Eesa M, Rempel JL, Thornton J, et al. Randomized assessment of rapid endovascular treatment of ischemic stroke. N Engl J Med. 2015;372:1019–30.
5. Berkhemer OA, Fransen PS, Beumer D, van den Berg LA, Lingsma HF, Yoo AJ, et al. A randomized trial of intraarterial treatment for acute ischemic stroke. N Engl J Med. 2015;372:11–20.
6. Chueh JY, Kuhn AL, Puri AS, Wilson SD, Wakhloo AK, Gounis MJ. Reduction in distal emboli with proximal flow control during mechanical thrombectomy: a quantitative in vitro study. Stroke. 2013;44:1396–401.
7. Gunning GM, McArdle K, Mirza M, Duffy S, Gilvarry M, Brouwer PA. Clot friction variation with fibrin content; implications for resistance to thrombectomy. J NeuroInterv Surg. 2017;10:34.
8. Ryan EA, Mockros LF, Weisel JW, Lorand L. Structural origins of fibrin clot rheology. Biophys J. 1999;77:2813–26.
9. Gralla J, Schroth G, Remonda L, Fleischmann A, Fandino J, Slotboom J, et al. A dedicated animal model for mechanical thrombectomy in acute stroke. Am J Neuroradiol. 2006;27:1357–61.
10. Chueh JY, Wakhloo AK, Hendricks GH, Silva CF, Weaver JP, Gounis MJ. Mechanical characterization of thromboemboli in acute ischemic stroke and laboratory embolus analogs. Am J Neuroradiol. 2011;32:1237–44.
11. Asakura F, Yilmaz H, Abdo G, Sekoranja L, San Millan D, Augsburger L, et al. Preclinical testing of a new clot-retrieving wire device using polyvinyl alcohol hydrogel vascular models. Neuroradiology. 2007;49:243–51.
12. Shah JV, Janmey PA. Strain hardening of fibrin gels and plasma clots. Rheol Acta. 1997;36:262–8.
13. Fitzgerald S, Dai D, Wang S, Douglas A, Kadirvel R, Layton KF, et al. Platelet-rich emboli in cerebral large vessel occlusion are associated with a large artery atherosclerosis source. Stroke. 2019;50:1907–10.
14. Siller-Matula JM, Plasenzotti R, Spiel AO, Quehenberger P, A Jilma B. Interspecies differences in coagulation profile. J Thromb Haemostas. 2008;100:397–404.
15. Duffy S, Farrell M, McArdle K, Thornton J, Vale D, Rainsford E, et al. Novel methodology to replicate clot analogs with diverse composition in acute ischemic stroke. J NeuroInterv Surg. 2017;9:486.
16. Slaboch CL, Alber MS, Rosen ED, Ovaert TC. Mechano-rheological properties of the murine thrombus determined via nanoindentation and finite element modeling. J Mech Behav Biomed Mater. 2012;10:75–86.
17. Krueger K, Deissler P, Coburger S, Fries JWU, Lackner K. How thrombus model impacts the in vitro study of interventional thrombectomy procedures. Investig Radiol. 2004;39:641–8.
18. Shao Q, Zhu L, Li T, Li L, Li D, Zhang J, et al. New method of thrombus preparation using a fluid model for evaluation of thrombectomy devices in a swine model. Thromb Res. 2014;134:1087–92.
19. PJC F. A study of artificial thrombi produced by a modification of chandler's method. Q J Exp Physiol Cogn Med Sci. 1959;44:377–84.
20. Robinson RA, Herbertson LH, Das SS, Malinauskas RA, Pritchard WF, Grossman LW. Limitations of using synthetic blood clots for measuring in vitro clot capture efficiency of inferior vena cava filters. Med Dev (Auckland, NZ). 2013;6:49–57.
21. Merritt W, Holter AM, Beahm S, Gonzalez C, Becker TA, Tabor A, et al. Quantifying the mechanical and histological properties of thrombus analog made from human blood for the creation of synthetic thrombus for thrombectomy device testing. J NeuroInterv Surg. 2018;10:1168.

22. Johnson S, Duffy S, Gunning G, Gilvarry M, McGarry JP, McHugh PE. Review of mechanical testing and modelling of thrombus material for vascular implant and device design. Ann Biomed Eng. 2017;45:2494–508.
23. Ashton JH, Vande Geest JP, Simon BR, Haskett DG. Compressive mechanical properties of the intraluminal thrombus in abdominal aortic aneurysms and fibrin-based thrombus mimics. J Biomech. 2009;42:197–201.
24. Krasokha N, Theisen W, Reese S, Mordasini P, Brekenfeld C, Gralla J, et al. Mechanical properties of blood clots – a new test method. Mater Werkst. 2011;41:1019–24.
25. Brown AEX, Litvinov RI, Discher DE, Purohit PK, Weisel JW. Multiscale mechanics of fibrin polymer: gel stretching with protein unfolding and loss of water. Science (New York, NY). 2009;325:741–4.
26. Saldívar E, Orje JN, Ruggeri ZM. Tensile destruction test as an estimation of partial proteolysis in fibrin clots. Am J Hematol. 2002;71:119–27.
27. Kim OV, Litvinov RI, Weisel JW, Alber MS. Structural basis for the nonlinear mechanics of fibrin networks under compression. Biomaterials. 2014;35:6739–49.
28. van Kempen THS, Donders WP, van de Vosse FN, Peters GWM. A constitutive model for developing blood clots with various compositions and their nonlinear viscoelastic behavior. Biomech Model Mechanobiol. 2016;15:279–91.
29. van Kempen THS, Peters GWM, van de Vosse FN. A constitutive model for the time-dependent, nonlinear stress response of fibrin networks. Biomech Model Mechanobiol. 2015;14:995–1006.
30. Riha P, Wang X, Liao R, F Stoltz J. Elasticity and fracture strain of whole blood clots. Clin Hemorheol Microcirc. 1999;21:45.
31. Weafer FM, Duffy S, Machado I, Gunning G, Mordasini P, Roche E, et al. Characterization of strut indentation during mechanical thrombectomy in acute ischemic stroke clot analogs. J Neurointerv Surg. 2019;11:891–7.
32. Vidmar J, Serša I, Kralj E, Popovič P. Unsuccessful percutaneous mechanical thrombectomy in fibrin-rich high-risk pulmonary thromboembolism. Thromb J. 2015;13:30.
33. Zaidat OO, Haussen DC, Hassan AE, Jadhav AP, Mehta BP, Mokin M, et al. Impact of stent retriever size on clinical and angiographic outcomes in the stratis stroke thrombectomy registry. Stroke. 2019;50:441–7.
34. Yuki I, Kan I, Vinters HV, Kim RH, Golshan A, Vinuela FA, et al. The impact of thromboemboli histology on the performance of a mechanical thrombectomy device. AJNR Am J Neuroradiol. 2012;33:643–8.
35. Shin JW, Jeong HS, Kwon HJ, Song KS, Kim J. High red blood cell composition in clots is associated with successful recanalization during intra-arterial thrombectomy. PLoS One. 2018;13:e0197492.
36. Nouh A, Mehta T, Hussain M, Song X, Ollenschleger M. Abstract tp210: histopathological evaluation of thrombus in acute stroke and correlation with stroke etiology. Stroke. 2017;48:ATP210.
37. Kaesmacher J, Boeckh-Behrens T, Simon S, Maegerlein C, Kleine JF, Zimmer C, et al. Risk of thrombus fragmentation during endovascular stroke treatment. AJNR Am J Neuroradiol. 2017;38:991–8.
38. Boeckh-Behrens T, Schubert M, Forschler A, Prothmann S, Kreiser K, Zimmer C, et al. The impact of histological clot composition in embolic stroke. Clin Neuroradiol. 2016;26:189–97.
39. Marder VJ, Chute DJ, Starkman S, Abolian AM, Kidwell C, Liebeskind D, et al. Analysis of thrombi retrieved from cerebral arteries of patients with acute ischemic stroke. Stroke. 2006;37:2086–93.
40. Nahirnyak VM, Yoon SW, Holland CK. Acousto-mechanical and thermal properties of clotted blood. J Acoust Soc Am. 2006;119:3766–72.
41. Liebeskind DS, Sanossian N, Yong WH, Starkman S, Tsang MP, Moya AL, et al. Ct and mri early vessel signs reflect clot composition in acute stroke. Stroke. 2011;42:1237–43.

42. Kim SK, Yoon W, Kim TS, Kim HS, Heo TW, Park MS. Histologic analysis of retrieved clots in acute ischemic stroke: correlation with stroke etiology and gradient-echo mri. Am J Neuroradiol. 2015;36:1756–62.
43. Laridan E, Denorme F, Desender L, Francois O, Andersson T, Deckmyn H, et al. Neutrophil extracellular traps in ischemic stroke thrombi. Ann Neurol. 2017;82:223–32.
44. De Meyer SF, Stoll G, Wagner DD, Kleinschnitz C. Von willebrand factor: an emerging target in stroke therapy. Stroke. 2012;43:599–606.
45. Fitzgerald ST, Wang S, Dai D, Douglas A, Kadirvel R, Gounis MJ, et al. Platelet-rich clots as identified by martius scarlet blue staining are isodense on ncct. J Neurointerv Surg. 2019;11:1145–9.
46. De Meyer SF, Andersson T, Baxter B, Bendszus M, Brouwer P, Brinjikji W, et al. Analyses of thrombi in acute ischemic stroke: a consensus statement on current knowledge and future directions. Int J Stroke. 2017;12:606–14.
47. Kirchhof K, Welzel T, Mecke C, Zoubaa S, Sartor K. Differentiation of white, mixed, and red thrombi: value of ct in estimation of the prognosis of thrombolysis—phantom study. Radiology. 2003;228:126–30.
48. Chandler A. In vitro thrombotic coagulation of the blood; a method for producing a thrombus. Lab Investig; a journal of technical methods and pathology. 1958;7:110–4.
49. Kan I, Yuki I, Murayama Y, Viñuela FA, Kim RH, Vinters HV, et al. A novel method of thrombus preparation for use in a swine model for evaluation of thrombectomy devices. Am J Neuroradiol. 2010;31:1741–3.
50. Yoh R, Matsumoto T, Sasaki J, Sohmura T. Biomimetic fabrication of fibrin/apatite composite material. J Biomed Mater Res A. 2008;87:222–8.
51. Haider T, Plasenzotti R, Bergmeister H, Mach G, Kleinpeter G, Aguilar-Perez M, et al. New mechanical thrombectomy model in the rabbit: a feasibility study. J Neurosci Methods. 2016;271:139–42.
52. van der Bom IM, Mehra M, Walvick RP, Chueh JY, Gounis MJ. Quantitative evaluation of c-arm ct cerebral blood volume in a canine model of ischemic stroke. AJNR Am J Neuroradiol. 2012;33:353–8.
53. Mehra M, Henninger N, Hirsch JA, Chueh J, Wakhloo AK, Gounis MJ. Preclinical acute ischemic stroke modeling. J Neurointerv Surg. 2012;4:307–13.
54. Gralla J, Schroth G, Remonda L, Fleischmann A, Fandino J, Slotboom J, et al. A dedicated animal model for mechanical thrombectomy in acute stroke. AJNR Am J Neuroradiol. 2006;27:1357–61.
55. Marosfoi MG, Korin N, Gounis MJ, Uzun O, Vedantham S, Langan ET, et al. Shear-activated nanoparticle aggregates combined with temporary endovascular bypass to treat large vessel occlusion. Stroke. 2015;46:3507–13.
56. Nurden AT. Thrombus stability on the vessel wall. Blood. 2008;112:4–5.
57. Randriamboavonjy V, Isaak J, Fromel T, Viollet B, Fisslthaler B, Preissner KT, et al. Ampk alpha2 subunit is involved in platelet signaling, clot retraction, and thrombus stability. Blood. 2010;116:2134–40.
58. Lishko VK, Burke T, Ugarova T. Antiadhesive effect of fibrinogen: a safeguard for thrombus stability. Blood. 2007;109:1541–9.
59. Calaminus SD, Auger JM, McCarty OJ, Wakelam MJ, Machesky LM, Watson SP. Myosiniia contractility is required for maintenance of platelet structure during spreading on collagen and contributes to thrombus stability. J Thromb Haemost. 2007;5:2136–45.
60. Andre P, Delaney SM, LaRocca T, Vincent D, DeGuzman F, Jurek M, et al. P2y12 regulates platelet adhesion/activation, thrombus growth, and thrombus stability in injured arteries. J Clin Invest. 2003;112:398–406.
61. Baumgartner HR, Sakariassen KS. Factors controlling thrombus formation on arterial lesions. Ann N Y Acad Sci. 1985;454:162–77.
62. Andrews RK, Berndt MC. Platelet physiology and thrombosis. Thromb Res. 2004;114:447–53.

63. Andrews RK, Berndt MC. Platelet adhesion: a game of catch and release. J Clin Invest. 2008;118:3009–11.
64. Blann AD, Lip GY. Virchow's triad revisited: the importance of soluble coagulation factors, the endothelium, and platelets. Thromb Res. 2001;101:321–7.
65. Ruggeri ZM. Von willebrand factor. J Clin Invest. 1997;100:S41–6.
66. Reininger AJ. Vwf attributes--impact on thrombus formation. Thromb Res. 2008;122(Suppl 4):S9–13.
67. Roquer J, Segura T, Serena J, Castillo J. Endothelial dysfunction, vascular disease and stroke: the artico study. Cerebrovasc Dis. 2009;27(Suppl 1):25–37.
68. Chen J, Lopez JA. Interactions of platelets with subendothelium and endothelium. Microcirculation. 2005;12:235–46.
69. Zhang ZG, Zhang L, Tsang W, Goussev A, Powers C, Ho KL, et al. Dynamic platelet accumulation at the site of the occluded middle cerebral artery and in downstream microvessels is associated with loss of microvascular integrity after embolic middle cerebral artery occlusion. Brain Res. 2001;912:181–94.
70. Christ KV, Turner KT. Methods to measure the strength of cell adhesion to substrates. J Adhes Sci Technol. 2010;24:2027–58.
71. Garcia AJ, Huber F, Boettiger D. Force required to break alpha5beta1 integrin-fibronectin bonds in intact adherent cells is sensitive to integrin activation state. J Biol Chem. 1998;273:10988–93.
72. Gallant ND, Michael KE, Garcia AJ. Cell adhesion strengthening: contributions of adhesive area, integrin binding, and focal adhesion assembly. Mol Biol Cell. 2005;16:4329–40.
73. Gutierrez E, Groisman A. Quantitative measurements of the strength of adhesion of human neutrophils to a substratum in a microfluidic device. Anal Chem. 2007;79:2249–58.
74. Thoumine O, Ott A. Comparison of the mechanical properties of normal and transformed fibroblasts. Biorheology. 1997;34:309–26.
75. Missirlis YF, Spiliotis AD. Assessment of techniques used in calculating cell–material interactions. Biomol Eng. 2002;19:287–94.
76. Thoumine O, Ott A, Louvard D. Critical centrifugal forces induce adhesion rupture or structural reorganization in cultured cells. Cell Motil Cytoskeleton. 1996;33:276–87.
77. Channavajjala LS, Eidsath A, Saxinger WC. A simple method for measurement of cell-substrate attachment forces: application to hiv-1 tat. J Cell Sci. 1997;110(Pt 2):249–56.
78. Chueh J, Kuhn AL, Mehra M, Feula G, Wakhloo AK, Gounis MJ. Abstract 3750: embolus adhesion to activated endothelium after embolization: a parameter to predict outcomes of mechanical thrombectomy in acute ischemic stroke. Stroke. 2012;43:A3750.
79. Nogueira RG, Jadhav AP, Haussen DC, Bonafe A, Budzik RF, Bhuva P, et al. Thrombectomy 6 to 24 hours after stroke with a mismatch between deficit and infarct. N Engl J Med. 2018;378:11–21.
80. Spiotta AM, Chaudry MI, Hui FK, Turner RD, Kellogg RT, Turk AS. Evolution of thrombectomy approaches and devices for acute stroke: a technical review. J Neurointerv Surg. 2015;7:2–7.
81. Flint AC, Cullen SP, Faigeles BS, Rao VA. Predicting long-term outcome after endovascular stroke treatment: the totaled health risks in vascular events score. AJNR Am J Neuroradiol. 2010;31:1192–6.
82. Kulcsar Z, Bonvin C, Pereira VM, Altrichter S, Yilmaz H, Lovblad KO, et al. Penumbra system: a novel mechanical thrombectomy device for large-vessel occlusions in acute stroke. AJNR Am J Neuroradiol. 2010;31:628–33.
83. Menon BK, Hill MD, Eesa M, Modi J, Bhatia R, Wong J, et al. Initial experience with the penumbra stroke system for recanalization of large vessel occlusions in acute ischemic stroke. Neuroradiology. 2011;53:261–6.
84. Chueh JY, Puri AS, Gounis MJ. An in vitro evaluation of distal emboli following lazarus cover-assisted stent retriever thrombectomy. J Neurointerv Surg. 2017;9:183–7.

85. Nguyen TN, Malisch T, Castonguay AC, Gupta R, Sun CH, Martin CO, et al. Balloon guide catheter improves revascularization and clinical outcomes with the solitaire device: analysis of the north american solitaire acute stroke registry. Stroke. 2013;45:141–5.
86. Nguyen TN, Castonguay AC, Nogueira RG, Haussen DC, English JD, Satti SR, et al. Effect of balloon guide catheter on clinical outcomes and reperfusion in trevo thrombectomy. J Neurointerv Surg. 2019;11:861–5.
87. Zaidat OO, Mueller-Kronast NH, Hassan AE, Haussen DC, Jadhav AP, Froehler MT, et al. Impact of balloon guide catheter use on clinical and angiographic outcomes in the stratis stroke thrombectomy registry. Stroke. 2019;50:697–704.
88. Menon BK, Sajobi TT, Zhang Y, Rempel JL, Shuaib A, Thornton J, et al. Analysis of workflow and time to treatment on thrombectomy outcome in the endovascular treatment for small core and proximal occlusion ischemic stroke (escape) randomized, controlled trial. Circulation. 2016;133:2279–86.
89. Velasco A, Buerke B, Stracke CP, Berkemeyer S, Mosimann PJ, Schwindt W, et al. Comparison of a balloon guide catheter and a non-balloon guide catheter for mechanical thrombectomy. Radiology. 2016;280:169–76.
90. Saedon M, Dilshad A, Tiivas C, Virdee D, Hutchinson CE, Singer DR, et al. Prospective validation study of transorbital doppler ultrasound imaging for the detection of transient cerebral microemboli. Br J Surg. 2014;101:1551–5.
91. Sarkar S, Ghosh S, Ghosh SK, Collier A. Role of transcranial doppler ultrasonography in stroke. Postgrad Med J. 2007;83:683–9.
92. Silbert BS, Evered LA, Scott DA, Rahardja S, Gerraty RP, Choong PF. Review of transcranial doppler ultrasound to detect microemboli during orthopedic surgery. AJNR Am J Neuroradiol. 2014;35:1858–63.
93. Vukovic-Cvetkovic V. Microembolus detection by transcranial doppler sonography: review of the literature. Stroke Res Treat. 2012;2012:382361.
94. Zolls S, Tantipolphan R, Wiggenhorn M, Winter G, Jiskoot W, Friess W, et al. Particles in therapeutic protein formulations, part 1: overview of analytical methods. J Pharm Sci. 2012;101:914–35.
95. Zolls S, Weinbuch D, Wiggenhorn M, Winter G, Friess W, Jiskoot W, et al. Flow imaging microscopy for protein particle analysis--a comparative evaluation of four different analytical instruments. AAPS J. 2013;15:1200–11.
96. Reynolds LO, Mohammad SF, Solen KA, Pantalos GM, Burns GL, Olsen DB. Light scattering detection of microemboli in an extracorporeal lvad bovine model. ASAIO Trans. 1990;36:M518–21.
97. Reynolds LO, Simon TL. Size distribution measurements of microaggregates in stored blood. Transfusion. 1980;20:669–78.
98. Reynolds LO, Solen KA, Mohammad SF, Pantalos GM, Kim J. Differential light scattering cuvettes for the measurement of thromboemboli in high shear blood flow systems. ASAIO Trans. 1990;36:M185–8.
99. Konstantopoulos K, Grotta JC, Sills C, Wu KK, Hellums JD. Shear-induced platelet aggregation in normal subjects and stroke patients. Thromb Haemost. 1995;74:1329–34.
100. Solen KA, Mohammad SF, Pijl AJ, Swier P, Monson RD, Olsen DB. Detection of microemboli by constant-pressure filtration during in vitro circulation of bovine and human blood. Artif Organs. 1990;14:466–70.
101. Swank RL, Roth JG, Jansen J. Screen filtration pressure method and adhesiveness and aggregation of blood cells. J Appl Physiol. 1964;19:340–6.
102. Zaidat OO, Castonguay AC, Linfante I, Gupta R, Martin CO, Holloway WE, et al. First pass effect: a new measure for stroke thrombectomy devices. Stroke. 2018;49:660–6.
103. Mordasini P, Frabetti N, Gralla J, Schroth G, Fischer U, Arnold M, et al. In vivo evaluation of the first dedicated combined flow-restoration and mechanical thrombectomy device in a swine model of acute vessel occlusion. AJNR Am J Neuroradiol. 2011;32:294–300.

104. Broussalis E, Trinka E, Hitzl W, Wallner A, Chroust V, Killer-Oberpfalzer M. Comparison of stent-retriever devices versus the merci retriever for endovascular treatment of acute stroke. AJNR Am J Neuroradiol. 2013;34:366–72.
105. Mendonca N, Flores A, Pagola J, Rubiera M, Rodriguez-Luna D, De Miquel MA, et al. Trevo versus solitaire a head-to-head comparison between two heavy weights of clot retrieval. J Neuroimaging. 2014;24:167–70.
106. Park H, Hwang GJ, Jin SC, Jung CK, Bang JS, Han MK, et al. A retrieval thrombectomy technique with the solitaire stent in a large cerebral artery occlusion. Acta Neurochir. 2011;153:1625–31.
107. Soize S, Kadziolka K, Estrade L, Serre I, Bakchine S, Pierot L. Mechanical thrombectomy in acute stroke: prospective pilot trial of the solitaire fr device while under conscious sedation. AJNR Am J Neuroradiol. 2013;34:360–5.
108. van der Marel K, Chueh JY, Brooks OW, King RM, Marosfoi MG, Langan ET, et al. Quantitative assessment of device-clot interaction for stent retriever thrombectomy. J Neurointerv Surg. 2016;8:1278.
109. Okawa M, Tateshima S, Liebeskind D, Rao N, Jahan R, Gonzalez N, et al. Early loss of immediate reperfusion while stent retriever in place predicts successful final reperfusion in acute ischemic stroke patients. Stroke. 2015;46:3266–9.
110. Korin N, Kanapathipillai M, Matthews BD, Crescente M, Brill A, Mammoto T, et al. Shear-activated nanotherapeutics for drug targeting to obstructed blood vessels. Science. 2012;337:738–42.
111. Saqqur M. Site of arterial occlusion identified by transcranial doppler predicts the response to intravenous thrombolysis for stroke. Stroke (1970). 2007;38:948.
112. De Silva DA. The benefits of intravenous thrombolysis relate to the site of baseline arterial occlusion in the echoplanar imaging thrombolytic evaluation trial (epithet). Stroke (1970). 2010;41:295.
113. Paciaroni M. Systemic thrombolysis in patients with acute ischemic stroke and internal carotid artery occlusion: the icaro study. Stroke. 2012;43:125.
114. Shi Z-S, Loh Y, Walker G, Duckwiler GR. Endovascular thrombectomy for acute ischemic stroke in failed intravenous tissue plasminogen activator versus non–intravenous tissue plasminogen activator patients. Revascularization and outcomes stratified by the site of arterial occlusions. Stroke. 2010;41:1185–92.
115. Mistry EA, Mistry AM, Nakawah MO, Chitale RV, James RF, Volpi JJ, et al. Mechanical thrombectomy outcomes with and without intravenous thrombolysis in stroke patients. A meta-analysis. Stroke. 2017;48:2450–6.
116. Fischer U, Kaesmacher J, Molina CA, Selim MH, Alexandrov AV, Tsivgoulis G. Primary thrombectomy in tpa (tissue-type plasminogen activator) eligible stroke patients with proximal intracranial occlusions. Stroke. 2018;49:265–9.
117. Kaesmacher J, Mordasini P, Arnold M, López-Cancio E, Cerdá N, Boeckh-Behrens T, et al. Direct mechanical thrombectomy in tpa-ineligible and -eligible patients versus the bridging approach: a meta-analysis. J Neurointerv Surg. 2019;11:20–27.
118. Fang J, Wan Y-L, Chen C-K, Tsui P-H. Discrimination between newly formed and aged thrombi using empirical mode decomposition of ultrasound b-scan image. Biomed Res Int. 2015;2015:9.
119. Minnerup J, Kleinschnitz C. Visualization of clot composition in ischemic stroke. Do we get what we see? Stroke. 2011;42:1193–4.
120. Huang CC, Chen PY, Shih CC. Estimating the viscoelastic modulus of a thrombus using an ultrasonic shear-wave approach. Med Phys. 2013;40:042901.
121. Schmitt C, Hadj Henni A, Cloutier G. Characterization of blood clot viscoelasticity by dynamic ultrasound elastography and modeling of the rheological behavior. J Biomech. 2011;44:622–9.

122. Riedel CH, Jensen U, Rohr A, Tietke M, Alfke K, Ulmer S, et al. Assessment of thrombus in acute middle cerebral artery occlusion using thin-slice nonenhanced computed tomography reconstructions. Stroke. 2010;41:1659–64.
123. Fujimoto M, Salamon N, Mayor F, Yuki I, Takemoto K, Vinters HV, et al. Characterization of arterial thrombus composition by magnetic resonance imaging in a swine stroke model. Stroke. 2013;44:1463–5.
124. Gasparian GG, Sanossian N, Shiroishi MS, Liebeskind DS. Imaging of occlusive thrombi in acute ischemic stroke. Int J Stroke. 2015;10:298–305.
125. Brinjikji W, Duffy S, Burrows A, Hacke W, Liebeskind D, Majoie CBLM, et al. Correlation of imaging and histopathology of thrombi in acute ischemic stroke with etiology and outcome: a systematic review. J NeuroInterv Surg. 2017;9:529–34.
126. Fogelson AL, Guy RD. Immersed-boundary-type models of intravascular platelet aggregation. Comput Methods Appl Mech Eng. 2008;197:2087–104.
127. Xie H, Kim K, Aglyamov SR, Emelianov SY, O'Donnell M, Weitzel WF, et al. Correspondence of ultrasound elasticity imaging to direct mechanical measurement in aging dvt in rats. Ultrasound Med Biol. 2005;31:1351–9.
128. Health CfDaR. Guidance for industry and fda staff pre-clinical and clinical studies for neurothrombectomy devices 2007.
129. Gu X, Qi Y, Erdman A, Li Z. The role of simulation in the design of a semi-enclosed tubular embolus retrieval. J Med Dev. 2017;11:021001-021001-021007.
130. Romero G, Higuera I, Martinez ML, Pearce G, Perkinson N, Roffe C, et al. Computational modeling of a new thrombectomy device for the extraction of blood clots. Adv Exp Med Biol. 2010:627–33.
131. Health CfDaR. Guidance for industry and fda staff - non-clinical engineering tests and recommended labeling for intravascular stents and associated delivery systems. 2010.

Chapter 3
Pediatric Acute Ischemic Stroke: Nuances for the Neurointerventionalist

Matias Negrotto, Ronil V. Chandra, and Todd A. Abruzzo

Introduction

Acute ischemic stroke (AIS) is unusual in childhood. Nevertheless, childhood AIS accounts for substantial mortality in the first two decades of life, and most survivors have long-term neurological impairment resulting in negative impact on quality of life for affected patients and their families. The relative rarity, age-related peculiarities, and the variety of manifested symptoms make the clinical diagnosis of pediatric AIS extremely difficult [1]. In particular, the disproportionately greater frequency of clinical stroke mimics presenting in children demands advanced neuroimaging studies for diagnostic confirmation and confounds the goal of rapid diagnosis of AIS. Most pediatric AIS patients are therefore ineligible for reperfusion with intravenous thrombolytic therapy by the time they come to diagnosis. Furthermore, pediatric protocols for intravenous thrombolytic therapy are not supported by clinical trial data and are lacking at most centers. The clinical outcomes of pediatric AIS are thus worsened by delayed diagnosis and lack of well-established, readily available treatment protocols.

Mechanical thrombectomy for adults with AIS is supported by multiple well-designed randomized clinical trials. Based on limited case series reported to date, and suboptimal study design, the quality of the data does not support level I

M. Negrotto (✉)
Hospital Maciel, Montevideo, Uruguay

R. V. Chandra
Monash Health and Monash University, NeuroInterventional Radiology, Melbourne, VIC, Australia

T. A. Abruzzo
Barrow Neurological Institute at Phoenix Children's Hospital, Phoenix, AZ, USA

University of Arizona College of Medicine, Phoenix, AZ, USA

Phoenix Children's Hospital, Phoenix, AZ, USA

F. K. Hui et al. (eds.), *12 Strokes*, https://doi.org/10.1007/978-3-030-56857-3_3

recommendations for endovascular intervention in pediatric AIS [2]. Nonetheless, a growing body of clinical data suggests that endovascular mechanical thrombectomy improves clinical outcomes in properly selected children with AIS due to large vessel occlusion [3]. Neuropediatric specialists remain concerned that endovascular interventions may cause harm in children with cerebral arteriopathies. Despite this, an increasing majority of neuropediatric specialists agree that endovascular interventions should be considered for pediatric AIS patients with large vessel occlusions on a case-by-case basis [4].

Epidemiology and Impact of Childhood AIS

In the population less than 18 years of age, the incidence of stroke is estimated at 4.6/100,000 person per year, which is greater than the incidence of leukemia or pediatric brain tumors. Approximately half of all pediatric stroke is ischemic, and half of ischemic stroke in the pediatric population occurs in the perinatal period. Perinatal stroke frequently manifests as periventricular leukomalacia (PVL) in premature neonates. PVL does not involve an arterial occlusive process but is the consequence of watershed injury in the immature brain subjected to a severe hemodynamic insult.

Non-perinatal pediatric AIS affects patients between 29 days and 18 years of age and has an incidence of 1–3 per 100,000 per year in Western developed countries [5, 6]. Non-perinatal pediatric AIS has a mortality of 3–6% (among the top 10 causes of death in children) [7] and is associated with significant neurological morbidity in 70% of affected patients. The majority of children with AIS experience life-long disability, and decreased quality of life [2], including long-term motor deficits in 65%, psychiatric illness in 50%, and epilepsy in one third [8].

In light of this, it is not surprising that pediatric AIS is associated with a high cost of care [9] and a significant impact on health care economics. The average adjusted 5-year cost of care is estimated to be $135,161 per pediatric patient. The annual cost of inpatient pediatric stroke care in the United States is estimated to be 42 million dollars [8].

Etiology of Childhood AIS

The common underlying causes of AIS in children differ from those observed in the adult population [5]. In clinical practice, a useful approach to the etiological differential diagnosis of AIS in a child is to group patients into one of three different categories: cardioembolic stroke, cervical artery dissection, and intracranial arteriopathy. This differentiates patients into easily recognized groups that are routed into distinct treatment pathways. Children with intracranial large vessel occlusions secondary to cardioembolism and cervical artery dissection are excellent candidates for endovascular mechanical revascularization. It is the opinion of the authors that children with intracranial arteriopathy are not likely to benefit from endovascular mechanical therapies. Furthermore, we believe that children with intracranial arteriopathy are specifically at higher risk of suffering serious procedure-related harm during endovascular mechanical revascularization.

Cardioembolic stroke accounts for approximately 30% of non-perinatal pediatric AIS. Most cases affect children with complex congenital heart disease, children undergoing transcatheter cardiac procedures, and children with acquired disorders of the myocardium or cardiac valves. Cyanotic cardiac lesions with right to left shunting (particularly uncorrected and in the perioperative period) and children supported by extra-corporeal circulatory assist devices have an especially high risk of stroke [6, 10–12].

Cervical artery dissection accounts for another 20% of non-perinatal pediatric AIS cases. Cervical artery dissection may be traumatic or non-traumatic. Non-traumatic cervical artery dissection is sometimes the result of a well-defined arteriopathy such as fibromuscular dysplasia, Loeys-Dietz, Marfans, and Ehlers-Danlos spectrum disorders. Some authors have estimated that specific extracranial arteriopathies account for as much as 7.5% of childhood stroke [13]. Childhood arteriopathies that have not been characterized as distinct entities account for some proportion of this group [14]. In children with non-traumatic vertebral artery dissection, a Bow Hunter's type syndrome must be considered and carefully evaluated [15].

Intracranial arteriopathy accounts for as much as 45% of non-perinatal pediatric AIS [16]. Sickle cell disease (SCD), which is responsible for 10% of non-perinatal pediatric AIS, is an important subgroup within this category. The majority of AIS cases in SCD are the result of an acquired multifocal intracranial steno-occlusive large vessel arteriopathy that has peak onset at 5 years of age [17–19]. The moyamoya arteriopathies are another subgroup within the intracranial arteriopathy category, which partially overlaps the SCD subgroup. The moyamoya subgroup is a heterogeneous group of disorders, all characterized by progressive bilateral occlusion of the carotid termini and/or their first-order branches. It is estimated that moyamoya arteriopathies account for 5–10% of childhood stroke [20].

The subgroup of intracranial arteriopathies known as the focal cerebral arteriopathies (FCAs) account for as much as 25% of non-perinatal pediatric AIS. This subgroup characteristically involves a monofocal steno-occlusive lesion of the intradural internal carotid artery and its first-order branches, most commonly the M1 segment of the middle cerebral artery (MCA). The FCA subgroup includes transient (transient cerebral arteriopathy of childhood) and progressive forms that are defined by clinical and imaging behavior over time. Recently, FCA has been differentiated into an intracranial arterial dissection (FCA-d) subgroup and an inflammatory subgroup (FCA-i) [21]. In patients with FCA-i, evidence suggests that an infectious or para-infectious process leads to localized vessel inflammation, mural swelling, luminal narrowing, and thrombus formation culminating in cerebral infarction. Postvaricella arteriopathy is a specific entity within this subgroup that occurs in children 2 to 10 years of age, weeks to months after an uncomplicated chickenpox infection due to reactivation of latent infection housed in trigeminal ganglia with transaxonal spread of reactivated virus to intracranial arteries through afferent nerve fibers and secondary infiltration of affected arteries with inflammatory cells [6].

Severe forms of hereditary thrombophilia such as homozygous factor V Leiden mutations and acquired prothrombotic states sometimes play an important role in the pathogenesis of pediatric cerebral sinovenous thrombosis. On the other hand, hereditary thrombophilia and acquired prothrombotic states are not considered to be an important primary driver of pediatric AIS. It is likely that prothrombotic states synergistically interact with otherwise subclinical arteriopathies to precipitate cerebral thromboembolism. Alternatively, a prothrombotic disorder may function as a cofactor to promote thromboembolism in a child with Bow Hunter's physiology and prolonged stasis of blood in an affected vertebral artery segment. As a general rule, coagulopathy plays a secondary adjunctive role to the primary pathology in pediatric AIS.

Clinical Presentation of Childhood AIS

The presentation of childhood AIS has similarities and differences compared with adult stroke. In adults, focal neurologic symptoms, such as sudden-onset hemiparesis with or without facial weakness and language problems, constitute the hallmark presenting features of stroke. Children may also present with focal neurologic symptoms. The study by Mallick et al. [22] found hemiparesis to be the most frequent presenting feature at 72%. Facial weakness and speech disturbances were present in 41% and 33%, respectively. However, focal neurologic symptoms occur less frequently in isolation. In 67% of children, diffuse neurologic symptoms, such as decreased consciousness, headache, vomiting, and papilledema, as well as seizures accompanied focal symptoms [5].

In most cases, clinical presentation of the child with AIS is non-specific. Stroke mimics including complicated migraine, seizures with post-ictal paralysis, central nervous system infection, central nervous system tumor, and sickle cell crisis with painful extremity are more common than AIS in the pediatric population [2]. All of these conditions may be very difficult or impossible to clinically differentiate from acute AIS in a child. Consequently, definitive diagnosis relies heavily on advanced neuroimaging studies. As a result, the diagnosis of AIS is often delayed in the pediatric population [1]. Although children are often brought in early after symptom onset (on average 1.7 hours after onset), there is a 12.7-hour median time to diagnosis, with >50% of diagnoses made >24 hours after arrival.

Neuroimaging of Acute AIS in Children

The clinical goal of acute neuroimaging is to confirm the diagnosis, to illuminate the etiology, and to establish eligibility for acute reperfusion therapy. Consequently, the imaging study must rapidly assess for intracranial hemorrhage, localize and quantify irreversible infarction (and reversible ischemia if possible), and identify intracranial large vessel occlusions. Overall, cerebral magnetic resonance imaging (MRI) is the preferred modality for the initial diagnosis of childhood AIS. It allows the confident diagnosis of infarction and accurate diagnosis of large vessel occlusion. A brain MRI with the following sequences is generally utilized for initial evaluation of children with suspected AIS – diffusion weighted imaging (DWI) completed in 1 minute, T2 fluid attenuated inversion recovery (FLAIR) imaging completed in 5 minutes, and time of flight (TOF) MR angiography completed in 6 minutes. This initial evaluation, often referred to as the "Acute Brain Attack" neuroimaging protocol, can be quickly performed in most children as young as 5 years of age without general anesthesia. In the majority of pediatric patients, this initial evaluation provides sufficient information to guide decisions about acute reperfusion therapies. Susceptibility weighted imaging (SWI) or gradient recalled echo (GRE) sequences can be quickly added if hemorrhage cannot be confidently excluded. In patients that do not require rapid transfer to a neurointerventional suite, additional sequences should be obtained to facilitate diagnosis. MR angiography and fat-suppressed T1-weighted imaging of the neck are useful to identify cervical artery dissection due to its sensitivity in the detection of intramural hematoma. MR venography, gadolinium-enhanced sequences, and flow sensitive arterial spin labeling (ASL) sequences are useful to refine the differential diagnosis and plan clinical management. Stroke mimics including migraine and seizures may be associated with reversible perfusion abnormalities on cerebral perfusion imaging studies.

Increasingly, at pediatric stroke centers, advanced perfusion imaging with dynamic susceptibility contrast or arterial spin labeling perfusion methods are being utilized to assist in reperfusion therapy decisions. Such utilization relies on extrapolation of principles learned from the treatment of stroke in adults because the quantitative perfusion metrics that define infarction, penumbra, and benign oligemia in children of different ages have not been established.

To assist in determining the presence of cervical artery dissection or intracranial arteriopathy, MR angiography of the brain and head and neck vessels is preferred over computed tomography angiography (CTA) due to radiation-related concerns. When MR techniques are utilized, fat-saturated T1-weighted sequences should be performed to increase the sensitivity for detection of intramural hematoma in cervical arterial dissection. Advanced MR vessel wall imaging techniques are useful in the differential diagnosis of intracranial arteriopathies, particularly in differentiating FCAi and FCAd.

Although digital subtraction angiography (DSA) is rarely necessary for diagnostic purposes in children, it remains the gold standard for the assessment of the cervical and cerebral vasculature. It is particularly useful in the definitive diagnosis of FCA and subtle arterial dissections. The luminal beading that is characteristic of FCAi is clearly delineated by DSA, but often below the detection threshold of CT and MR imaging (Fig. 3.1). Small intimal flaps missed by CT and MR imaging are easily detected by DSA (Fig. 3.2). In children, a false-positive diagnosis of dissection on CT angiography is sometimes caused by extreme pulsatility and elasticity

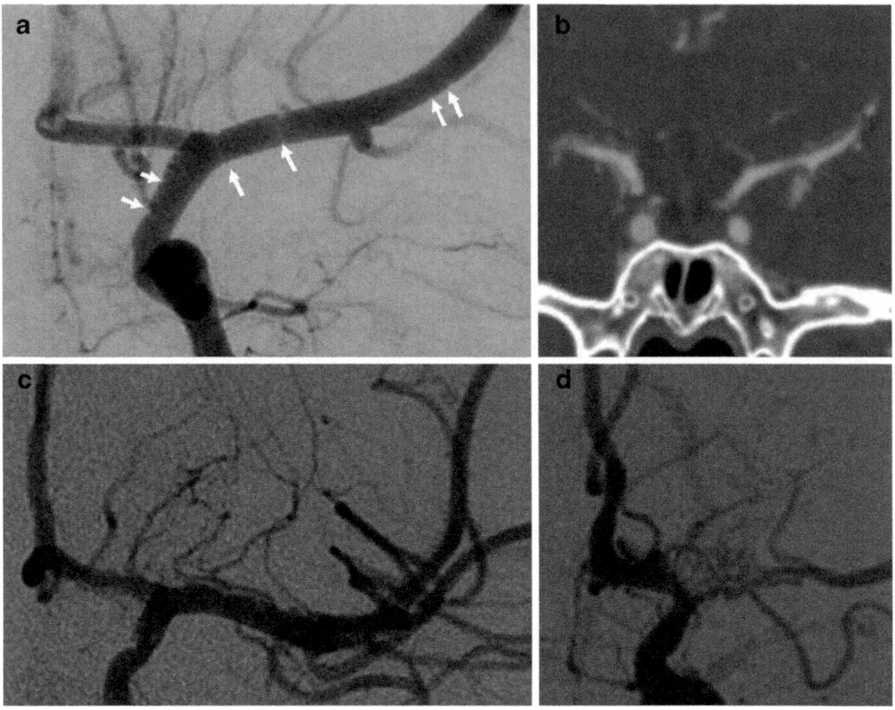

Fig. 3.1 (**a**, **b**) Typical DSA findings of FCAi in a 9 year-old male presenting with acute left middle cerebral artery territory infarction (**a**). Note the series of concentric linear ring-like constrictions along the intradural left internal carotid artery (ICA) and proximal left middle cerebral artery. Coronal reformatted CT angiography in the same patient fails to demonstrate the diagnostic features. DSA in another child with FCAi involving the left ICA, A1, and M1 (**c**). DSA findings in another child with FCAd (**d**)

of the cervical arteries (Fig. 3.3). DSA should be considered where diagnostic uncertainty persists after MRA or CTA. In patients with segmental narrowing of cortical branch arteries, intra-arterial vasodilator infusion during the DSA study can differentiate reversible vasoconstriction from non-constrictive arteriopathies. Serial imaging of arteriopathies to monitor for progression or recurrent events is best performed with MRI. Vessel wall imaging (VWI) may be a useful tool in assessing wall enhancement associated with inflammatory vasculopathies and vasculitides [23].

Medical Management of Acute AIS in Children

With the lack of data driving the development of clinical practice guidelines, there are no level 1 recommendations offered by the American Heart Association (AHA) for pediatric acute stroke care [2]. Despite substantial advances in pediatric stroke

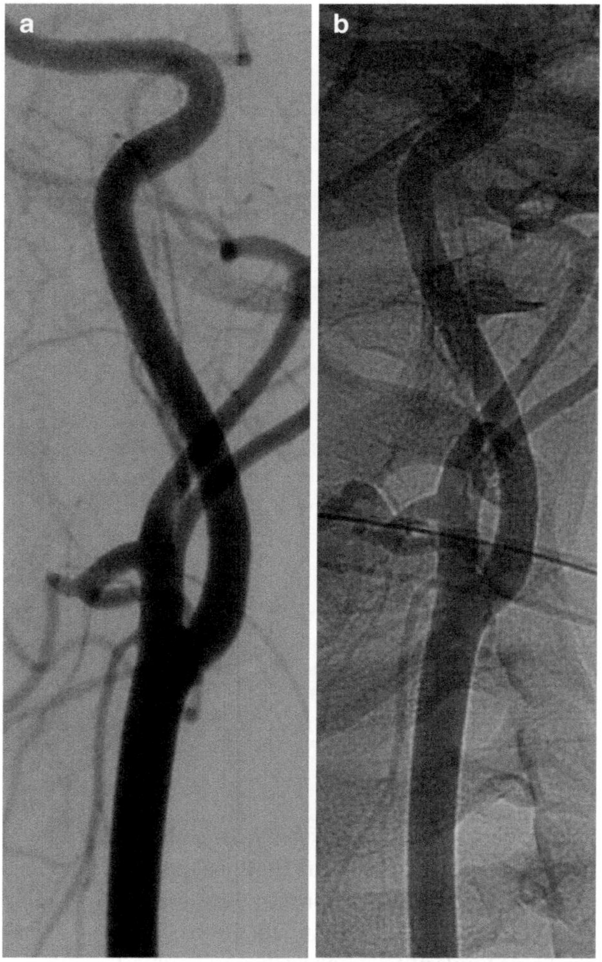

Fig. 3.2 A 9-year-old male with acute stroke (same patient shown in Fig. 3.1a, b) incorrectly diagnosed with cervical left ICA dissection due to artifact caused by marked ICA pulsatility on CTA (**a**). DSA and un-subtracted companion imaging confirmed absence of cervical ICA dissection (**b**)

research and clinical care, many unanswered questions remain concerning both acute treatment and secondary stroke prevention. Consequently, treatment recommendations are mainly extrapolated from studies on the adult population [1]. As a general rule, AHA guidelines recommend conservative management of childhood stroke (e.g., control fever, maintain good oxygenation, blood pressure, and glucose levels), and provide guidelines for antiplatelet or anticoagulation therapy, left to the clinician's discretion if they are to be used [24].

Intravenous (IV) thrombolytic therapy with tissue-type plasminogen activator (tPA) has been shown to significantly benefit adults with acute AIS when administered within 4.5 hours of stroke onset [25–27]. Recent studies suggest that properly selected adult stroke patients identified by cerebral perfusion imaging may benefit from IV thrombolytic therapy administered within 9 hours of stroke onset, or within 4.5 hours of a wake up stroke [28, 29]. Whether and how to apply this therapy in

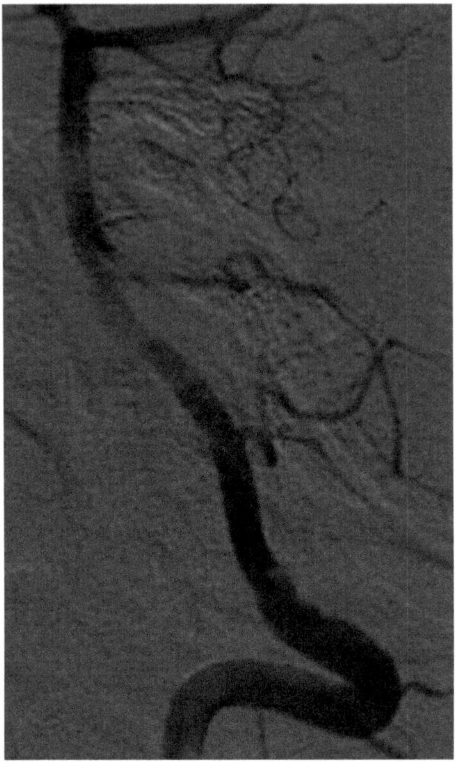

Fig. 3.3 A 15-year-old boy with recurrent posterior circulation strokes eventually found to be the result of Bow Hunter's syndrome due to vertebral artery impingement by a ponticulus posticus. DSA clearly shows subtle dissection of V3 segment of vertebral artery missed by multiple MR and CT angiography imaging studies

childhood remains controversial. In childhood stroke, the emergence of specialized pediatric stroke expertise, institutional pathways, and increased access to rapid stroke neuroimaging makes IV thrombolytic therapy for children potentially feasible [6].

Although level 2 recommendations for IV tPA exist for selected children with stroke secondary to cerebral venous sinus thrombosis, all randomized controlled trials for IV tPA in acute AIS have excluded patients <18 years of age [2]. The National Institutes of Health (NIH)-funded *Thrombolysis in Pediatric Stroke Study* (TIPS) was the only prospective clinical trial of IV tPA in children with acute AIS [30, 31]. Although the study was closed because of low patient enrollment, the multidisciplinary TIPS investigators succeeded in establishing systems for the evaluation and care of children with hyperacute AIS [31]. In the absence of clinical trial data, a consensus opinion suggests that when intravenous tPA is considered in children, the adult dose of 0.9 mg/kg may be used. It is noted that this is most likely a conservative dose given developmental differences in plasminogen levels may actually make the effective dose for children higher [32].

The first-line management of acute AIS in patients with SCD includes supplemental oxygen, hydration with intravenous D5 1/2 normal saline and rapid blood transfusion to a hemoglobin S of <30%, and total hemoglobin level of 10–11 g/dL. There is some evidence that thrombolytic therapy may be beneficial for acute AIS in adults with SCD.

Anticoagulation is recommended for secondary stroke prevention in children with cardioembolic stroke, cervical artery dissection, and arteriopathy. Historically the moyamoya arteriopathies (MMAs) were excluded, but preliminary data suggest a benefit in selected patients with MMA. Steroids are currently under investigation as a therapeutic agent in children with FCA-i.

Rationale for Mechanical Thrombectomy in Children with Acute AIS

Multiple RCTs show that mechanical endovascular thrombectomy (EVT) substantially increases disability-free survival in adults with AIS. Consequently, guidelines for the management of adults with AIS emphatically stress EVT as a first-line therapy in eligible patients with large vessel occlusions (LVOs). In contrast, published guidelines for treatment of pediatric AIS with mechanical thrombectomy are ambiguous due to a paucity of supporting high-quality scientific evidence. In 2015, AHA guidelines [33] for the early management of acute AIS stated that EVT with stent retrievers may be reasonable for some patients <18 years of age if initiated within 6 hours of symptom onset, acknowledging that the benefits and risks are not established. In 2018, the updated guidelines did not introduce any changes to this statement [27]. In the absence of randomized clinical trial data, one rational approach to the problem is to compare clinical outcomes in pediatric AIS patients treated with mechanical thrombectomy to clinical outcomes in a cohort of historical controls treated with standard of care. Since the standard of care for acute AIS in children is limited to supportive management, natural history outcomes are suitable for comparison.

Published studies show that the clinical outcome of untreated AIS in the pediatric population is generally poor, particularly in patients with cardiogenic strokes involving large portions of the MCA territory. Although most published pediatric AIS studies do not systemically report the results of vascular imaging studies, infarctions covering a majority of the MCA territory are most consistent with LVO, particularly in patients with cardiogenic stroke. The authors consider a large MCA territory infarction in a child with cardiogenic stroke to be a surrogate marker of LVO. Consequently, the literature indicates that acute pediatric AIS secondary to LVO is highly likely to end in a poor clinical outcome if only supportive care is administered. In unselected pediatric stroke patients, the majority of which have mild strokes, the likelihood of a poor clinical outcome is in the range of 40%. In children with acute LVO affecting the MCA territory, the likelihood of a poor clinical outcome is in the range of 70%.

Having established that the natural history of acute pediatric AIS with LVO is generally associated with a poor clinical outcome, it is necessary to determine if EVT is feasible, safe, and associated with better clinical outcomes than would otherwise be expected for the untreated natural history. In 2005, the first reported case of an early stent retriever used in a child with a basilar artery occlusion resulted in an excellent clinical result with the reversal of a patient with locked-in

Table 3.1 Consideration of thrombectomy according to AIS etiology

Etiology	Plan
Cardioembolic – 30%	Consider thrombectomy
Cervical dissection – 20%	Consider thrombectomy/stent/angioplasty
Intracranial arteriopathy – 45% (SCD, FCA)	No accepted endovascular treatment
Moyamoya – 5–10%	No accepted endovascular treatment

syndrome [34]. However, most early clinical reports of EVT for acute AIS used outdated modalities (intra-arterial thrombolysis) and ineffective first-generation devices [2]. These cases were associated with low rates of technically successful recanalization, and less than satisfactory clinical outcomes. More recent reports using modern revascularization technologies have shown high rates of successful reperfusion (~ 90%), and most patients show an improvement in neurological deficit after thrombectomy. The proportion with excellent clinical outcomes is significantly better than expected natural history outcomes [3]. Moreover, the literature shows that EVT with modern revascularization technologies is safe, with a low rate of peri-interventional complications, and low rates of symptomatic intracranial hemorrhage [35]. Observational data thus support the utilization of EVT to improve clinical outcomes in properly selected pediatric AIS patients. Familiarity with non-embolic causes of pediatric large vessel occlusions is necessary to appropriately recognize the pathology and plan accordingly (Table 3.1). It is important to engage in interdisciplinary partnerships with experienced pediatric stroke providers and neurointerventional teams to establish consensus-based best practices prior to offering mechanical thrombectomy in order to minimize adverse outcomes [36, 37].

Technical Aspects of EVT in Pediatric AIS

Pediatric neuroscience specialists have expressed many concerns about the application of transcatheter revascularization therapies to children with acute AIS. One concern is that the underlying vascular pathology may be too dangerous for mechanical instrumentation. Opponents of EVT cite the high incidence of dissecting steno-occlusive and inflammatory cerebral arteriopathies in children with AIS and express concerns that affected intracranial vessels are too vulnerable to perforation and rupture. The authors agree that indiscriminate application of mechanical devices to high-risk "arteriopathic vessels" does involve excessive and unjustified risk. On the other hand, embolic intracranial LVO, which accounts for a significant proportion of non-perinatal pediatric AIS cases, can be safely and effectively treated by EVT.

Another concern that pediatric specialists have raised is that the amount of procedure-related contrast media is too high for small children. The position of the authors is that contrast nephropathy is not a clinically significant problem in the pediatric population when patients receive adequate intraoperative and postoperative hydration. This fundamental holds true over a wide range of contrast loads in excess of 6 ml/Kg particularly at the rate of administration that is typical for neurointerventional practice. Furthermore, only small amounts of contrast are necessary in the relatively short EVT procedures for pediatric AIS.

Another concern that pediatric specialists often express is that the procedure-related radiation exposure is dangerous for small children. The authors assert that EVT procedures are very short and exposure rates are very low using modern equipment and technique. Moreover, these concerns are generally outweighed by the potential benefit from reperfusion therapy in well-selected pediatric patients who will benefit from neurological recovery and prevention of long-term disability.

In 2019, the AHA published a scientific statement on stroke in children and neonates [6]. The report stated that it is reasonable to limit EVT to "larger children" with persistent NIHSS score of 6 or more with confirmed LVO (Table 3.2). The authors emphasized that smaller children may be more vulnerable to vascular injury at the arterial access site and the intracranial treatment site due to small size and fragility of the vessels, in addition to a higher tendency toward vasospasm.

In the vast majority of pediatric patients, the common femoral artery will be the access artery of choice for EVT. Femoral artery diameter correlates closely with age and height. The incidence of procedure-related femoral artery thrombosis and its outcome correlates with the size of the indwelling arterial introducer sheath and the duration of the procedure. Since EVT procedures are usually very short by most standards, access strategies can usually be safely adjusted to facilitate success even in very young patients. Table 3.3 summarizes example access strategies for different age groups and compatible intracranial revascularization devices – though it is worth noting that these devices are subject to regional availability, and new devices are becoming available with similar ID, OD, and material characteristics and may represent valid alternative device choices.

Table 3.2 AHA scientific statement on endovascular thrombectomy in children [6]

Persistent disabling neurological deficits (e.g., Pediatric NIH Stroke Scale score ≥6 at the time of intervention or higher if DAWN trial criteria are being applied).
Radiographically confirmed cerebral large artery occlusion.
Larger children because of concerns about introducing catheters into small groin and cerebral arteries and size-based limitations on contrast dye and radiation exposure.
Treatment decision made in conjunction with neurologists with expertise in the treatment of children with stroke.
Intervention performed by an endovascular surgeon with experience in both treating children and performing thrombectomy in adult stroke patients.

Table 3.3 Access approaches and revascularization device compatibility chart. Stryker Neurovascular, Fremont, CA; Medtronic Neurovascular, Irvine, CA; Penumbra, Alameda, CA

Age group	Transfemoral-carotid access	Compatible stent-retriever and microcatheter delivery options	Compatible thromboaspiration options
1–3 years	Long 5 F sheath extended from transfemoral arterial access site into carotid artery Medtronic Asahi Fubuki™ sheath	Trevo XP ProVue™ stent-retriever [3 mm × 20 mm, 4 mm × 20 mm, 6 mm × 25 mm] Stryker Trevo Pro 14™ microcatheter [157 cm, 2.0 F distal tip, 2.4 F proximal shaft] Medtronic Solitaire X™ stent-retriever [4 mm × 20/40 mm, 6 mm × 20/40 mm] Penumbra Velocity™ microcatheter [160 cm, 2.6 F distal tip, 2.95 F proximal shaft] Medtronic Phenom 21™ microcatheter [160 cm, 2.3 F distal tip, 2.6 F proximal shaft]	Penumbra 3 MAX™ tapered thromboaspiration catheter [0.043″ → 0.035″]- 3.8 F distal tip Penumbra 4 MAX™ straight thromboaspiration catheter [0.041″]- 4.1 F distal tip
≥4 years	Long 6 F sheath extended from transfemoral arterial access site into carotid artery Penumbra Neuron MAX™	*Trevo XP ProVue™ stent-retriever* [3 mm × 20 mm, 4 mm × 20 mm, 6 mm × 25 mm] Stryker Trevo Pro 14™ microcatheter [157 cm, 2.0 F distal tip, 2.4 F proximal shaft]*Medtronic Solitaire X™ stent-retriever* [4 mm × 20/40 mm, 6 mm × 20/40 mm] Penumbra Velocity™ microcatheter [160 cm, 2.6 F distal tip, 2.95 F proximal shaft] Medtronic Phenom 21™ microcatheter [160 cm, 2.3 F distal tip, 2.6 F proximal shaft]	Penumbra 3 MAX™ tapered thromboaspiration catheter [0.043″ → 0.035″]- 3.8 F distal tip Penumbra 4 MAX™ straight thromboaspiration catheter [0.041″]- 4.1 F distal tip Penumbra 4 MAX™ tapered thromboaspiration catheter [0.064″ → 0.041″]- 4.3 F (1.43 mm) distal 20 cm Penumbra JET D™ thromboaspiration catheter[0.054″ → 0.064″]- 4.9 F (1.65 mm) distal 20 cm Penumbra ACE 60™, ACE 64™, ACE 68™, JET7™ thromboaspiration catheters

Our experience shows that some pre-school children, 2 to 5 years of age, can be safely treated using modern adult embolectomy devices and techniques (Fig. 3.4). Using modified techniques and devices we have successfully performed mechanical embolectomy in children as young as 14 months of age (Fig. 3.4). The reason for this is that although the major intracranial arteries of the circle of Willis do not reach full

Fig. 3.4 (**a-h**)

Patient	Pretreatment DSA figures	Posttreatment DSA figures	Transfemoral arterial access	Carotid access	Revascularization approach	Number of passes	Technical result
(1) A 15-year-old female with congenital heart disease and acute heart failure presents with intracranial ICA occlusion	a	b	9F sheath	6 F Neuron MAX	1. ADAPT with ACE68 2. SOLUMBRA with ACE68 + 4 mm × 40 mm Solitaire Platinum	2	mTICI 2b
(2) A 6-year-old female with Fontan circulation awaiting heart transplant presents with acute left M1 occlusion	c	d	6 F Neuron MAX	6 F Neuron MAX extended from femoral access site	ADAPT with 5 MAX ACE	1	mTICI 2b
(3) A 14-month-old male with acute intraoperative M1 occlusion during preoperative embolization of choroid plexus carcinoma	e	f	5F sheath	5 F Envoy	1. 135 cm 0.027" Hi Flo Renegade with syringe aspiration used to revascularize M1 2. ADAPT technique using Penumbra 0.026″ reperfusion catheter with vacuum pump suction used to revascularize each M2 division	3	mTICI 2b
(4) 4-year-old female with Berlin heart awaiting second heart transplant found to have intracranial ICA occlusion on CT, CTA, and CTP performed because of seizures	g	h	6 F Neuron MAX	6 F Neuron MAX extended from femoral access site	1.ADAPT with ACE68 2. SOLUMBRA with ACE68 + 4 *mm* × 40 *mm Solitaire* Platinum 3. SOLUMBRA with ACE68 + 4 mm × 40 mm Solitaire Platinum 4. SOLUMBRA with ACE68 + Penumbra 3D Separator	4	mTICI 2b *Blood transfusion required to replace blood losses during revascularization. Verapamil required to manage vasospasm

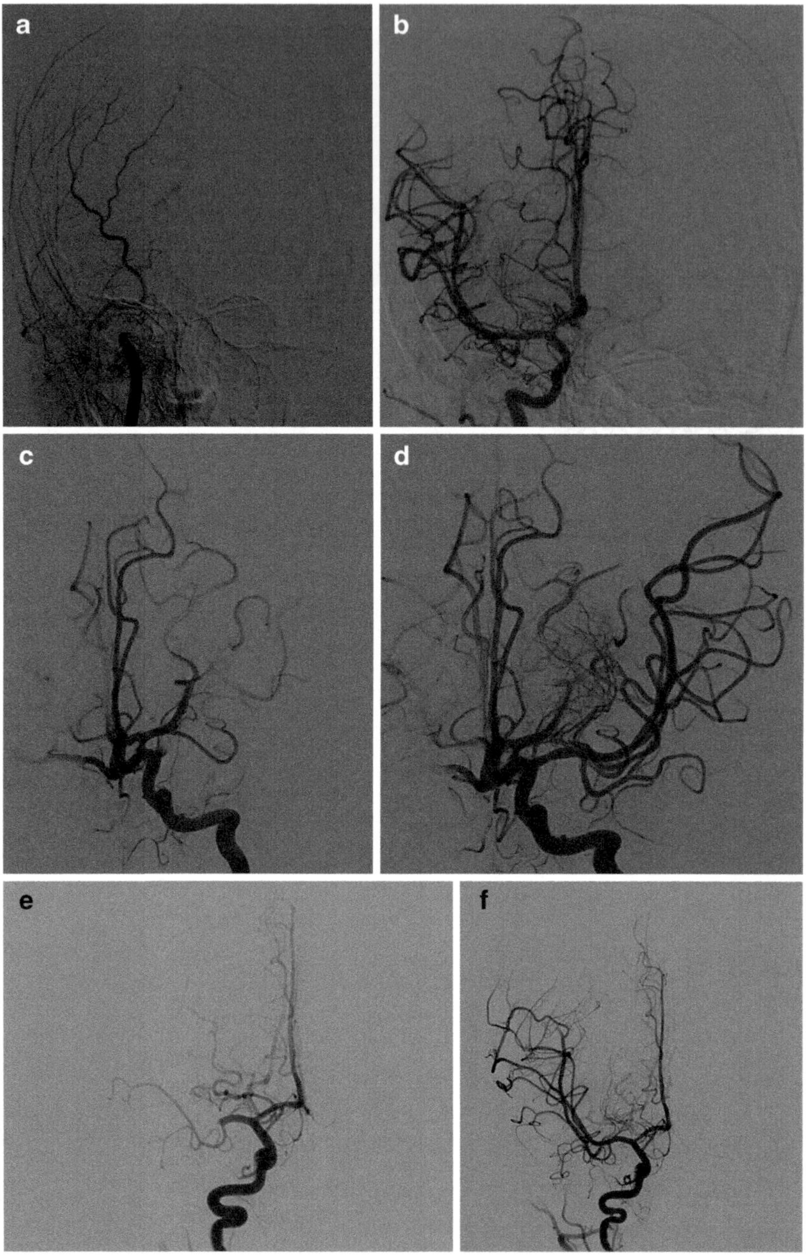

Fig. 3.4 (**i–l**) CT perfusion imaging (**i**, **j**) in a 4-year-old female with Berlin heart awaiting second heart transplant (patient #4 in table above) shows predicted core infarction in red (cerebral blood flow </=30% of contralateral normal) and penumbra in green (TTP >/= 6 seconds). It is notable that unaffected left posterior cerebral artery territory shows quantitative perfusion levels in the penumbral range, likely due to chronically reduced tissue perfusion in this child with severely depressed cardiac function. CT imaging obtained 48 hours after revascularization (**k**, **l**) demonstrates that CT perfusion imaging overestimated the patient's core infarction

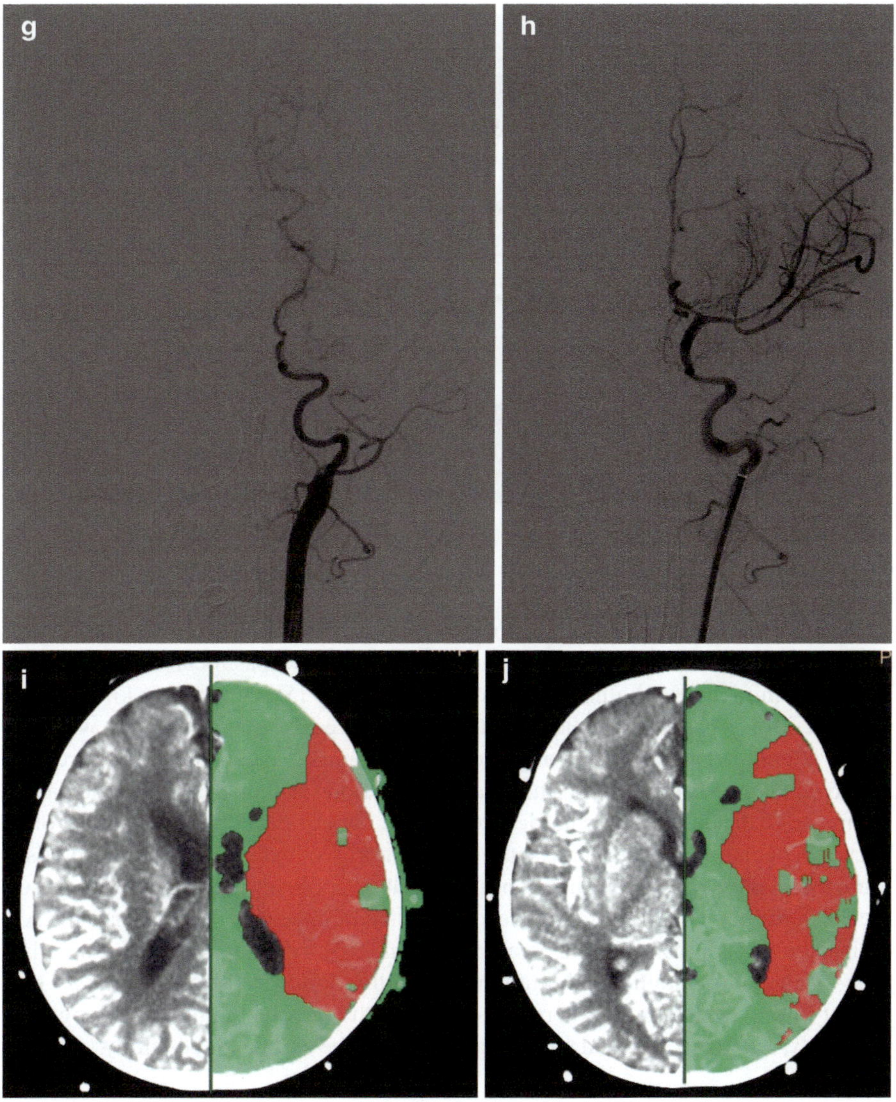

Fig. 3.4 (continued)

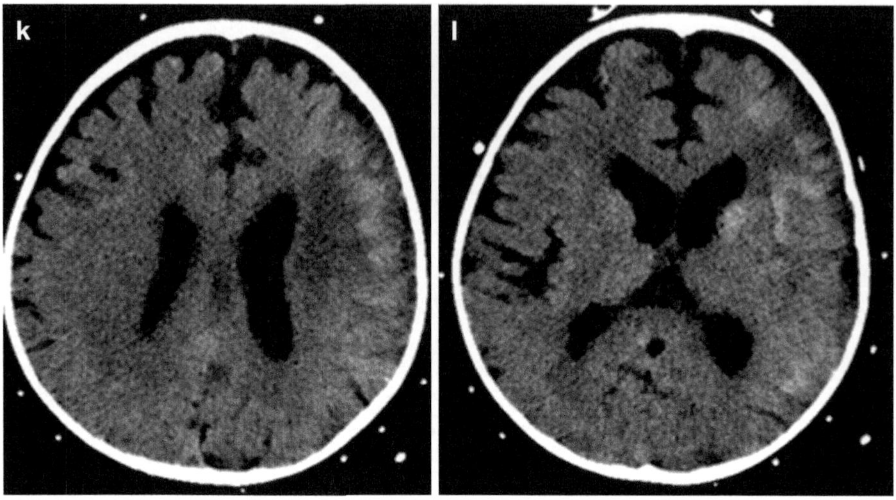

Fig. 3.4 (continued)

adult size until 12–14 years of age, most growth is completed by 2 to 5 years of age (Fig. 3.5). In children as young as 3 months of age, vasospasm can be safely managed with intra-arterial boluses of verapamil up to 100 micrograms per kilogram.

After EVT procedures, pediatric patients should receive supportive care with particular attention to optimization of glycemia, euvolemia, oxygenation, blood pressure and to prevent and correct hyperthermia and infections. Although there are no data to demonstrate the benefit of pediatric stroke units, care of pediatric AIS patients often occurs in pediatric intensive care settings. A minority of patients may develop raised intracranial pressure, which should prompt early supportive care and early neurosurgical referral for consideration of decompressive craniectomy, particularly for AIS patients with malignant middle cerebral arterial territory infarction. Given the plasticity of the young brain, rehabilitation for children following stroke can likely lead to vast improvements in long-term outcomes, with a favorable impact on long-term morbidity, quality of life, and emotional health for the child and the family [1].

Imaging Selection of Children for Endovascular Thrombectomy

In contrast to adults with suspected AIS, where CT and CTA are often used for first-line imaging, children presenting with acute neurological deficits are best imaged with MRI and MRA. This is because there is a high prevalence of stroke mimics that are indistinguishable from early AIS on CT. CT has been reported to miss as many as 47% of AIS later confirmed by MR imaging in children. Most pediatric medical centers have "rapid stroke MR imaging protocols" that can be performed in awake

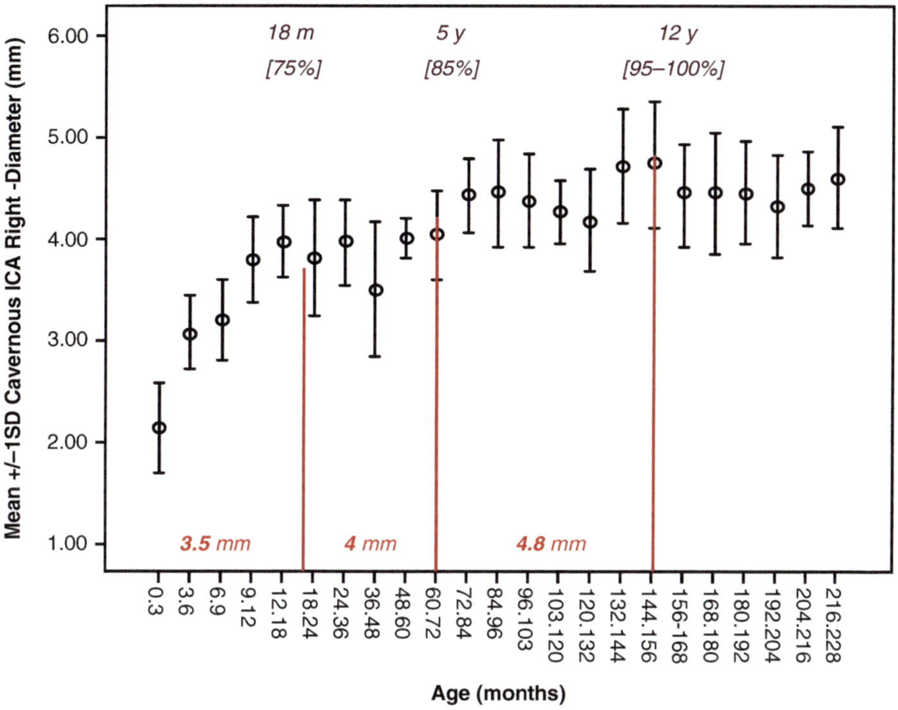

Fig. 3.5 Diameter of the cavernous segment of the internal carotid artery (ICA) as a function of age for 318 pediatric subjects without stroke, cerebrovascular disease, or vascular risk factors. ICA diameters were measured on axial and coronal T2-weighted images of the brain obtained for evaluation of trauma, headaches, or hearing loss. The mean ICA diameter for all patients within a given age range is indicated as a circle, and error bars show + and – one standard deviation. The growth curve is divided into 3 growth regions by 3 red lines. The subject's age, and the percent of fully mature ICA diameter in the plateau of the curve corresponding to each of the red lines, is annotated above each red line. The measured ICA diameter corresponding to each of the red lines is indicated in red text to the left of each read line

children in 12 minutes or less. Such protocols are usually limited to a DWI sequence, a T2 FLAIR sequence, a hemorrhage-sensitive sequence such as gradient echo or susceptibility weighted imaging, and a time-of-flight MRA sequence. It should be noted that MR imaging is contraindicated in patients with extracorporeal circulatory assist devices and some types of implantable devices.

One of the greatest challenges involved with EVT in the pediatric population concerns the implementation of perfusion imaging-based patient selection. Experience has shown that perfusion imaging biomarkers of infarction and ischemia are altered by patient age and chronically impaired cardiopulmonary function. In particular, profoundly altered cerebral perfusion may be present in children with Fontan circulation or children requiring prolonged support from extracorporeal circulatory assist devices such as a Berlin heart. Furthermore, CT perfusion thresholds, which predict infarction in adults, may be different in the pediatric brain (Fig. 3.4i–l). Consequently, for accurate core infarct assessment, DWI is preferred. In addition, direct translation of adult Tmax threshold values may be misleading for estimation of penumbra in childhood AIS (Fig. 3.4i–l). It may be prudent to weight clinical assessment and relative perfusion measures to estimate the territory at risk.

A general approach to imaging-based patient selection should begin with exclusion of patients with malignant core infarctions that are likely to render revascularization futile and potentially harmful. Rankin shift analysis in two recent large adult cohorts shows thrombectomy is beneficial in adults with core infarctions <100 ml [38]. Assuming that 100 ml is roughly 40% of the adult MCA territory, ASPECT score of 6, this translates to an adjusted core infarct volume of 70–80 ml in children 5 to 10 years of age [39].

The quantitative cerebral perfusion imaging metrics, which define penumbral tissue fated to infarction in the absence of revascularization therapy, are under investigation. One study reported that the results of DSC cerebral perfusion imaging correlated with cardiac status in five children with LVO strokes. In one child with heart failure, symptomatic cerebral ischemia correlated with a Tmax >6 seconds, but in two children without cardiac insufficiency, symptomatic cerebral ischemia correlated with a Tmax >4 seconds. One explanation for the findings is that the brains of younger, rapidly growing children with normal cardiopulmonary function demand a higher perfusion relative to adults due to increased metabolic activity in the developing brain. Neuronal metabolic activity may be adapted to a lower perfusion level in children with chronically impaired cardiopulmonary function. Patient selection will improve with advances in imaging biomarker research and new trials such as the PETITE trial (Pediatric Endovascular Therapy after Imaging in acuTE stroke).

Conclusion

Level 1 evidence for the effectiveness of pediatric stroke intervention remains unavailable, and, due to the heterogeneity of stroke causation and prevalence of mimics, an efficient randomized trial will be difficult to perform. However, the presentation of a child with a large vessel occlusion will undoubtedly present in major comprehensive stroke centers with increasing frequency. Familiarity with non-embolic causes of pediatric large vessel occlusions will guide the interventionalist in interpreting real-time imaging on non-invasive imaging and catheter angiography to appropriately recognize the pathology and plan accordingly. The role of catheter-based therapy in many of the non-embolic causes of vessel occlusion is presently limited, but there are numerous case series indicating feasibility and safety in the interventional treatment of large vessel embolic occlusions and dissection. Until such time that more substantial trial data are available, individual treatment plans should be made on a case-by-case basis.

References

1. Rosa M, De Lucia S, Rinaldi VE, Le Gal J, Desmarest M, Veropalumbo C, et al. Pediatric arterial ischemic stroke: acute management, recent advances and remaining issues. Ital J Pediatr. 2015;41:95.
2. Cobb MI, Laarakker AS, Gonzalez LF, Smith TP, Hauck EF, Zomorodi AR. Endovascular therapies for acute ischemic stroke in children. Stroke. 2017;48:2026–30.
3. Sporns PB, Kemmling A, Hanning U, Minnerup J, Strater R, Niederstadt T, et al. Thrombectomy in childhood stroke. J Am Heart Assoc. 2019;8:e011335.
4. Wilson JL, Eriksson CO, Williams CN. Endovascular therapy in pediatric stroke: utilization, patient characteristics, and outcomes. Pediatr Neurol. 2017;69:87–92.
5. Gonzalez–Odriozola R, Rawie E, Parmar HA, Rivas–Rodriguez F. Arterial ischemic stroke in the pediatric population. Neurographics. 2019;9(6):395–404.
6. Ferriero DM, Fullerton HJ, Bernard TJ, Billinghurst L, Daniels SR, DeBaun MR, et al. Management of stroke in neonates and children. A scientific statement from the American Heart Association/American Stroke Association. Stroke. 2019;50:e51–96.
7. Powers WJ, Rabinstein AA, Ackerson T, Adeoye OM, Bambakidis NC, Becker K, et al. Guidelines for the early management of patients with acute ischemic stroke: 2019 update to the 2018 guidelines for the early management of acute ischemic stroke. Stroke. 2019;50:e344–418.
8. Gardner MA, Hills NK, Sidney S, et al. The 5-year direct medical cost of neonatal and childhood stroke in a population-based cohort. Neurology. 2010;74:372–37.
9. Lo W, Zamel K, Ponnappa K, et al. The cost of pediatric stroke care and rehabilitation. Stroke. 2008;39:161–5.
10. Lo W, Stephens J, Fernandez S. Paediatric stroke in the United States and the impact of risk factors. J Child Neurol. 2009;24:194–203.
11. Fox C, Fullerton H. Recent advances in childhood arterial ischemic stroke. Curr Atheroscler Rep. 2010;12:217–24.
12. Fox CK, Sidney S, Fullerton HJ. Community-based case-control study of childhood stroke risk associated with congenital heart disease. Stroke. 2015;46:336–40.
13. Rafay MF, Armstrong D, Deveber G, Domi T, Chan A, MacGregor DL. Craniocervical arterial dissection in children: clinical and radiographic presentation and outcome. J Child Neurol. 2006;21:8–16.
14. DeVela G, Taylor JM, Zhang B, Linscott LL, Chen AM, Karani KB, et al. Quantitative arterial tortuousity suggest arteriopathy in children with cryptogenic stroke. Stroke. 2018;49(4):1011–4.
15. Rollins NK, Braga B, Hogge A, Beavers S, Dowling M. Dynamic arterial compression in pediatric vertebral arterial dissecion. Stroke. 2017;48(4):1070–3.
16. Wintermark M, Hills NK, deVeber GA, Barkovich AJ, Elkind MS, Sear K, et al. Arteriopathy diagnosis in childhood arterial ischemic stroke: results of the vascular effects of infection in pediatric stroke study. Stroke. 2014;45:3597–605.
17. Adams RJ, McKie VC, Hsu L, Files B, Vichinsky E, Pegelow C, et al. Prevention of a first stroke by transfusions in children with sickle cell anemia and abnormal results on transcranial Doppler ultrasonography. N Engl J Med. 1998;339:5–11.
18. Kassim AA, Galadanci NA, Pruthi S, De Baun MR. How I treat acute stroke and long-term management in sickle cell disease. Blood. 2015;125:3401–10.
19. Lee MT, Piomelli S, Granger S, Miller ST, Harkness S, Brambilla DJ, et al. Stroke prevention trial in sickle cell anemia (STOP): extended follow-up and final results. Blood. 2006;108(3):847–52.
20. Scott RM, Smith ER. Moyamoya disease and moyamoya syndrome. N Engl J Med. 2009;360:1226–37.
21. Wintermark M, Hills NK, DeVeber GA, Barkovich AJ, Bernard TJ, Friedman NR, et al. Clinical and imaging characteristics of arteriopathy subtypes in children with arterial ischemic stroke: results of the VIPS study. AJNR Am J Neuroradiol. 2017;38:2172–9.

22. Mallick AA, Ganesan V, Kirkham FJ, Fallon P, Hedderly T, McShane T, et al. Childhood arterial ischaemic stroke incidence, presenting features, and risk factors: a prospective population-based study. Lancet Neurol. 2014;13(1):35–43.
23. Stence NV, Pabst LL, Hollatz AL, Mirsky DM, Herson PS, Poisson S, et al. Predicting progression of intracranial arteriopathies in childhood stroke with vessel wall imaging. Stroke. 2017;48(8):2274–7.
24. Roach ES, Golomb MR, Adams R, Biller J, Daniels S, Deveber G, et al. American Heart Association Stroke Council; Council on Cardiovascular Disease in the young. Management of stroke in infants and children: a scientific statement from a Special Writing Group of the American Heart Association Stroke Council and the Council on Cardiovascular Disease in the young. Stroke. 2008;39:2644–91.
25. Goyal M, Menon BK, van Zwam WH, Dippel DW, Mitchell PJ, Demchuk AM, et al. Endovascular thrombectomy after large-vessel ischaemic stroke: a meta-analysis of individual patient data from five randomised trials. Lancet. 2016;387:1723–31.
26. Saver JL. Time is brain–quantified. Stroke. 2006;37:263–6.
27. Powers WJ, Rabinstein AA, Ackerson T, Adeoye OM, Bambakidis NC, Becker K, Biller J, et al. 2018 guidelines for the early management of patients with acute ischemic stroke: a guideline for healthcare professionals from the American Heart Association/ American Stroke Association. Stroke. 2018;49:e233–4.
28. Ma H, Campbell BCV, Parsons MW, Churilov L, Levi CR, Hsu C, et al. Thrombolysis guided by perfusion imaging up to 9 hours after onset of stroke. N Engl J Med. 2019;380(19):1795–803.
29. Thomalla G, Simonsen CZ, Boutitie F, Andersen G, Berthezene Y, Cheng B, et al. MRI-guided thrombolysis for stroke with unknown time of onset. N Engl J Med. 2018;379(7):611–22.
30. Lee S, Heit JJ, Albers GW, Wintermark M, Jiang B, Bernier E, et al. Neuroimaging selection for thrombectomy in pediatric stroke: a single-center experience. J NeuroIntervent Surg. 2019;11:940–6.
31. Rivkin MJ, deVeber G, Ichord RN, Kirton A, Chan AK, Hovinga CA, et al. Thrombolysis in pediatric stroke study. Stroke. 2015;46:880–5.
32. Rivkin MJ, Bernard TJ, Dowling MM, Amlie-Lefond C. Guidelines for urgent management of stroke in children. Pediatr Neurol. 2016;56:8–17.
33. Powers WJ, Derdeyn CP, Biller J, Coffey CS, Hoh BL, Jauch EC, et al. 2015 American Heart Association/American Stroke Association focused update of the 2013 guidelines for the early management of patients with acute ischemic stroke regarding endovascular treatment. Stroke. 2015;46:3020–35.
34. Zaidat OO, Tolbert M, Smith TP, Alexander MJ. Primary endovascular therapy with clot retrieval and balloon angioplasty for acute basilar artery occlusion. Pediatr Neurosurg. 2005;41(6):323–7.
35. Satti S, Chen J, Sivapatham T, Jayaraman M, Orbach D. Mechanical thrombectomy for pediatric acute ischemic stroke: review of the literature. J Neurointervent Surg. 2017;9(8):732–7.
36. Ellis MJ, Amlie-Lefond C, Orbach DB. Endovascular therapy in children with acute ischemic stroke: review and recommendations. Neurology. 2012;79(13 Supplement 1):S158–64.
37. Buompadre MC, Andres K, Slater LA, Mohseni-Bod H, Guerguerian AM, Branson H, et al. Thrombectomy for acute stroke in childhood: a case report, literature review, and recommendations. Pediatr Neurol. 2017;66:21–7.
38. Sarraj A, Savitz S, Pujara D, Kamal H, Carroll K, Shaker F, et al. Endovascular thrombectomy for acute ischemic strokes: current US access paradigms and optimization methodology. Stroke. 2020;50:1207–17.
39. Phan TG, Donnan GA, Wright PM, Reutens DC. A digital map of middle cerebral artery infarcts associated with middle cerebral artery trunk and branch occlusions. Stroke. 2005;36(5):986–91.

Chapter 4
ELVO in Urban Areas: Evolution of Stroke Systems of Care

Johanna T. Fifi and Jacob Morey

Introduction

Endovascular therapy (EVT) is now the standard of care for emergent large vessel occlusion (ELVO) acute ischemic stroke (AIS) in the early time window following positive outcomes from multiple randomized trials [1]. Furthermore, based on the results of the DWI or CTP Assessment with Clinical Mismatch in the Triage of Wake-Up and Late-Presenting Strokes Undergoing Neurointervention with Trevo (DAWN) [2] and Endovascular Therapy Following Imaging Evaluation for Ischemic Stroke (DEFUSE 3) trials [3], guidelines for the treatment of patients with ELVO AIS now recommend an extended time window for EVT up to 24 hours after onset [1]. This extended window for stroke thrombectomy also expands the number of patients who qualify for treatment, but time to treatment continues to be critical to patient outcome. An analysis on Solitaire with the Intention for Thrombectomy as Primary Endovascular Treatment (SWIFT PRIME) data found patients with a last known well to reperfusion time of less than 150 minutes had 91% estimated probability of functional independence. The probability of a good outcome decreased by 10% over the next hour and 20% after each subsequent hour [4]. Therefore, timely and direct access to thrombectomy is important for outcome in ELVO stroke.

Stroke systems of care were developed in the prior decades to optimize the timely delivery of intravenous (IV) tissue plasminogen activator (tPA) in the first 3 hours after stroke onset [5]. This required development and geographic distribution of certified Primary Stroke Centers (PSC) able to perform neuroimaging and deliver tPA. Comprehensive Stroke Centers (CSC) were then created for more specialized

J. T. Fifi (✉)
Department of Neurology and Neurosurgery, Mount Sinai Health System, New York, NY, USA

J. Morey
Icahn School of Medicine at Mount Sinai, New York, NY, USA

F. K. Hui et al. (eds.), *12 Strokes*, https://doi.org/10.1007/978-3-030-56857-3_4

care often involving neurosurgical or neurointerventional procedures. The more recent development has been the creation of another level of certification for thrombectomy-capable hospitals (TSC). Recent guidelines estimate at least 1500 PSCs in the United States, with about 200 CSCs [6], and the number of TSC-type hospitals is growing. Despite the fact that many CSCs and TSC-type hospitals are localized to urban areas, access to EVT for many patients in urban settings is challenging. Strategies to improve timely access to EVT are necessary and optimal implementation of stroke systems of care will vary depending on geography and population density.

Stroke services in urban areas face unique challenges to coordination of care and timely treatment of patients with EVT. A challenge to minimizing onset-to-treatment times in urban environments is that patient transfer is often subject to gridlock and prone to delay. These obstacles are especially problematic in New York City, which has the largest population and highest population density of any major city in the United States. Onset-to-door times are a critical area of improvement in stroke care, as prehospital delays are the most common cause of patients missing the therapeutic window for IV-tPA, with only 20–25% of patients presenting to the emergency department within 3 hours of stroke onset [7, 8]. Since the demonstration of overwhelming efficacy of EVT, many urban health-care systems, from the EMS to the hospital and hospital network level, have rapidly transformed to care for the ELVO patient importantly under the guidance of state and local regulations and stakeholder groups.

Historic Stroke Care Delivery Models

The two most common models of stroke care delivery, "drip and ship" and "mothership," have their roots in IV-tPA protocols [5, 9]. Initially IV-tPA was available only in largely academic stroke centers with significant resources for the comprehensive care of the stroke patient's entire clinical course from the emergency department (ED) through rehabilitation. However, in order to allow for this time-sensitive treatment to be brought into the community, more hospitals became equipped to deliver IV-tPA in the ED followed by transfer. This "drip and ship" model allowed community hospitals to quickly administer the time-sensitive tPA to AIS patients and then immediately transport them to a more advanced medical center for comprehensive stroke care including EVT. In the mothership model, stroke patients are instead transported directly to a CSC, which minimizes delays surrounding transfer between hospitals. The drip and ship model worked well for IV-tPA administration, enlarging the patient pool eligible for stroke therapy [10]. However, EVT often necessitates a transfer to a comprehensive center before initiation. There is growing evidence that transfer is associated with worse outcome in ELVO patients. In the urban setting, there are typically several EVT-capable centers frequently in close proximity while PSCS will be distributed throughout the city, often creating disparate geographical, and sometimes socioeconomic, access to care within the same urban area. The paradigm shift to EVT has created a strong impetus for stroke systems of care to adjust to meet patient's needs. Strategies to increase access are discussed below.

Prehospital Triage

The delays to EVT in the drip and ship model have led to a recommendation by the AHA/ASA (American Heart Association/American Stroke Association) Mission Lifeline algorithm to consider direct transport to CSCs, bypassing a PSC, if the additional travel time is less than 15 minutes [11, 12]. Recent implementation of prehospital triage has included a 30-minute bypass window in large cities such as Los Angeles [13] and New York City. More recent guidelines have suggested further evidence is needed to establish optimal time parameters [6]. Evidence in favor of the mothership model is accumulating for select patients, especially in cases of efficient prehospital stratification of patients with high clinical suspicion for LVO [14, 15]. Probability models and prediction models suggest the relative benefit of the mothership model over drip and ship is based on distance between PSC and CSC as well as fast door-to-needle times at the CSC [16, 17]. The mothership model in this context requires field triaging of the patient, typically via clinical examination and standardized scales administered by first responders. Prehospital triage of ELVO stroke and bypass to stroke centers capable of thrombectomy has been initiated in several regions across the United States, including New York City. This type of triage appears well-suited for urban areas where bypass distances and times will be small for the majority of patients compared with rural or remote areas where thrombectomy centers can be hundreds of miles away. There is concern for delay of initiation of IV-tPA in eligible patients when bypassing a PSC. However, recent studies in Providence, Rhode Island, and Los Angeles, California, have demonstrated that faster door-to-IV-tPA times at CSCs mitigate any delay in time to IV-tPA when bypass is performed [13, 18]. The RACECAT trial based in Barcelona and Catalonia is currently ongoing and directly compares these two models [19].

The decision for direct transport to a CSC is based on protocols utilizing various prehospital stroke severity scales that vary greatly in sensitivity and specificity from 49% to 91% and 40% to 94%, respectively [20]. Among other factors, this means that a significant proportion of patients will still present to PSCs. Algorithm for the evaluation and triage of patients in the prehospital setting is the perfect problem for computer-aided solutions. The development of machine learning software for such finite parts of the problem such as ELVO detection by video examination of the patient to GPS-aided routing of the ambulance is currently ongoing. The accuracy of prehospital triage is also likely to increase with new technology, such as portable, non-invasive ELVO detection visors and mobile stroke units. This is an active field of research and device development [21–23].

Mobile Interventional Stroke Teams

Despite prehospital triage, some pockets of large urban areas are without timely access to a TSC or CSC. Transformation of certain PSCs to include interventional capability has occurred over the last few years. There are still unanswered questions on how these facilities fit into the model with CSCs present. A further alternative model to drip and ship has also developed wherein the interventional team based at a large-volume CSC covers an integrated system by traveling to the patient for EVT performed at a PSC or TSC [24]. This type of model is likely best suited to urban environments where travel time between multiple centers can be shorter as compared with rural areas. Instead of the patient transferring to the CSC, a Mobile Interventional Stroke Team (MIST) travels from the CSC to treat the patient at the PSC or TSC. One form of a MIST, as described in the literature from New York City, consists of an attending neurointerventionalist physician, a fellow or assistant, and radiologic technologist. Use of a MIST allows patients to receive IV-tPA and medical management while the MIST is mobilized and reduces risks and delays inherent inpatient transfers. Since 2016, similar models to the MIST (nine total) have been proposed with inter-hospital transfers of an endovascular-trained attending physician [24–31]. The majority of these models utilize ground transportation, with air being less common, and are primarily located in Germany, Japan, and New York City (USA). Helistroke has also been described in the literature and involves transporting a neurointerventionalist to the patient via helicopter, which may further expand application of the "trip and treat" paradigm [30, 31]. All relevant published reports demonstrated a reduction in the initial door-to-puncture time, with the New York trip and treat model publishing an onset-to-treatment time that was 79 minutes faster than drip and ship [32]. One advantage of this model is born out as more and more patients qualify for endovascular treatment for stroke, and growing case volume taxes bed capacity at CSCs. Furthermore, this model allows a single neurointerventional team to expand coverage across multiple hospitals potentially saving costs and concentrating procedural experience. The MIST model currently exists alongside and complements EMS triage, mothership, and DS models creating a more complete stroke care system.

Mobile Stroke Units

First pioneered in Germany and introduced in the United States in the city of Houston, a Mobile Stroke Unit (MSU) allows stroke patients to be diagnosed and treated with IV-tPA en route to the hospital [33, 34]. The MSU is a specialized ambulance equipped with a CT scanner, laboratory testing, and tPA. The ambulance is staffed by a radiology technologist and paramedics and has either a vascular neurologist on board or has telestroke capacity. Studies have demonstrated that MSUs are associated with faster times to treatment with tissue plasminogen activator compared with conventional ambulance transport followed by tPA delivered in emergency departments [33]. A recent publication looking at the MSU out of NewYork-Presbyterian in New York City demonstrated that faster times hold true even in dense urban areas [35]. Despite, the ambulance pick-up location often being in close proximity to several designated stroke centers, the MSU was able to deliver tPA 29.7 minutes faster than conventional ambulance transport. An additional step of performance of CT angiography in the scanner can accurately identify ELVO patients and triage them in the field for delivery to CSC [36]. The capability for CTA varies in the MSUs in service today. One hurdle is the need for on-board power generation and additional size and weight of the ambulance. While in use in various cities around the United States and Europe, the cost-effectiveness of the MSU and potential for universal availability are still being studied [37].

Conclusions

Health-care systems in urban regions have incorporated a broad range of models into their stroke systems of care to minimize times to treatment. The high population density, relatively close proximity of hospitals, and inefficiencies in patient transfer associated with traffic congestion make traditional "drip and ship" prone to treatment delays. No one model is sufficient in these complex environments, and the best solution is likely one that allows and integrates various pathways for getting the patient to the treatment. The systems implemented include prehospital triage, mothership, MIST models, and rapid stroke transfer, including drip and ship. MSUs incorporating specialized stroke ambulances have also been introduced. Systems of stroke care have continued to evolve rapidly over the past few years, and, in a large urban environment, coordination and cooperation between existing multiple hospital systems, government agencies, professional organizations, and other stakeholders for each region will be key to improving efficiencies and access to this revolutionary therapy for the larger population.

References

1. Powers WJ, Rabinstein AA, Ackerson T, Adeoye OM, Bambakidis NC, Becker K, et al. Guidelines for the early management of patients with acute ischemic stroke: 2019 update to the 2018 guidelines for the early management of acute ischemic stroke: a guideline for healthcare professionals from the American Heart Association/American Stroke Association. Stroke. 2019;50:e344–418.
2. Albers GW, Marks MP, Kemp S, Christensen S, Tsai JP, Ortega-Gutierrez S, et al. Thrombectomy for stroke at 6 to 16 hours with selection by perfusion imaging. N Engl J Med. 2018;378:708–18.

3. Nogueira RG, Jadhav AP, Haussen DC, Bonafe A, Budzik RF, Bhuva P, et al. Thrombectomy 6 to 24 hours after stroke with a mismatch between deficit and infarct. N Engl J Med. 2018;378:11–21.
4. Goyal M, Jadhav AP, Bonafe A, Diener H, Mendes Pereira V, Levy E, et al. Analysis of workflow and time to treatment and the effects on outcome in endovascular treatment of acute ischemic stroke: results from the swift prime randomized controlled trial. Radiology. 2016;279:888–97.
5. Merino JG, Silver B, Wong E, Foell B, Demaerschalk B, Tamayo A, et al. Extending tissue plasminogen activator use to community and rural stroke patients. Stroke. 2002;33:141–6.
6. Adeoye O, Nystrom KV, Yavagal DR, Luciano J, Nogueira RG, Zorowitz RD, et al. Recommendations for the establishment of stroke systems of care: a 2019 update. Stroke. 2019;50:e187–210.
7. Kleindorfer D, Kissela B, Schneider A, Woo D, Khoury J, Miller R, et al. Eligibility for recombinant tissue plasminogen activator in acute ischemic stroke - a population-based study. Stroke. 2004;35:E27–9.
8. Barber PA, Zhang J, Demchuk AM, Hill MD, Buchan AM. Why are stroke patients excluded from tpa therapy? An analysis of patient eligibility. Neurology. 2001;56:1015–20.
9. Rymer MM, Thurtchley D, Summers D. Stroke MABSI. Expanded modes of tissue plasminogen activator delivery in a comprehensive stroke center increases regional acute stroke interventions. Stroke. 2003;34:E58–60.
10. Sheth KN, Smith EE, Grau-Sepulveda MV, Kleindorfer D, Fonarow GC, Schwamm LH. Drip and ship thrombolytic therapy for acute ischemic stroke: use, temporal trends, and outcomes. Stroke. 2015;46:732–9.
11. Adeoye O, Nyström KV, Yavagal DR, Luciano J, Nogueira RG, Zorowitz RD, et al. Recommendations for the establishment of stroke systems of care: a 2019 update. Stroke. 2019;50:e187–210.
12. Severity-based stroke triage algorithm for EMS. AHA/ASA on-line published guidelines under Mission Lifeline Stroke, 2018.
13. Bosson N, Gausche-Hill M, Saver JL, Sanossian N, Tadeo R, Clare C, et al. Increased access to and use of endovascular therapy following implementation of a 2-tiered regional stroke system. Stroke. 2020;51(3):908–13.
14. Stiell IG, Clement CM, Campbell K, Sharma M, Socha D, Sivilotti ML, et al. Impact of expanding the prehospital stroke bypass time window in a large geographic region. Stroke. 2017;48:624–30.
15. Schlemm E, Ebinger M, Nolte CH, Endres M, Schlemm L. Optimal transport destination for ischemic stroke patients with unknown vessel status: use of prehospital triage scores. Stroke. 2017;48:2184–91.
16. Milne MS, Holodinsky JK, Hill MD, Nygren A, Qiu C, Goyal M, et al. Drip 'n ship versus mothership for endovascular treatment: modeling the best transportation options for optimal outcomes. Stroke. 2017;48:791–4.
17. Holodinsky JK, Williamson TS, Kamal N, Mayank D, Hill MD, Goyal M. Drip and ship versus direct to comprehensive stroke center: conditional probability modeling. Stroke. 2017;48:233–8.
18. Jayaraman MV, Hemendinger ML, Baird GL, Yaghi S, Cutting S, Saad A, et al. Field triage for endovascular stroke therapy: a population-based comparison. J Neurointerv Surg. 2019;12:neurintsurg-2019-015033.
19. Abilleira S, Perez de la Ossa N, Jimenez X, Cardona P, Cocho D, Purroy F, et al. Transfer to the local stroke center versus direct transfer to endovascular center of acute stroke patients with suspected large vessel occlusion in the catalan territory (racecat): study protocol of a cluster randomized within a cohort trial. Int J Stroke. 2019;14:734–44.
20. Krebs W, Sharkey-Toppen TP, Cheek F, Cortez E, Larrimore A, Keseg D, et al. Prehospital stroke assessment for large vessel occlusions: a systematic review. PrehospEmerg Care. 2018;22:180–8.

21. Kellner CP, Sauvageau E, Snyder KV, Fargen KM, Arthur AS, Turner RD, et al. The vital study and overall pooled analysis with the vips non-invasive stroke detection device. J Neurointerv Surg. 2018;10:1079–84.
22. Yaeger KA, Shoirah H, Kellner CP, Fifi J, Mocco J. Emerging technologies in optimizing pre-intervention workflow for acute stroke. Neurosurgery. 2019;85:S9–s17.
23. Helwig SA, Ragoschke-Schumm A, Schwindling L, Kettner M, Roumia S, Kulikovski J, et al. Prehospital stroke management optimized by use of clinical scoring vs mobile stroke unit for triage of patients with stroke: a randomized clinical trial. JAMA Neurol. 2019;76:1484.
24. Wei D, Oxley TJ, Nistal DA, Mascitelli JR, Wilson N, Stein L, et al. Mobile interventional stroke teams lead to faster treatment times for thrombectomy in large vessel occlusion. Stroke. 2017;48:3295–300.
25. Brekenfeld C, Goebell E, Schmidt H, Henningsen H, Kraemer C, Tebben J, et al. "Drip-and-drive": shipping the neurointerventionalist to provide mechanical thrombectomy in primary stroke centers. J Neurointerv Surg. 2018;10:932–6.
26. Osanai T, Ito Y, Ushikoshi S, Aoki T, Kawabori M, Fujiwara K, et al. Efficacy of 'drive and retrieve' as a cooperative method for prompt endovascular treatment for acute ischemic stroke. J Neurointerv Surg. 2019;11:757–61.
27. Uchiyama N, Misaki K, Mohri M, Kamide T, Hirota Y, Higashi R, et al. Treatment result in the initial stage of Kanazawa mobile embolectomy team for acute ischemic stroke. Neurol Med Chir (Tokyo). 2016;56:737–44.
28. Seker F, Fiehler J, Möhlenbruch MA, Heimann F, Flottmann F, Ringleb PA, et al. Time metrics to endovascular thrombectomy in 3 triage concepts. Stroke. 0:STROKEAHA.119.027050.
29. Seker F, Mohlenbruch MA, Nagel S, Ulfert C, Schonenberger S, Pfaff J, et al. Clinical results of a new concept of neurothrombectomy coverage at a remote hospital-"drive the doctor". Int J Stroke. 2018;13:696–9.
30. Hui FK, El Mekabaty A, Schultz J, Hong K, Horton K, Urrutia V, et al. Helistroke: Neurointerventionalist helicopter transport for interventional stroke treatment: proof of concept and rationale. J Neurointerv Surg. 2018;10:225–8.
31. Kraus F, Hubert G, Friedrich B, Maegerlein C, Hohenbichler K, Hubert N, et al. Abstract 30: safety and feasibility of the "flying intervention team" model for endovascular thrombectomy in rural areas: pilot phase. Stroke. 2019;50:A30.
32. Wei D, Oxley TJ, Nistal DA, Mascitelli JR, Wilson N, Stein L, et al. Mobile interventional stroke teams lead to faster treatment times for thrombectomy in large vessel occlusion. Stroke. 2017;48:3295.
33. Ebinger M, Winter B, Wendt M, Weber JE, Waldschmidt C, Rozanski M, et al. Effect of the use of ambulance-based thrombolysis on time to thrombolysis in acute ischemic stroke: a randomized clinical trial. JAMA. 2014;311:1622–31.
34. Bowry R, Parker S, Rajan SS, Yamal JM, Wu TC, Richardson L, et al. Benefits of stroke treatment using a mobile stroke unit compared with standard management: the best-msu study run-in phase. Stroke. 2015;46:3370–4.
35. Kummer BR, Lerario MP, Hunter MD, Wu X, Efraim ES, SalehiOmran S, et al. Geographic analysis of mobile stroke unit treatment in a dense urban area: the New York City metronome registry. J Am Heart Assoc. 2019;8:e013529.
36. Kettner M, Helwig SA, Ragoschke-Schumm A, Schwindling L, Roumia S, Keller I, et al. Prehospital computed tomography angiography in acute stroke management. Cerebrovasc Dis. 2017;44:338–43.
37. Fassbender K, Grotta JC, Walter S, Grunwald IQ, Ragoschke-Schumm A, Saver JL. Mobile stroke units for prehospital thrombolysis, triage, and beyond: benefits and challenges. Lancet Neurol. 2017;16:227–37.

Chapter 5
Surviving Large Vessel Occlusions in Uruguay: Current Challenges and Solutions

Roberto Crosa

Uruguay is a relatively small South American country (175,215 km^2). It lies between Argentina and Brazil, in one of the most flagrantly unequal regions of the world, from an economical and cultural point of view. Taking into account its geography, its demography, its culture, and its health system, it should be a model for successful stroke treatment in the region and the world at large, but in these last years, the country has been going in the wrong direction. Consider demography: the number of inhabitants is just over 3.4 million and the percentage of elderly population is one of the highest in this part of the world (more than half the population is over 50 years of age). In addition, nearly half the population of the country lives in the capital, Montevideo (metropolitan area: approximately 530 km^2) (Fig. 5.1). Currently, life expectancy for both sexes is 76.5 years [1]. From the geographical point of view, Uruguay is an extended plain with some hills, with no outstanding landforms. The climate is subtropical, with no dangerous weather events.

As to cultural level, the United Nations rates it as the second Latin American country regarding easy access to education with a literacy rate of 98.5%. Education in Uruguay is secular, free, and compulsory. University is free as well.

The health system reunites a public and a private sector, both ruled by the guidelines of the Ministry of Public Health. Our country defines the right to health as an essential human right and a public resource; the government and the State are held responsible for health and this responsibility cannot be delegated. According to this definition, the State and the government must ensure that the health needs of every inhabitant are completely covered, regardless of his personal ability to pay (law 18211). The system for the transportation of patients in critical condition is always provided with physicians, most of them emergency specialists. The rate of available ambulances is quite acceptable for this region. Uruguay also disposes of a broad experience regarding the management of hemorrhagic or ischemic stroke patients in

R. Crosa (✉)
Médica Uruguaya, CEN Neuro Endovascular Center, Montevideo, Uruguay

F. K. Hui et al. (eds.), *12 Strokes*, https://doi.org/10.1007/978-3-030-56857-3_5

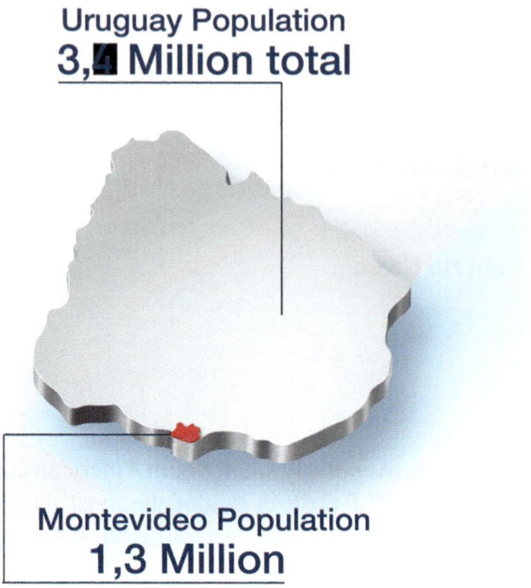

Fig. 5.1 Map of Uruguay with comparative populations for Montevideo (1.3 million) and the whole country (3.4 million)

intensive care and emergency care and can offer a center for mechanical thrombectomy that was a model for Latin America and a pioneer in this medical area.

For all these reasons, it would stand to reason that implementation of universal access to all forms of stroke treatment should be relatively straightforward in Uruguay. However, despite all those positive factors, the results of stroke treatment are paradoxically quite unsatisfactory. According to PAHO stroke mortality in Uruguay is one of the highest in Latin America [2]. The main cause of death in Uruguay for both sexes is stroke, with a rate of 74.6 per 100,000 inhabitants, which is far higher than the rates of other countries in the same region of the world. Stroke is one of the leading causes of severe disability, loss of healthy life years, and years of life lost on account of premature death.

The reason for these statistics is easily discovered: there are no campaigns of health promotion to educate the population about stroke and the recognition of its symptoms. That is why by and large the population of Uruguay cannot identify stroke symptoms. On the other hand, the health system operates separately, in a disjointed manner. For example, transportation systems, whether public or private, do not follow the same stroke protocol. Each facility decides priorities according to its protocol, without input from the Ministry of Public Health. There are practically no centers offering stroke patients all forms of prompt study and treatment for this epidemic. In Uruguay a stroke patient has more chances to be admitted into a hospital devoid of protocol for the prompt care of this disease (on account of lack of specialists, no access to emergency CT angiography, and no possibility of treatment with r-tPA or thrombectomy) than to be hospitalized in a center offering comprehensive stroke management.

These difficulties, which may seem to be beyond the understanding of people used to patient-centered thinking, have nevertheless spurred our imagination and resulted in some techniques that have solved difficult cases and have been accepted internationally, as outlined in the following illustrative cases:

Case Illustration 1

The year was 2016. In our hospital center we had developed a protocol for acute management of ischemic stroke according to the last evidence presented at the AHA [3]. We had successfully treated scores of patients with mechanical thrombectomy following those guidelines. We operated within a private system, with no State support whatever, and activated the protocol if the patient chanced to arrive in the therapeutic window. It was a matter of luck.

We were dining with colleagues from the 2nd International Stroke Course in Montevideo, Professor Alex Spiotta, MD (Charleston, USA), and W. Casagrande, MD (Buenos Aires, Argentina), sitting next to me, when the protocol was activated for a stroke patient 2 hours after onset, with a proximal occlusion of right M1 confirmed by CT angiogram (CTA). At this untimely moment, I explained the situation and left, although I was president of the congress. To their credit both colleagues decided to join me, in an effort to learn about stroke treatment in a country unfamiliar to them. The patient was an obese 57-year-old man with hypertension and dyslipidemia. He had right facial deviation, right gaze deviation, and left hemiparesis. His NIHSS amounted to 12 and he had an early ALBERTA score of 10. The patient had exclusion criteria for r-tPA, so he went directly to the angiographic suite we had inaugurated the previous year, where we had a last-generation angiography system, the first in Uruguay to be exclusively dedicated to neurologic procedures. With the patient under conscious sedation, we were able to reach the occlusion site at right M1, and we tried to perform mechanical thrombectomy with a stent retriever, using Solitaire (Covidien) FR 4 × 20. We could not aspirate because no aspiration system had been authorized for use in Uruguay at that time. After several passes (three tries with Solitaire FR) without noticeable effects, Dr. Spiotta decided to make a drawing of a possible way to dislodge this resilient clot which adhered so firmly to the M1 endothelium. Very quickly and racing against time, he proposed using Y-stenting [4]. I must say I was by no means convinced and feared we would only damage the artery further, but the patient was getting worse and we decided to act. I put a Solitaire stent in the upper branch of M2 toward M1 with a Catch SR stent inside it and then inserted it in the lower branch, covering the lesion. The whole system was removed and aspiration was performed by means of the guide catheter. I was surprised to see complete recanalization of M1 with a normal anterograde flow (Fig. 5.2). TICI score amounted to 3. Having performed this feat, born of a combination of the creative intelligence of colleagues I admire and the local lack of resources, we were surprised to see that many colleagues all round the world had began to use this technique in case of failure of better-known methods. It involves

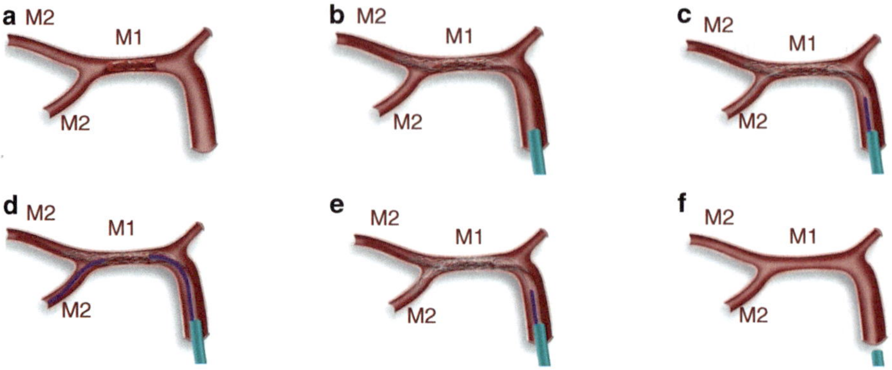

Fig. 5.2 (**a**)Thrombus occluding M1. (**b**) Solitaire FR stent (Medtronic) is deployed from upper branch of M2 toward M1. (**c**) A microguide catheter is inserted through the Solitaire FR stent toward the lower branch of M2. (**d**) A microcatheter containing a Catch stent (BALT) has been inserted from the lower branch of M2. (**e**) The Catch stent is deployed from M2 to M1, forming aY. (**f**) The Y-stent was retrieved, the whole clot was extracted, and the vessel recovered its permeability

the addition of extra technical challenges, but in spite of that in expert hands we have not seen complications.

Case Illustration 2

A 61-year-old female patient consulted at another center and was diagnosed with ischemic stroke. This center performs neither CTA nor mechanical thrombectomy and has no Stroke Unit. On admittance, the patient had an NIHSS of 8. CT was performed and hemorrhagic stroke was ruled out. Therefore r-tPA was started, 2 hours after onset of symptoms. When administration of r-tPA finished (3 hours after onset), the neurologist suggested “waiting for the drug to take effect.” The patient did not improve at all; in fact she worsened. Her relatives wanted to try another method and exerted pressure on the attending physicians, who consulted us. We suggested CTA at that center, but were denied that possibility, because although they have the technology their technicians do not work on call. At that stage, survival of the patient being our priority, we decided that it would be better to send her over to our comprehensive center, which is 700 meters away from their facility. Transport was delayed for 1 hour because “no ambulances were available.” When the patient arrived, 5.5 hours had elapsed since onset and NIHSS increased to 10. Internal carotid occlusion was confirmed. The clot was T-shaped and was located at the distal segment of the internal carotid, extending to proximal segments of A1 and M1. The patient had atrial fibrillation and had been treated with warfarin but her compliance had been poor. We tried to perform a thrombectomy, first with a Solitaire FR 6 × 20 stent and later with an FR 4 × 20 (Medtronic). The carotid segment and

A1 were recanalized, but not the M1 segment. We noticed that while the 4 × 20 stent was deployed, M1 was reperfused but on withdrawing the stent it became occluded again. Six hours and 20 minutes had elapsed since onset of symptoms. We decided to change to an AB Solitaire 4 × 20 detachable stent, we deployed it, and the vessel restored recanalization as before. We then decided to detach the stent and start anti-aggregation therapy on the patient. The outcome was hugely satisfactory in spite of everything that had happened. But this was not the only time we chose to leave the deployed stent in M1 and not the only one to have the very good results shown in Fig. 5.3.

Five years have gone by, anecdotes (good and bad) and experience have accumulated and the different governments have disregarded scientific evidence and also the factual evidence of the democratization of access to health that the

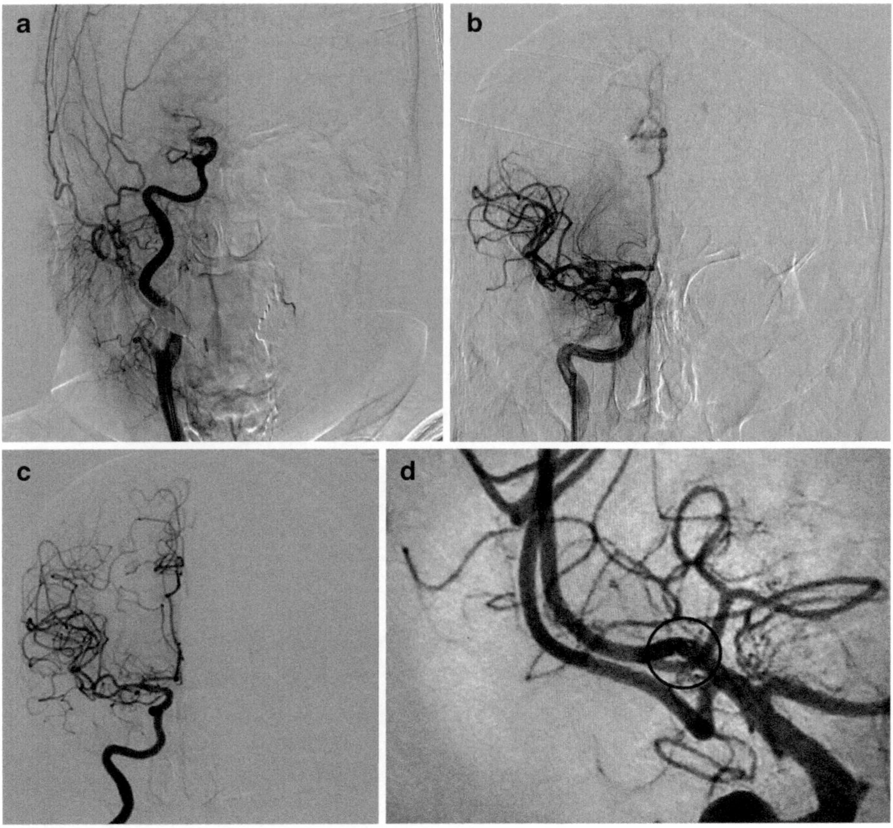

Fig. 5.3 61-year-old female patient. Hypertension, chronic atrial fibrillation, under treatment with warfarin and diltiazem, bad adherence to treatment. Door-to-puncture time 244 min, NIHSS 10. Diagnostic angiography at (**a**) shows tandem occlusion, while (**b**) demonstrates mTICI 3 reperfusion after mechanical thrombectomy and stent deployment in the M1 segment. Note previous stenosis at the initial segment of M1. One year later, follow-up conventional angiography in (**c**). Functional outcome was excellent. Distal mark of the stent is evident in (**d**)

implementation of such protocols mean. A foundation has emerged (APECV), supported by 34,000 people who promote and demand a general access to education on stroke, as well as viable and timely means of transportation and treatment of stroke patients. We have come to realize that these therapies cannot be made available to the whole population through individual efforts. It must be done through the development of intelligent systems as a State policy, in order to achieve national solutions for this serious situation.

At this moment Uruguay is undergoing a political change and we hope the medical situation will change as well. The mechanisms are not operating yet but there is an agreement to consider stroke as an epidemic requiring high priority. A specialized unit will be implemented in the Ministry of Public Health, whose goals will be to teach the population how to recognize stroke symptoms, to organize an orderly and coordinated system for transportation where the protocol will give first priority to stroke, and to create model centers offering ALL the possible forms of study and treatment in real time (Fig. 5.4). Should this initiative succeed, Uruguay will serve as the model and inspiration for the remainder of Latin America, as is evident in many other aspects.

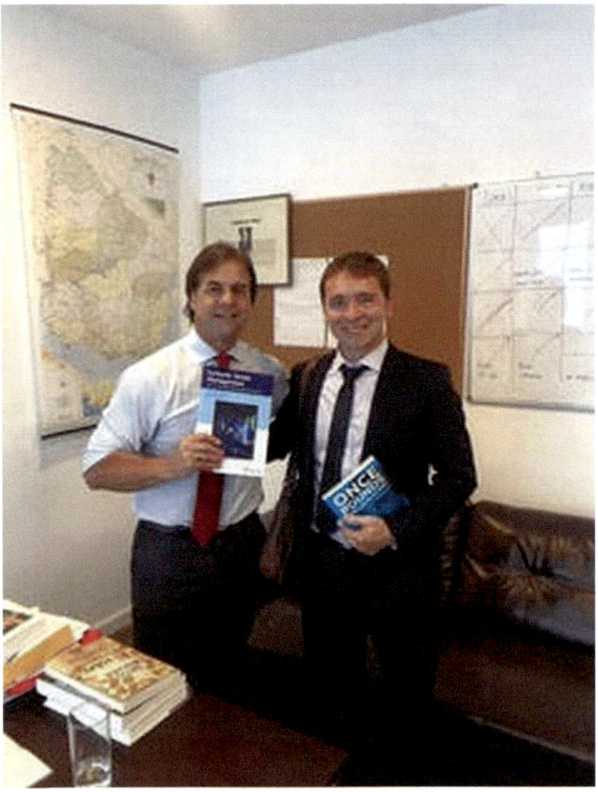

Fig. 5.4 Dr. Crosa, Director of the Endovascular Center (CEN) in Montevideo visits President-elect Dr. Luis Lacalle Pou in his office

References

1. Instituto Nacional de Estadística de Uruguay. Datos socio-demográficos. Disponible en: http://www.ine.gub.uy/socio-demograficos/proyecciones2008.asp.
2. Source:PAHO https://www.paho.org/uru/index.php?option=com_content&view=article&id=844:la-opsoms-insta-a-las-personas-en-las-americas-a-chequear-su-presion-arterial-para-prevenir-infartos-y-accidentes-cerebrovasculares&Itemid=451.
3. Powers J, Derdeyn CP. 2015 American Heart Association/American Stroke Association focused update of the 2013 guidelines for the early management of patients with acute ischemic stroke regarding endovascular treatment. Stroke. 2015;46:3020–35.
4. Crosa R, Spiotta A. "Y stent retriever": a new technique for refractory large-vessel occlusion? J Neurosurg. 2017; https://doi.org/10.3171/2016.12.JNS161233.

Chapter 6
Direct to Angiography—An Emerging Paradigm in Large Vessel Occlusion Stroke: Rationale, Feasibility, and Preliminary Results

Tudor G. Jovin

Introduction

Acute ischemic stroke (AIS) is a neurological emergency characterized by cessation of cerebral blood flow due to arterial occlusion, resulting in rapid loss of neurons in the territory supplied by the occluded vessel and consequent cerebral infarction. Large vessel occlusion (LVO) [1], defined as internal carotid artery (ICA), middle cerebral artery (MCA) M1 and M2 segments, and basilar artery (BA) occlusion, causes approximately one-third of ischemic stroke but accounts for more than 60% of morbidity and 90% of mortality due to AIS [2]. Thus, LVO stroke constitutes prognostically the most severe form of AIS with outcomes that to date have only been shown to be improved by timely reperfusion of the ischemic brain. This can be accomplished either with intravenous therapy (using lytic drugs such as tissue plasminogen activator [t-PA] or tenecteplase [TNK]) or with endovascular therapy (EVT), typically in the form of mechanical thrombectomy.

"Direct to Angiography" (DTA) is a recently coined term used to describe a time-efficient method of delivery of LVO stroke patients directly to the neuro-angiography suite without valuable time spent on additional evaluations including neuroimaging studies in the emergency department. This new approach may be employed both in transferred cases from a non-thrombectomy-capable stroke center (nTSC) to the thrombectomy-capable stroke center (TSC) and in directly presenting cases to the

T. G. Jovin (✉)
Cooper University Hospital, Professor of Neurology, Cooper Medical School of Rowan University, Pittsburgh, PA, USA
e-mail: jovin-tudor@cooperhealth.edu

F. K. Hui et al. (eds.), *12 Strokes*, https://doi.org/10.1007/978-3-030-56857-3_6

TSC. The primary rationale for DTA is to significantly reduce the time elapsed between hospital arrival and achievement of successful brain reperfusion. To better understand the rationale for this emerging approach, it is useful to review the importance of time, the role of imaging, the utility of the emergency room evaluation, and existing models of triage and transfer of LVO strokes.

Why Is Time Important?

Time and Outcomes

The time-dependent benefit demonstrated by the National Institute of Neurological Disorders and Stroke (NINDS) IV tissue plasminogen activator (t-PA) trial brought about a paradigm shift in the treatment of acute ischemic stroke [3]. Time became a fundamental patient selection criterion for reperfusion therapy as early reperfusion has long been considered a vital factor in achieving favorable outcomes as exemplified by the widespread use of the aphorism, "time is brain." In 2015, five landmark randomized controlled trials demonstrated the superiority of EVT over medical therapy alone (which included intravenous thrombolysis in eligible patients) for LVO stroke [4–8], leading to a dramatic change in the landscape of acute reperfusion therapy for AIS. An individual-level meta-analysis of these five trials (HERMES) in which the vast majority of patients were treated in the 0–6-hour time window confirmed that thrombectomy is a highly effective treatment, with a number-needed-to-treat (NNT) of less than 5 to obtain an independent level of functioning at 3 months post-stroke [9]. Further knowledge gained from this meta-analysis revealed that similar to the benefit conferred by intravenous t-PA for stroke, the benefit of thrombectomy in non-selected patients is exquisitely time-dependent. The magnitude of the treatment effect is strongly correlated to the time from stroke onset to reperfusion and treatment benefit can no longer be demonstrated with high degree of certainty after 7.3 hours after stroke onset [10]. There are abundant data confirming the impact of time on outcomes post-thrombectomy [10–13]. On average, in the setting of an LVO stroke, 2 million neurons are lost per minute, and the earlier blood flow is restored to the brain, the higher the likelihood of a good clinical outcome [14]. The HERMES collaborators reported that for every 100 patients treated, every 15 min of earlier reperfusion results in a 2.5% higher chance of achieving independence in activities of daily living [10]. Retrospective data suggest that every minute of delay to recanalization leads to the reduction of 4.2 days of disability-free survival [15].

Heterogeneity in Stroke Pathophysiology

Two years after the publication of the early time window trials, the DAWN and DEFUSE-3 trials led to a dramatic expansion of the therapeutic time window for thrombectomy, with benefit demonstrated up to 24 hours from stroke onset [16, 17]. These trials, however, were highly selective with regard to inclusion criteria and only enrolled patients with "mismatch" (i.e., small infarct volumes in the presence of large areas at risk) presenting >6 hours after the patient was last seen well (TLSW).

The seemingly difficult-to-reconcile discrepancy between the finding of a strong relationship between timing of reperfusion and outcomes in the early time window and the finding of strong benefit from thrombectomy in the late time window can be explained by patient selection with respect to speed of infarct progression. Whereas the early time window trials enrolled largely unselected patients, the late time window trials restricted enrollment to "slow progressors," a term derived from the recognition of two distinct phenotypes with respect to infarct growth rate following proximal large vessel occlusion, the "slow" and "fast progressors" [18]. At a cellular level, the corresponding rate of neuronal loss following vessel occlusion has been described to be highly variable, ranging from <35,000 to >27 million neurons per minute [19]. The variability in the rate of infarct growth in the setting of LVO is highly dependent on the individual degree of leptomeningeal collateral blood flow [20–22]. Not surprisingly, leptomeningeal collaterals have also been shown to be an independent predictor of good outcome in LVO stroke [23]. Factors influencing the presence and extent of collaterals and consequent susceptibility to ischemic damage include genetic factors; physiologic parameters such as blood pressure, body position, CO2, temperature, and glucose; and demographics [18]. Long-standing intracranial stenosis can lead to the development of more extensive collaterals but comorbidities promoting its development (e.g., hypertension, diabetes) are associated with impaired collateral blood flow during acute stroke [24, 25]. Cerebral edema has also been shown to impair blood flow through collateral vessels, and this may explain the decreased final infarct size seen in studies evaluating sulfonylurea use for the reduction of cerebral edema [26].

When patients with M1 MCA occlusion are defined as fast progressors if harboring an infarct in the MCA territory greater than 70 ml within 6 hours of TLSW and slow progressors if their infarct is less than 30 ml beyond 6 hours of TLSW, about 50% of LVO strokes can be described as "slow progressors" and 25% can be described as "fast progressors" [27]. This latter category of individuals with acute stroke due to LVO experiences rapid infarct growth and represents the most sensitive group with respect to delays in time to recanalization [28]. The identification of predictive biomarkers for the rate of stroke progression is an active area of research. One recent study which utilized sequential brain MRI studies in patients with LVO strokes showed that an initial infarct growth rate of <4.1 ml/hr and core volume of <19.9 ml detected on MRI at a median of 5 hours post-TLSW had high accuracy in predicting an infarct core of <50 ml at 24 hours post-stroke onset and thus having a higher likelihood of good outcome with thrombectomy [29].

Time and Neuroimaging

Current AHA/ASA guidelines recommend the use of neuroimaging to select patients for thrombectomy according to time window. In the 0–6-hour window, head CT and CT angiography alone are deemed sufficient, but in the 6–24-hour window, advanced imaging with CT perfusion or MRI is recommended to select patients with small infarct volume and large tissue at risk (mismatch) [30].

What Is the Role of the Emergency Department?

Evaluation and Emergency Care

Acute ischemic stroke patients, either presenting directly to the thrombectomy center or transferred from another hospital, are routinely admitted to the emergency department (ED). There, they undergo a focused evaluation to rule out immediately life-threatening conditions that may be associated with acute stroke such as acute cardiac or respiratory failure, severe hyper- or hypotension, etc. Another critical element of the initial stroke patient evaluation is the National Institutes of Health Stroke Scale (NIHSS) score which can determine the likelihood of stroke as presenting diagnosis and, by measuring the degree of stroke severity, also determine the likelihood of large vessel occlusion given that higher NIHSS scores reflect a higher likelihood of large vessel occlusion [31].

Neuroimaging for IV t-PA and Thrombectomy Eligibility

Acute clinical evaluation is typically followed by relevant neuroimaging, which is comprised at most centers of head CT, with or without CT angiography. Alternatively, MRI-based imaging (MRI and MR angiography) is used instead at some centers although its use even at the most efficient centers is associated with significant additional delays compared to CT. This, along with implanted devices or other metallic structures that constitute absolute contraindications to MRI use, represents the main disadvantage of MRI use in acute stroke. Originally, the main goal of acute imaging was to rule out intracerebral hemorrhage for the purpose of administering IV t-PA. However, since the advent of thrombectomy as standard of care in LVO stroke, imaging has been increasingly utilized to assess for thrombectomy eligibility by confirming the presence of an LVO, by ruling out a large infarction and by confirming the presence of reversible ischemic tissue. While the exclusion of intracerebral hemorrhage is the only prerequisite with respect to IV t-PA administration, all other neuroimaging studies are essentially performed for screening purposes with the ultimate goal of accurately identifying patients considered ineligible for thrombectomy for the purpose of excluding them from angiography. Furthermore, stroke patients transferred to thrombectomy-capable stroke center (TSC) from a non-thrombectomy-capable stroke center (nTSC) routinely undergo repeat evaluation and neuroimaging upon arrival in the TSC emergency department prior to activation of the thrombectomy team. Oftentimes, repeat imaging occurs despite already having established thrombectomy eligibility at the referring hospital with the justification that the imaging study obtained at the referring hospital no longer accurately reflects tissue viability status [32].

What Are the Pitfalls of the Current Approach?

Multi-step Approach and Time Delay

Current intrahospital stroke systems at most hospitals continue to reflect a workflow that is designed around IV t-PA administration. Emergency department evaluation and treatment by ED physicians and nurses, along with head CT performed in the ED CT scanner and (if available) emergent evaluation by a neurologist, represent the typical steps preceding IV t-PA administration, followed at some centers by additional imaging and admission to a specialized care unit. Despite the widespread adoption of thrombectomy, stroke systems of care have lagged behind in the evolution of workflow paradigms best suited to the particular aspects of endovascular therapy and continue to use approaches that lend themselves to delays in thrombectomy initiation including a serial rather than parallel workflow typically pursued at most centers. First, the patient is evaluated in the ED, head CT is obtained, IV t-PA is administered if appropriate, and, in many instances, only subsequently the patient undergoes further imaging (CTA,CTP,MRI, MRA) to assess for thrombectomy eligibility which is primarily determined by the presence of LVO and by exclusion of a large infarct. If the patient is then deemed eligible, transfer to the angio-suite for thrombectomy ensues. This serial, multi-step approach often results in significant time delays [33].

Large Ischemic Core Volume in the Early Time Window

A long-held belief among stroke experts has been that reperfusion of large volumes of infarcted brain tissue is detrimental to patient's outcomes due to the development of symptomatic intracerebral hemorrhage, malignant edema, or other reperfusion-related deleterious effects. Important unresolved questions related to this concept include the definition of large infarct and the accuracy of available imaging-based tools for infarct measurement. While definitive evidence against a net detrimental effect of reperfusion is still lacking, the results of recent studies have shed considerable doubt on its validity as to date no category of patients defined by imaging or otherwise has been found to be harmed by thrombectomy.

Most commonly used imaging-based methods to estimate the ischemic core in LVO stroke patients are non-contrast CT, CT perfusion, and MRI. The score of 7 on the Alberta Stroke Program Early CT Score (ASPECTS) [34] as baseline infarct volume threshold associated with benefit from reperfusion was initially described in the first-generation endovascular trials [35, 36]. However, advances in technology and workflow have shifted this cut-off to lower values. Indeed, in the initial HERMES collaborator's publication, a statistically significant benefit from mechanical thrombectomy could be demonstrated using an ASPECTS cut-off of 6 and above. Subsequent to this publication, in the prospective study ETIS [37], Panni et al. reported a rate of good outcome, defined as a modified Rankin Scale (mRS) score of 0–2 at 3 months, of 32% in the subgroup of patients with ASPECTS of 4–5. Similarly, analysis of patients with ASPECTS 0–5, who underwent thrombectomy in the BEYOND-SWIFT registry, showed that 40% had favorable outcome (mRS 0–3) at 90 days [38]. These outcome rates are superior to what would be expected in non-treated LVO stroke patients with similar baseline ASPECTS scores.

CT perfusion is considered superior to non-contrast CT in its ability to estimate the core although some studies have shown that with respect to its ability to estimate a large infarct (> 70 ml), a non-contrast CT cut-off of <7 is equivalent to CT perfusion when compared to the gold standard of DWI MRI [39]. Furthermore, in the era of modern thrombectomy, with fast and complete reperfusion achieved in an increasingly higher proportion of patients, CT perfusion-derived thresholds defining infarct are being redefined and seem to be a "moving target." Indeed, as early as 2015, d'Esterre et al. showed that the cerebral blood flow (CBF) thresholds defining infarct were dependent on both the timing of reperfusion relative to the CT perfusion study and on the timing of reperfusion relative to the stroke symptom onset [40]. These findings were confirmed by Qiu et al. based on patients from the HERMES database [41]. Earlier reperfusion necessitates lower CBF thresholds in order to estimate infarct volume with same accuracy as those used in patients who achieve reperfusion later. However, even with these adjustments, thresholds used for infarct measurement on CTP are far from being 100% reliable.

Improvements in stroke systems of care, coupled with advances in thrombectomy technology, make it likely that high-quality reperfusion will be achieved earlier and earlier in the future. As such, it is not clear that the thresholds defining infarct on CT perfusion are ever going to have sufficient accuracy. Indeed, the final infarct volumes in patients who undergo successful reperfusion are not uncommonly shown to be smaller than predicted by CT perfusion imaging on the pre-thrombectomy CTP.

DWI MRI is widely considered as the most precise method for core estimation in clinical practice but it is associated with significant delays. Furthermore, even though superior to all other imaging modalities in clinical use, MRI is also prone to inaccurate characterization of the infarcted brain especially in the context of reperfusion. The earlier the pre-reperfusion MRI scan is performed relative to ischemia onset and the faster reperfusion occurs following completion of the MRI scan, the higher the likelihood that the DWI lesion noted on the initial MRI scan will no longer be demonstrated on a follow-up MRI scan. This phenomenon, termed DWI reversibility, has been noted to occur in up to a quarter of patients with acute stroke [42].

Data from HERMES collaboration indicate strong signals of benefit in favor of thrombectomy in patients with large (>70 ml) and even very large (>100 ml) baseline infarct volumes [43]. Thus, both the limitations of CTP or MRI in accurately measuring the core and the lack of convincing evidence of lack of benefit (or harm) with thrombectomy in patients with large core measured by these imaging modalities call into question the utility of advanced imaging (CTP or MRI) in determining thrombectomy eligibility in the early time window.

Perhaps the most compelling data showing the benefit of EVT, even in patients with large baseline infarcts, come from the expanded dataset making up the HERMES collaboration which included seven randomized endovascular stroke trials showing superiority of EVT plus best medical therapy (that included IV lysis in eligible patients) over best medical therapy alone [4–8, 44, 45]. Although most of the participating trial's protocols largely excluded patients with large baseline infarctions, some of these patients were inadvertently enrolled due to lack of recognition of large infarcts on initial imaging by local investigators. In a meta-analysis of these trials, of the 1764 patients enrolled, 126 underwent thrombectomy with core lab-adjudicated baseline ASPECTS <5 on CT (61 patients) or MRI (65 patients) [46]. Both in the MRI and CT groups there was a trend in favor of benefit with EVT, while in the combined analysis of CT- or MRI–imaged patients the benefit from EVT reached statistical significance (OR 2.15, 95% CI 1.06–4.37). Additionally, in 228 patients with evidence of hypodensity involving greater than one-third of the MCA territory, another measure of large baseline infarct, benefit from EVT was also demonstrated (OR 1.70, 95%CI 1.04–2.78) [46]. Using the same expanded HERMES dataset, similar results were seen on a CT perfusion-based analysis of patients with large core infarcts (>70 ml and even >100 ml) with no significant reduction in absolute treatment effect with EVT and no net signals of harm despite a higher incidence of sICH in the thrombectomy group compared to controls [43]. Findings from these studies suggest that patients with LVO who have large baseline infarcts are likely to benefit from EVT compared to medical treatment alone and that although a large baseline infarct represents a prognostic factor, it does not represent a treatment effect modifier.

Efforts to identify patients with large baseline infarcts for the purpose of exclusion from thrombectomy may lack justification not only due to the observed strong trends of benefit but also because in patients presenting in the early time window, the prevalence of large infarctions without significant salvageable tissue is exceedingly low, as demonstrated by the 95% of patients who had mismatch by SWIFT PRIME criteria and by the 78% of patients who had large penumbral volumes (>60 ml) in the HERMES collaboration-derived CT perfusion-based study [43]. In fact, the prevalence of large infarcts (ASPECTS 0–5) has been estimated to be no more than about 15% of patients with M1 MCA occlusion presenting within 6 hours after last seen well [38] while within the first 3 hours after symptom onset the prevalence of ASPECTS 0–5 in patients with MCA occlusion is 4% [47]. As such, not only there is no evidence to suggest a lack of benefit of EVT for LVO strokes with large baseline core infarcts, but also the prevalence of large infarcts in the early time window is low.

The Tradeoff Between Advanced Imaging and Delays in Time to Reperfusion

Advanced imaging requires not an insignificant time for completion. In SWIFT PRIME, the median time from start of CT to post-processing of CT perfusion imaging was 24 min while MRI-based selection was associated with a delay from door to groin puncture of a median of 16 min compared to CT-based selection [48]. Considering that based on data derived from HERMES every 15 min of delay in reperfusion results in a 3.9% lower chance of reduction in disability, if the delay in reperfusion caused by CTP in SWIFT PRIME was a conservative 15 min, this delay translates into 3.9% higher chance of disability in those patients who achieved reperfusion in the interventional arm of the trial. The delays incurred by advanced imaging can be inferred from the fact that in DAWN and DEFUSE-3, studies with protocol requirements of advanced imaging (CT perfusion or MRI), median ED arrival-to-groin puncture times were 109 and 112 min, respectively, compared to 89 min in the ESCAPE trial, 60 min in the ESCAPE NA-1 trial, and 60 min in the ARISE II study [5, 16, 17, 49, 50], none of which required advanced imaging. The limited usefulness of advanced imaging in the early time window is reflected in the AHA guidelines which endorse thrombectomy as level I evidence only for patients harboring an LVO and a limited core volume defined as an ASPECT score >5 [30] . However, based on data published after the publication of the AHA guidelines, in the early time window (0–6 hours), following exclusion of intracerebral hemorrhage (typically accomplished with a non-contrast head CT), it is justified to question the necessity for patient selection for thrombectomy based on any baseline infarct size.

Is Vessel Imaging Always Necessary?

Currently, the vast majority of stroke centers still perform a CT angiogram in a conventional CT scanner to confirm the presence of large vessel occlusion prior to the decision to proceed with transport to the angiography suite. Studies examining workflow efficiency in intrahospital systems of care have shown that when only a plain CT (showing arterial thrombus) is utilized in lieu of the standard CTA for the purposes of large vessel occlusion diagnosis, the time required for imaging decreases by an average of 28 min and the time elapsed from hospital presentation to access site puncture times decreased by 36 min [51]. Thus, in situations when there is an a priori high likelihood of large vessel occlusion, forgoing of the CTA and transport directly to the angiography suite after the initial head CT may save substantial time to brain reperfusion. Although a combination of findings on a plain CT combined with clinical information is likely to result in highest yield for prediction of LVO, an NIHSS cut-off of 10 or above has been shown to predict the presence of LVO with 80% accuracy in the early time window [52].

In the cardiology literature, the well-known entity of myocardial infarction with non-obstructive coronary arteries (MINOCA) is characterized by patent coronary arteries during emergent cardiac catheterization despite clinical, electrocardiographic, and biomarker features consistent with myocardial infarction. The finding of MINOCA is encountered with a frequency of 5–25% and typically results in no coronary intervention at the time of the emergent cardiac catheterization procedure [53]. However, despite this non-insignificant frequency of instances where an emergent cardiac catheterization in a patient with acute myocardial infarction results in no intervention, it is the standard of care in virtually all cardiac catheterization laboratories across the world to assess coronary patency via emergent coronary angiography without prior non-invasive studies (coronary CTA or MRI). The widely accepted fact among cardiologists that substantial savings in time to reperfusion for the entire population of reperfusion candidates are likely to offset any negative repercussions of invasive angiography in the minority of patients of reperfusion candidates who have patent arteries in the setting of myocardial infarction should equally apply in the setting of acute stroke. Therefore, it is reasonable to question the need for non-invasive vessel imaging prior to transfer to the neuro-angiography suite when the pre-test probability of large vessel occlusion is high and thus the likelihood of no intervention is low. The threshold for what constitutes an acceptable likelihood of patent vessel on angiography is likely to vary depending on resources available at each individual stroke center. However, based on cardiology data, a 15–20% such likelihood may represent a reasonable trade-off between the increase in necessary cath lab resources and the clinical benefit derived from timelier reperfusion associated with this approach. Furthermore, recent advances in flat panel angiography technology have made possible identification of both intracranial hemorrhage and presence of large vessel occlusion on the angiography table which represents a non-invasive way of answering the questions relevant for triage of LVO patients in the most time-efficient manner [54]. Flat panel CT and CTA, obtained by low-dose contrast injection to create CTA-like images, demonstrated high accuracy in their respective ability to rule out hemorrhage and detect LVO in the neuro-angiography suite [55, 56].

Cost Considerations

In the era of increased cost awareness related to healthcare utilization, economic considerations should also be taken into account when assessing the overall value of a DTA approach. At a first glance, the DTA approach requires a higher level of resources compared to the conventional approach. However, there is a decrease in cost associated with bypassing the CTA and other advanced imaging for all patients and a decrease in healthcare cost associated with earlier brain reperfusion. Because earlier reperfusion leads to lower infarct volumes and infarct volume is the main driver of hospitalization costs in LVO stroke patients [57], earlier reperfusion leads to lower hospitalization costs. In addition the economical benefit of reperfusion therapy has been shown to translate beyond the acute hospitalization [58]. Therefore, the cost reduction associated with a DTA approach which will lead to intervention and earlier reperfusion in a majority of patients without additional CTA or CTP must be weighed against the increase in cost associated with the performance of cerebral angiography with findings of no occlusion in a minority of patients.

Thus, if assumed conservatively that in the 0–6-hour time window an NIHSS cut-off of 10 and above predicts the presence of treatable large vessel occlusion 80% of the time; that patients with largest baseline infarcts, which constitute a minority, are not harmed by thrombectomy; and that forgoing of any type of CT or MRI imaging prior to transfer to the angiography suite (because intracerebral hemorrhage has been already performed at the transferring hospital or will be performed with flat panel detector in the angiography suite), then per hundred evaluated patients, a direct to angio approach saves on average 45 min to reperfusion for 80 patients and saves 100 CTAs or CTPs at the expense of 20 negative angiograms (conventional or flat panel CTA).

How to Address Time Delays in the Emergency Department?

Existing Transfer Paradigms

Most transfer paradigms currently in use include transfer of patients from site of stroke onset (home or field) to the emergency room at the non-thrombectomy center or at the thrombectomy center (either directly or via the non-thrombectomy center or via the mobile stroke unit, an increasingly utilized transfer modality). These are portrayed in Fig. 6.1 in black arrows and are indirect ways of patient transfer to the angio-suite.

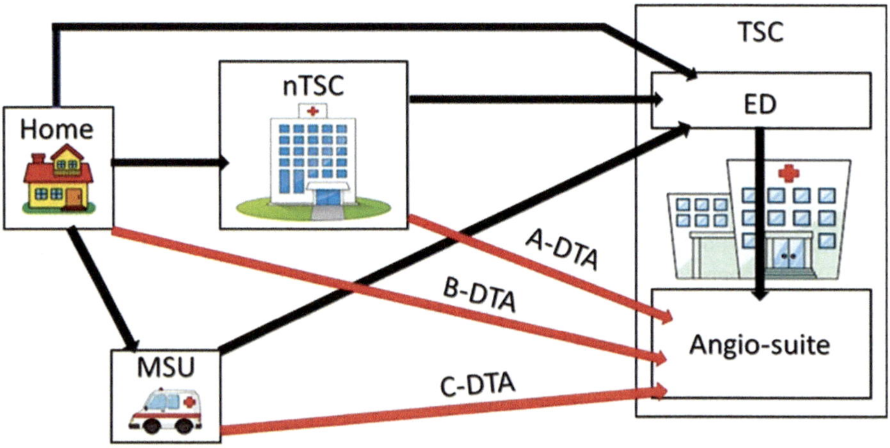

Fig. 6.1 Triage and transfer paradigms. nTSC non-thrombectomy-capable stroke center, TSC thrombectomy-capable stroke center, ED emergency department, MSU mobile stroke unit, DTA Direct to Angiography

Bypassing the Emergency Department: Direct to Angiography

Given that emergency department admission leads to time delays, a novel way of transferring patients directly to the angio-suite involves bypassing the emergency department. Broadly, three types of Direct to Angiography pathway may occur—Route ADTA, ED at non-thrombectomy-capable center to angio-suite at TSC; Route BDTA, home or field direct to angio-suite at TSC; or Route CDTA, home or field to mobile stroke unit (MSU) to thrombectomy center angio-suite at TSC (red arrows in Fig. 6.1).

Initial Experience with Direct to Angiography (Table 6.1)

Several single-center series have reported their experiences with Direct to Angiography. All studies have reported significant reductions in door-to-groin puncture time using the Direct to Angiography approach [32, 59–63]. Jadhav et al. reported a time saving of 1 hour using the Direct to Angiography approach [32]. Across studies, median door-to-groin puncture times in the DTA paradigm were between 16 and 33 min and clinical benefit compared to historical controls was observed in three of these studies [60, 61, 63] (Table 6.1). Other studies did not

Table 6.1 Published experience regarding the DTA approach

Author group	Publication date	Method of screening	Sample size of DTA patients (vs. non-DTA)	False-positive angio-suite activations	Door-to-puncture time	Outcome
Jadhav et al.	May 2017	Transferred patients with confirmed LVO and/or NIHSS ≥9	111 (vs. 150)	6.3% - Vessel open	22 min vs. 81 min ($p = 0.001$)	90-day mRS 0–2 44% vs. 43% (but more patients with large infarcts treated in DTA group)
Psychogios et al.	October 2017	Direct and transferred patients NIHSS ≥10	30 (vs. 44)	13.5% -hemorrhage 13.5% -Todd's paralysis	20.5 min vs. 54.5 min ($p < 0.01$)	Not available
Ribo et al.	March 2018	Direct and transferred patients NIHSS ≥10	40 (vs. 161)	7.5% - hemorrhage 17.5% - open vessels	17 min vs. 60 min ($p < 0.01$)	Early improvement 49% vs. 24% ($p < 0.01$)

(continued)

Table 6.1 (continued)

Author group	Publication date	Method of screening	Sample size of DTA patients (vs. non-DTA)	False-positive angio-suite activations	Door-to-puncture time	Outcome
Mendez et al.	September 2018	Direct admissions RACE ≥4 and NIHSS >10	79 (vs. 145)	7.2% - open vessels	16 min vs. 70 min ($p < 0.01$)	90-day mRS 0–2 41% vs. 28% ($p = 0.05$)
Brehm et al.	July 2019	Transferred patients with confirmed LVO and NIHSS >7	15 (vs. 23)	None	24 min vs. 53 min ($p < 0.01$)	Mortality 27% vs. 17% (0.14)
Bouslama et al.	June 2019	Direct and transferred patients with (flat panel angio-suite vs. ED)	61 (vs. 156)	None	33 min vs. 55 min ($p < 0.01$)	90-day mRS 0–2 45% vs. 41% ($p = 0.68$)
Requena et al.	May 2020	Direct and transferred patients AIS patients within 6 hours of onset with RACE score ≥4 and/or NIHSS >10	174 (vs. 175)	Not applicable (case controlled study of patients undergoing EVT)	16 min vs. 70 min ($p < 0.01$)	90-day mRS 0–2 43% vs. 29% ($p = 0.01$)

DTA indicates Direct to Angiography, *LVO* large vessel occlusion, *NIHSS* National Institutes of Health Stroke Scale, *mRS* modified Rankin Scale, *RACE* Rapid Arterial oCclusion Evaluation, *AIS* acute ischemic stroke, *ASPECTS* Alberta Stroke Program Early CT Score, *ED* emergency department

report significant improvement in outcomes via the DTA approach compared to historical controls highlighting the importance of trials utilizing active controls in this area. Nonetheless, these data uniformly point toward substantial gains in door to access site puncture while demonstrating that the DTA approach is feasible and safe. Furthermore, recent data suggest that patients who stand most to benefit from a DTA approach are those who present to the thrombectomy center in the earliest time window (0–3 hours) [63].

Practical Considerations of Bypassing the Emergency Department

Evaluation and Emergency Care

Evaluation and treatment of stroke-related acute medical complications begin in the ambulance, the MSC, or the ED of the nTSC. To decrease time delays, ED care can be bypassed and initial in-hospital care can be provided in the neuro-angiography suite at the thrombectomy center. For judicious use of resources, only patients with high likelihood of LVO and those deemed to be most sensitive to time delays (NIHSS >9 presenting within 6 hours of TLSW) will be evaluated under the DTA model. Ideally, the mandatory (according to US law—EMTALA) [64] ED evaluation for patients presenting directly to a thrombectomy-capable center should occur very rapidly either by the patient passing through (without stopping) in the ED or by the patient being evaluated by ED staff in the angiography suite in those cases where the angiography suite is in close proximity to the ED.

IV t-PA

A majority of LVO stroke patients present beyond the 4.5-hour time window for t-PA administration. Of the LVO strokes presenting within this window, a large percentage are transferred from an NTSC [65] and can receive IV t-PA there while transfer is being coordinated. The same holds true for patients being transferred from home or the field using a mobile stroke unit. Hence, Direct to Angiography from an NTSC or MSU (Fig. 6.1, Route ADTA and CDTA) is feasible for most patients who are treated with IV t-PA.

In cases of t-PA-eligible thrombectomy candidates who present directly to a TSC (the minority of patients in the USA [65], bypassing the emergency department is dependent on the feasibility of obtaining acute brain imaging to rule out intracranial hemorrhage without stopping in the ED. Neuro-angiography suites that are equipped with multi-detector flat panel CT imaging can serve as a single location where imaging, t-PA administration, and endovascular therapy for LVO can all be performed without intrahospital time delays [59]. This would enable Route BDTA on Fig. 6.1 (home or field to angio-suite). It has been shown that administration of IV t-PA based on flat panel CT technology has a similar safety profile to IV t-PA treatment when hemorrhage is excluded with conventional CT scanners [62]. Furthermore, the need for IV thrombolytic administration in IV thrombolysis-eligible thrombectomy candidates presenting directly to a TSC has been called into question, and recent randomized trials showed no difference in outcomes when IV t-PA is administered prior to thrombectomy compared to thrombectomy without prior IV t-PA [66, 67]. If this finding is confirmed by other ongoing randomized trials, in the future IV thrombolysis may no longer be indicated for thrombectomy candidates presenting directly to TSC, and thus, the issue of ruling out intracerebral hemorrhage for the purpose of IV thrombolysis administration may become moot.

Conclusions

Acute stroke due to large vessel occlusion is a prognostically ominous stroke subset with clinical outcomes that to date have only been shown to be improved by reperfusion therapy in the form of IV thrombolysis, endovascular thrombectomy, or a combination of both. Multiple randomized trials have shown that thrombectomy with or without IV thrombolysis is associated with the strongest clinical response in LVO stroke and that the benefit of this approach is exquisitely time dependent especially in the early time window (0–6 hours). Therefore, system-based approaches aiming at reducing times from stroke onset to reperfusion have been a priority in the quest to improve acute stroke care. The Direct to Angiography (DTA) suite represents a new paradigm which aims to dramatically reduce reperfusion times through bypass of conventional pathways for early-presenting LVO stroke patients and consists of clinical and imaging evaluation on the angiography table using either no additional imaging (in the case of transferred patients) or flat panel technology (in case of patients presenting directly to a thrombectomy-capable center) (Table 6.2). This model relies on emerging data suggesting that knowledge of baseline infarct volume may no longer be necessary for patient selection in the early time window and that the presence of LVO can be estimated with high likelihood either based on the NIHSS or even more accurately with a flat panel CTA performed after patient arrival in the angiography suite. DTA has been shown to be feasible and safe and is associated with significant decreases in time to treatment initiation. There are logistical challenges in adopting this model, but preliminary experience has shown that most if not all of them can be overcome. Because of these challenges, widespread implementation of this concept akin to the cardiology model for STEMI is unlikely to occur without level I evidence. Therefore, planned randomized trials will need to clarify whether the substantial time savings associated with this approach will ultimately translate into clinical benefits.

Table 6.2 Conventional neuroimaging and alternatives under DTA approach

Role	Prevalence of specific condition	Conventional imaging modalities	Alternatives under DTA approach: Transfers (nTSC/MSU) (Route ADTA/CDTA on Fig. 6.1)	Alternatives under DTA approach: Direct (home/field) (Route BDTA on Fig. 6.1)
Rule out intracranial hemorrhage	~13% of all strokes have intracranial haemorrhage [68]	Head CT (preferred) MRI (more time consuming)	Can be done in non-thrombectomy centers/MSU	Can be done with multi-detector flat panel angio-suite
Rule out absence of LVO	~20% of all strokes [69] and ~80% of strokes with NIHSS score >9 have LVO [31, 70]	CTA (preferred) MRA	Can be done in nTSC/MSU	Flat panel CTA DSA LVO screening tools to enrich population with LVO (RACE scale >5 NIHSS >9) [31, 70, 71] Alternative tools include EEG [72], transcranial Doppler [73], infrared spectroscopy [74], and accelerometers [75] to reduce rate of patent vessels on angio
Rule out large infarct	Prevalence is low in 0–6-hour time window (10–15%)	Head CT CTP/MRI	Can be done in nTSC/MSU by ASPECTS Due to core growth during transfer and significant delays CTP/MRI not recommended at nTSC/MSU	Flat panel ASPECTS Unclear if exclusion from thrombectomy is even necessary based on recent data randomized trials in progress
Rule out absence of mismatch	~95% of LVO strokes have mismatch in the 0–6-hour window [43]	CTP/MRI	Due to core growth during transfer and significant delays, not recommended at nTSC/MSU	Flat panel CTP for patients beyond 6 hours No longer considered necessary in the 0–6-hour time window No evidence for lack of benefit in patients without mismatch

ED indicates emergency department, *nTSC* non-thrombectomy-capable stroke center, *MSU* mobile stroke unit, *CT* computed tomography, *LVO* large vessel occlusion, *CTA* computed tomography angiography, *MRA* magnetic resonance angiography, *DSA* digital subtraction angiography, *CTP* computed tomography perfusion, *MRI* magnetic resonance imaging, *ASPECTS* Alberta Stroke Program Early CT Score

References

1. González RG, Furie KL, Goldmacher GV, Smith WS, Kamalian S, Payabvash S, et al. Good outcome rate of 35% in IV-tPA-treated patients with computed tomography angiography confirmed severe anterior circulation occlusive stroke. Stroke. 2013;44(11):3109–13.
2. Malhotra K, Gornbein J, Saver JL. Ischemic strokes due to large-vessel occlusions contribute disproportionately to stroke-related dependence and death: a review. Front Neurol. 2017;8:651.
3. National Institute of Neurological Disorders and Stroke rt-PA Stroke Study Group. Tissue plasminogen activator for acute ischemic stroke. N Engl J Med. 1995 14;333(24):1581–7.
4. Jovin TG, Chamorro A, Cobo E, de Miquel MA, Molina CA, Rovira A, et al. Thrombectomy within 8 hours after symptom onset in ischemic stroke. N Engl J Med. 2015;372(24):2296–306.
5. Goyal M, Demchuk AM, Menon BK, Eesa M, Rempel JL, Thornton J, et al. Randomized assessment of rapid endovascular treatment of ischemic stroke. N Engl J Med. 2015;372(11):1019–30.
6. Berkhemer OA, Fransen PSS, Beumer D, van den Berg LA, Lingsma HF, Yoo AJ, et al. A randomized trial of intraarterial treatment for acute ischemic stroke. N Engl J Med. 2015;372(1):11–20.
7. Campbell BCV, Mitchell PJ, Kleinig TJ, Dewey HM, Churilov L, Yassi N, et al. Endovascular therapy for ischemic stroke with perfusion-imaging selection. N Engl J Med. 2015;372(11):1009–18.
8. Saver JL, Goyal M, Bonafe A, Diener H-C, Levy EI, Pereira VM, et al. Stent-retriever thrombectomy after intravenous t-PA vs. t-PA alone in stroke. N Engl J Med. 2015;372(24):2285–95.
9. Goyal M, Menon BK, van Zwam WH, Dippel DWJ, Mitchell PJ, Demchuk AM, et al. Endovascular thrombectomy after large-vessel ischaemic stroke: a meta-analysis of individual patient data from five randomised trials. Lancet. 2016;387(10029):1723–31.
10. Saver JL, Goyal M, van der Lugt A, Menon BK, Majoie CBLM, Dippel DW, et al. Time to treatment with endovascular thrombectomy and outcomes from ischemic stroke: a meta-analysis. JAMA. 2016;316(12):1279–88.
11. He AH, Churilov L, Mitchell PJ, Dowling RJ, Yan B. Every 15-min delay in recanalization by intra-arterial therapy in acute ischemic stroke increases risk of poor outcome. Int J Stroke. 2015;10(7):1062–7.
12. Alawieh A, Vargas J, Fargen KM, Langley EF, Starke RM, De Leacy R, et al. Impact of procedure time on outcomes of thrombectomy for stroke. J Am Coll Cardiol. 2019;73(8):879–90.
13. Jahan R, Saver JL, Schwamm LH, Fonarow GC, Liang L, Matsouaka RA, et al. Association between time to treatment with endovascular reperfusion therapy and outcomes in patients with acute ischemic stroke treated in clinical practice. JAMA. 2019;322(3):252–63.
14. Saver JL. Time is brain--quantified. Stroke. 2006;37(1):263–6.
15. Meretoja A, Keshtkaran M, Tatlisumak T, Donnan GA, Churilov L. Endovascular therapy for ischemic stroke: save a minute-save a week. Neurology. 2017;88(22):2123–7.
16. Nogueira RG, Jadhav AP, Haussen DC, Bonafe A, Budzik RF, Bhuva P, et al. Thrombectomy 6 to 24 hours after stroke with a mismatch between deficit and infarct. N Engl J Med. 2018;378(1):11–21.
17. Albers GW, Marks MP, Kemp S, Christensen S, Tsai JP, Ortega-Gutierrez S, et al. Thrombectomy for stroke at 6 to 16 hours with selection by perfusion imaging. N Engl J Med. 2018;378(8):708–18.
18. Rocha M, Jovin TG. Fast versus slow progressors of infarct growth in large vessel occlusion stroke: clinical and research implications. Stroke. 2017;48(9):2621–7.
19. Desai SM, Rocha M, Jovin TG, Jadhav AP. High variability in neuronal loss. Stroke. 2019;50(1):34–7.
20. Jung S, Gilgen M, Slotboom J, El-Koussy M, Zubler C, Kiefer C, et al. Factors that determine penumbral tissue loss in acute ischaemic stroke. Brain. 2013;136(Pt 12):3554–60.
21. Zhang H, Prabhakar P, Sealock R, Faber JE. Wide genetic variation in the native pial collateral circulation is a major determinant of variation in severity of stroke. J Cereb Blood Flow Metab. 2010;30(5):923–34.

22. Campbell BCV, Christensen S, Tress BM, Churilov L, Desmond PM, Parsons MW, et al. Failure of collateral blood flow is associated with infarct growth in ischemic stroke. J Cereb Blood Flow Metab. 2013;33(8):1168–72.
23. Lima FO, Furie KL, Silva GS, Lev MH, Camargo ECS, Singhal AB, et al. The pattern of leptomeningeal collaterals on CT angiography is a strong predictor of long-term functional outcome in stroke patients with large vessel intracranial occlusion. Stroke. 2010;41(10):2316–22.
24. Chan S-L, Sweet JG, Bishop N, Cipolla MJ. Pial collateral reactivity during hypertension and aging: understanding the function of collaterals for stroke therapy. Stroke. 2016;47(6):1618–25.
25. Letourneur A, Roussel S, Toutain J, Bernaudin M, Touzani O. Impact of genetic and renovascular chronic arterial hypertension on the acute spatiotemporal evolution of the ischemic penumbra: a sequential study with MRI in the rat. J Cereb Blood Flow Metab. 2011;31(2):504–13.
26. Simard JM, Yurovsky V, Tsymbalyuk N, Melnichenko L, Ivanova S, Gerzanich V. Protective effect of delayed treatment with low-dose glibenclamide in three models of ischemic stroke. Stroke. 2009;40(2):604–9.
27. Rocha M, Desai SM, Jadhav AP, Jovin TG. Prevalence and temporal distribution of fast and slow progressors of infarct growth in large vessel occlusion stroke. Stroke. 2019;50(8):2238–40.
28. Ribo M, Molina CA, Cobo E, Cerdà N, Tomasello A, Quesada H, et al. Association between time to reperfusion and outcome is primarily driven by the time from imaging to reperfusion. Stroke. 2016;47(4):999–1004.
29. González RG, Silva GS, He J, Sadaghiani S, Wu O, Singhal AB. Identifying severe stroke patients likely to benefit from thrombectomy despite delays of up to a day. Sci Rep. 2020;10(1):4008.
30. Powers WJ, Rabinstein AA, Ackerson T, Adeoye OM, Bambakidis NC, Becker K, et al. Guidelines for the early management of patients with acute ischemic stroke: 2019 update to the 2018 guidelines for the early management of acute ischemic stroke: a guideline for healthcare professionals from the American Heart Association/American Stroke Association. Stroke. 2019;50(12):e344–418.
31. Heldner MR, Zubler C, Mattle HP, Schroth G, Weck A, Mono M-L, et al. National Institutes of Health stroke scale score and vessel occlusion in 2152 patients with acute ischemic stroke. Stroke. 2013;44(4):1153–7.
32. Jadhav AP, Kenmuir CL, Aghaebrahim A, Limaye K, Wechsler LR, Hammer MD, et al. Interfacility transfer directly to the neuroangiography suite in acute ischemic stroke patients undergoing thrombectomy. Stroke. 2017;48(7):1884–9.
33. Aghaebrahim A, Streib C, Rangaraju S, Kenmuir CL, Giurgiutiu D-V, Horev A, et al. Streamlining door to recanalization processes in endovascular stroke therapy. J Neurointerv Surg. 2017;9(4):340–5.
34. Barber PA, Demchuk AM, Zhang J, Buchan AM. Validity and reliability of a quantitative computed tomography score in predicting outcome of Hyperacute stroke before thrombolytic therapy. ASPECTS Study Group. Alberta stroke Programme early CT score [Internet]. Lancet (London, England). 2000; [cited 2020 May 19]. Available from: https://pubmed.ncbi.nlm.nih.gov/10905241/?from_term=ASPECTS+score+2000&from_pos=1.
35. Kimura K, Iguchi Y, Shibazaki K, Terasawa Y, Inoue T, Uemura J, et al. Large ischemic lesions on diffusion-weighted imaging done before intravenous tissue plasminogen activator thrombolysis predicts a poor outcome in patients with acute stroke. Stroke. 2008;39(8):2388–91.
36. Hill MD, Rowley HA, Adler F, Eliasziw M, Furlan A, Higashida RT, et al. Selection of acute ischemic stroke patients for intra-arterial thrombolysis with pro-Urokinase by using ASPECTS [Internet]. Stroke. 2003; [cited 2020 May 19]. Available from: https://pubmed.ncbi.nlm.nih.gov/12843342/.
37. Panni P, Gory B, Xie Y, Consoli A, Desilles J-P, Mazighi M, et al. Acute stroke with large ischemic core treated by thrombectomy. Stroke. 2019;50(5):1164–71.
38. Kaesmacher J, Chaloulos-Iakovidis P, Panos L, Mordasini P, Michel P, Hajdu SD, et al. Mechanical thrombectomy in ischemic stroke patients with Alberta stroke program early computed tomography score 0-5. Stroke. 2019;50(4):880–8.

39. Demeestere J, Garcia-Esperon C, Garcia-Bermejo P, Ombelet F, McElduff P, Bivard A, et al. Evaluation of hyperacute infarct volume using ASPECTS and brain CT perfusion core volume. Neurology. 2017;88(24):2248–53.
40. d'Esterre CD, Boesen ME, Ahn SH, Pordeli P, Najm M, Minhas P, et al. Time-dependent computed tomographic perfusion thresholds for patients with acute ischemic stroke. Stroke. 2015;46(12):3390–7.
41. Qiu W, Kuang H, Lee TY, Boers AM, Brown S, Muir K, et al. Confirmatory study of time-dependent computed tomographic perfusion thresholds for use in acute ischemic stroke. Stroke. 2019;50(11):3269–73.
42. Nagaraja N, Forder JR, Warach S, Merino JG. Reversible diffusion-weighted imaging lesions in acute ischemic stroke: a systematic review. Neurology. 2020;94(13):571–87.
43. Campbell BCV, Majoie CBLM, Albers GW, Menon BK, Yassi N, Sharma G, et al. Penumbral imaging and functional outcome in patients with anterior circulation ischaemic stroke treated with endovascular thrombectomy versus medical therapy: a meta-analysis of individual patient-level data. Lancet Neurol. 2019;18(1):46–55.
44. Bracard S, Ducrocq X, Mas JL, Soudant M, Oppenheim C, Moulin T, et al. Mechanical thrombectomy after intravenous alteplase versus alteplase alone after stroke (THRACE): a randomised controlled trial. Lancet Neurol. 2016;15(11):1138–47.
45. Muir KW, Ford GA, Messow C-M, Ford I, Murray A, Clifton A, et al. Endovascular therapy for acute ischaemic stroke: the Pragmatic Ischaemic Stroke Thrombectomy Evaluation (PISTE) randomised, controlled trial. J Neurol Neurosurg Psychiatry. 2017;88(1):38–44.
46. Román LS, Menon BK, Blasco J, Hernández-Pérez M, Dávalos A, Majoie CBLM, et al. Imaging features and safety and efficacy of endovascular stroke treatment: a meta-analysis of individual patient-level data. Lancet Neurol. 2018;17(10):895–904.
47. Tsivgoulis G, Saqqur M, Sharma VK, Lao AY, Hoover SL, Alexandrov AV. Association of Pretreatment ASPECTS scores with tPA-induced arterial recanalization in acute middle cerebral artery occlusion. J Neuroimaging. 2008;18(1):56–61.
48. Goyal M, Jadhav AP, Bonafe A, Diener H, Mendes Pereira V, Levy E, et al. Analysis of workflow and time to treatment and the effects on outcome in endovascular treatment of acute ischemic stroke: results from the SWIFT PRIME randomized controlled trial. Radiology. 2016;279(3):888–97.
49. Zaidat Osama O, Hormozd B, Marc R, Saver Jeffrey L, Mattle Heinrich P, René C, et al. Primary results of the multicenter ARISE II study (analysis of revascularization in ischemic stroke with EmboTrap). Stroke. 2018;49(5):1107–15.
50. Hill MD, Goyal M, Menon BK, Nogueira RG, McTaggart RA, Demchuk AM, et al. Efficacy and safety of nerinetide for the treatment of acute ischaemic stroke (ESCAPE-NA1): a multicentre, double-blind, randomised controlled trial. Lancet [Internet]. 2020. [cited 2020 Feb 24];0(0). Available from: https://www.thelancet.com/journals/lancet/article/PIIS0140-6736(20)30258-0/abstract.
51. Atchaneeyasakul K, Tipirneni A, Khandelwal P, Saini V, Ronca R, Lord S, et al. Utilizing CT with maximum intensity projection reconstruction bypassing CTA improves time to groin puncture in large vessel occlusion stroke thrombectomy. Interv Neurol. 2017;6(3–4):147–52.
52. Martins-Filho RK do V, Dias FA, Alves FFA, Camilo MR, Barreira CMA, Libardi MC, et al. Large vessel occlusion score: a screening tool to detect large vessel occlusion in the acute stroke setting. J Stroke Cerebrovasc Dis. 2019;28(4):869–75.
53. Scalone G, Niccoli G, Crea F. Editor's choice- pathophysiology, diagnosis and management of MINOCA: an update. Eur Heart J Acute Cardiovasc Care. 2019;8(1):54–62.
54. Leyhe JR, Tsogkas I, Hesse AC, Behme D, Schregel K, Papageorgiou I, et al. Latest generation of flat detector CT as a peri-interventional diagnostic tool: a comparative study with multidetector CT. J Neurointerv Surg. 2017;9(12):1253–7.
55. Heran NS, Song JK, Namba K, Smith W, Niimi Y, Berenstein A. The utility of DynaCT in neuroendovascular procedures. Am J Neuroradiol. 2006;27(2):330–2.

56. Namba K, Niimi Y, Song JK, Berenstein A. Use of Dyna-CT angiography in neuroendovascular decision-making. Interv Neuroradiol. 2009;15(1):67–72.
57. Streib CD, Rangaraju S, Campbell DT, Winger DG, Paolini SL, Zhang AJ, et al. Infarct volume predicts hospitalization costs in anterior circulation large-vessel occlusion stroke. AJNR Am J Neuroradiol. 2019;40(1):51–8.
58. Shireman TI, Wang K, Saver JL, Goyal M, Bonafé A, Diener H-C, et al. Cost-effectiveness of solitaire stent retriever thrombectomy for acute ischemic stroke: results from the SWIFT-PRIME trial (solitaire with the intention for thrombectomy as primary endovascular treatment for acute ischemic stroke) [Internet]. Stroke. 2017; [cited 2020 May 19]. Available from: https://pubmed.ncbi.nlm.nih.gov/28028150/.
59. Psychogios M-N, Behme D, Schregel K, Tsogkas I, Maier IL, Leyhe JR, et al. One-stop management of acute stroke patients: minimizing door-to-reperfusion times. Stroke. 2017;48(11):3152–5.
60. Ribo M, Boned S, Rubiera M, Tomasello A, Coscojuela P, Hernández D, et al. Direct transfer to angiosuite to reduce door-to-puncture time in thrombectomy for acute stroke. J Neurointerv Surg. 2018;10(3):221–4.
61. Mendez B, Requena M, Aires A, Martins N, Boned S, Rubiera M, et al. Direct transfer to Angio-suite to reduce workflow times and increase favorable clinical outcome: a case-control study. Stroke. 2018;49(11):2723–7.
62. Brehm A, Tsogkas I, Maier IL, Eisenberger HJ, Yang P, Liu J-M, et al. One-stop management with perfusion for transfer patients with stroke due to a large-vessel occlusion: feasibility and effects on in-hospital times. AJNR Am J Neuroradiol. 2019;40(8):1330–4.
63. Manuel R, Marta O, Álvaro G-T, Noelia R-V, Matías D, Jesús J, et al. Time matters. Stroke. 0(0):STROKEAHA.119.028586.
64. Zibulewsky J. The emergency medical treatment and active labor act (EMTALA): what it is and what it means for physicians. Proc (Bayl Univ Med Cent). 2001;14(4):339–46.
65. Rinaldo L, Brinjikji W, McCutcheon BA, Bydon M, Cloft H, Kallmes DF, et al. Hospital transfer associated with increased mortality after endovascular revascularization for acute ischemic stroke. J Neurointerv Surg. 2017;9(12):1166–72.
66. Yang P, Zhang Y, Zhang L, Zhang Y, Treurniet KM, Chen W, et al. Endovascular thrombectomy with or without intravenous Alteplase in acute stroke. N Engl J Med. 2020;382(21):1981–93.
67. Suzuki K, Kimura K, Takeuchi M, Morimoto M, Kanazawa R, Kamiya Y, et al. The randomized study of endovascular therapy with versus without intravenous tissue plasminogen activator in acute stroke with ICA and M1 occlusion (SKIP study). Int J Stroke. 2019;14(7):752–5.
68. Benjamin EJ, Virani SS, Callaway CW, Chamberlain AM, Chang AR, Cheng S, et al. Heart disease and stroke statistics-2018 update: a report from the American Heart Association. Circulation. 2018;137(12):e67–492.
69. Lakomkin N, Dhamoon M, Carroll K, Singh IP, Tuhrim S, Lee J, et al. Prevalence of large vessel occlusion in patients presenting with acute ischemic stroke: a 10-year systematic review of the literature. J Neurointerv Surg. 2019;11(3):241–5.
70. Smith Eric E, Kent David M, Bulsara Ketan R, Leung Lester Y, Lichtman Judith H, Reeves Mathew J, et al. Accuracy of prediction instruments for diagnosing large vessel occlusion in individuals with suspected stroke: a systematic review for the 2018 guidelines for the early management of patients with acute ischemic stroke. Stroke. 2018;49(3):e111–22.
71. de la Ossa NP, Carrera D, Gorchs M, Querol M, Millán M, Gomis M, et al. Design and validation of a prehospital stroke scale to predict large arterial occlusion: the rapid arterial occlusion evaluation scale [Internet]. Stroke. 2014; [cited 2020 May 20]. Available from: https://pubmed.ncbi.nlm.nih.gov/24281224/.
72. EEG controlled triage in the ambulance for acute ischemic stroke - full text view - ClinicalTrials.gov [Internet]. [cited 2020 May 20]. Available from: https://clinicaltrials.gov/ct2/show/NCT03699397.

73. Antipova D, Eadie L, Macaden AS, Wilson P. Diagnostic value of transcranial ultrasonography for selecting subjects with large vessel occlusion: a systematic review. Ultrasound J. 2019;11(1):29.
74. Giacalone G, Zanoletti M, Re R, Germinario B, Contini D, Spinelli L, et al. Time-domain near-infrared spectroscopy in acute ischemic stroke patients. Neurophotonics [Internet]. 2019 [cited 2020 May 20];6(1). Available from: https://www.ncbi.nlm.nih.gov/pmc/articles/PMC6365799/.
75. UCSF. UCSF ischemic stroke trial: head pulse for ischemic stroke detection [Internet]. [cited 2020 May 20]. Available from: https://clinicaltrials.ucsf.edu/trial/NCT03824496.

Part II
Techniques

Chapter 7
Thrombectomy Techniques: Stent Retriever – Balloon Guide

Dennys Reyes, Italo Linfante, and Guilherme Dabus

Introduction

Mechanical thrombectomy has emerged as a powerful treatment modality for acute ischemic stroke from large vessel occlusion. Several recent randomized controlled clinical trials (RCTs) have demonstrated the effectiveness of mechanical thrombectomy with stent retrievers compared to IV tPA or best medical management [1–3]. Furthermore, approximately 40% of patients suffering from a large vessel occlusion arrive to the emergency department more than 6 hours after symptom onset making them not eligible for IV tPA. In these cases, if a large vessel occlusion is the culprit, mechanical thrombectomy is the only treatment available. Endovascular therapy has also been demonstrated to be effective in selected cases presenting from 6 to 24 hours after symptom onset according to the recent data from DEFUSE and DAWN clinical trials [1, 2].

Various techniques are used to maximize the results of mechanical thrombectomy with stent retrievers, including proximal flow arrest with balloon guide catheter (BGC), conventional large-bore proximal catheter (CGC), or combination with local aspiration through a large-bore distal catheter positioned at the clot interface (aspiration-retriever technique for stroke [ARTS]) [4]. A recent publication from the NASA registry reported comparable results from the ARTS and BGC techniques in regard of the time from arterial puncture to reperfusion [4].

D. Reyes · I. Linfante · G. Dabus (✉)
Interventional Neuroradiology and Neuroendovascular Surgery, Miami Cardiac & Vascular Institute, Baptist Neuroscience Center, Miami, FL, USA
e-mail: GuilhermeD@baptisthealth.net

F. K. Hui et al. (eds.), *12 Strokes*, https://doi.org/10.1007/978-3-030-56857-3_7

Data on Balloon Guide Catheter

Mechanical thrombectomy recanalization results using the combination of BGC and stent retriever have been consistently reported from 65% to almost 90% according to multiple RCTs [3]. A recent study also demonstrated the benefit of BGC compared to non-BGC to reduce distal embolization during thrombus aspiration under flow arrest. Time from arterial puncture to reperfusion or end of procedure has been found to be shorter for the BGC and ARTS techniques when compared to CGC technique [4]. The overall mean procedure time can be significantly shorter for BGC-treated stroke patients when compared to those treated with non-BGC techniques based on a meta-analysis study [5].

Despite similar amount of passes in a study evaluating recanalization results after mechanical thrombectomy while comparing BGC and non-BGC techniques, the thrombolysis in cerebral infarction (TICI) 3 or 2b recanalization scores were higher for patients treated with BGC with less frequent findings for distal embolization [6]. The use of BGC technique has higher odds of first-pass recanalization as well as lower need for additional passes resulting in higher TICI 3 or 2b/3 scores, good clinical outcome (mRS < 2), and lower mortality odds [5, 7]. Additionally, not using BGC mechanical thrombectomy techniques carries an increased risk of poor outcome (modified Rankin Scale, mRS > 2) as demonstrated by the data from the North America Solitaire Stent Retriever Acute Stroke (NASA) registry [8] despite having similar occurrence of distal emboli and emboli to new territory. Additionally, the NASA registry has demonstrated that the use of BCG resulted in more TICI 3 recanalization and lower NIHSS at discharge [8].

The recently described first-pass effect (FPE) is the result of a single thrombectomy device pass achieving complete recanalization [9]. A recent study demonstrated that FPE is an independent predictor of good clinical outcome and that FPE is more frequently associated with the use of BGC and the use of BGC was shown to be an independent predictor of FPE [9].

Recent data from the TRACK registry demonstrated that despite the fact that time from symptom onset to groin puncture being longer in the BGC group (357 vs. 319 min, $P = 0.06$) and that no difference in reperfusion time, first-pass effect, number of passes, or rescue therapy was seen comparing BGC to non-BGC groups, TICI 2b/3 scores were higher in the BGC cohort (84% vs. 75.5%, $P = 0.01$). Furthermore, good clinical outcome at 3 months was superior in patients with BGC (57% vs. 40%, $P = 0.0004$) with a lower mortality rate (13% vs. 23%, $P = 0.008$). In the multivariate analysis, BGC use was an independent predictor of good clinical outcome (OR 2, 95% CI 1.3 to 3.1, $P = 0.001$) [10].

Large-bore balloon guide catheters can also be used to support distal catheters for combined proximal and distal aspiration. Unfortunately, most of the new larger distal aspiration catheters will not be compatible with most BGC. The operator should be aware of this incompatibility and plan accordingly. Another use of BGC is what has been described as simple aspiration with balloon catheter technique (simple ABC technique). This technique has been used for proximal internal carotid

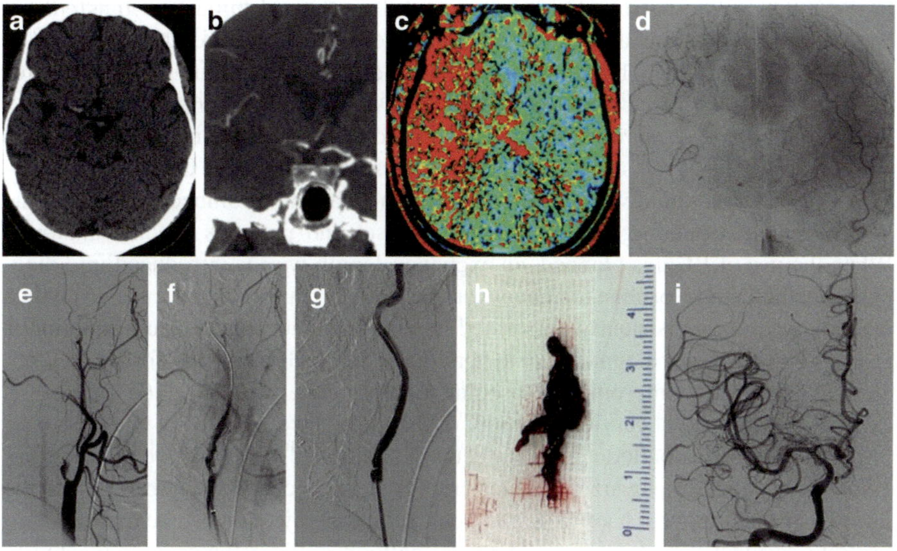

Fig. 7.1 Patient in the late 40s who presented with right MCA syndrome and had an NIHSS of 15. CT, CTA, and CTP revealed intracranial large vessel occlusion with clot extending from the ICA into the M1 and A1 ("T" occlusion) with a large area of elevated mean transit time (**a**–**c**, respectively). Left ICA angiography demonstrated poor collaterals to the right MCA territory (**d**). There was collusion of the cervical right ICA immediately distal to the origin which was severely stenotic (**e**). Angioplasty was performed (**f**). The BCG was then advanced into the proximal RICA where the balloon was inflated and vigorous aspiration performed with a 60-cc syringe (**g**). A large clot was aspirated which completely blocked the BGC requiring it to be removed (**h**). Follow-up angiography demonstrated successful intracranial reperfusion (TICI 2B) (**i**)

artery occlusion and it is useful in removing large amount of thrombus, shortening procedure time, and providing an easy pathway to shift for either stent retriever or ADAPT techniques [11]. Also remote aspiration thrombectomy in large vessel occlusion of supraclinoid internal carotid artery through balloon guide catheter positioned at the cervical segment has been reported [12] (Fig. 7.1).

Stent Retriever – Balloon Guide Catheter Technique

Appropriate consenting process remains an important first step in this emergent situation while a patient is suffering from acute ischemic stroke such as a large vessel occlusion. This implies the emergency in discussing the rationale, risk, and benefits of the endovascular therapy typically with a family member over the phone or in person. This first process establishes expectations for recanalization and potential good clinical outcome but also treatment failure and complications.

The use of anesthesia for mechanical thrombectomy remains debatable depending on the preference of the neuro-interventionalist and the patient's clinical status.

In our practice, most stroke treatments are still performed through a transfemoral approach, leaving transradial or transcarotid access to selective cases. Access to common femoral artery by using a modified Seldinger technique is the most frequent scenario with placement of either an 8 or a 9 French arterial sheath. A 5 French Berenstein 2 catheter is typically introduced and selective catheterization with angiography of the suspected occluded vessel is performed. Once there is confirmation of intracranial vessel occlusion, the mechanical thrombectomy technique is determined depending on the occluded vessel and patient's specific anatomy. When the use of BGC is planned, an exchange-length wire is introduced into diagnostic catheter and exchange maneuver performed. In our experience exchange maneuver can be consistently performed in less than 30 seconds. Another option is to use longer 125-cm diagnostic catheters inside the BGC allowing for direct catheterization of the compromised vascular territory. The balloon guide catheter is carefully positioned at cervical segment of the internal carotid artery with aid of its introducer. Rarely a balloon guide catheter is positioned within the vertebral artery given the reduced lumen size of the artery. Once the exchange-length wire and the introducer are removed, back flow and gentle contrast injection can be used to demonstrate cervical vessel patency. Then the balloon guide catheter is connected to continuous heparinized saline while preventing air emboli from the lines. Manual injections through the balloon guide catheter at this point will not only confirm successful positioning of the catheter but also the presence of continuous flow, demonstrate no injury of the vessel intima during the exchange and better opacification of the cervical and cranial vessels, and serve to determine working AP and lateral projections and confirm the location of the vessel occlusion.

In the scenario of internal carotid occlusion extending from the cervical level, a simple aspiration through the balloon catheter technique (simple ABC) can be used as a starting point especially if the tip of the catheter is well positioned facing the thrombus. In this scenario, the balloon is inflated and vigorous aspiration is performed through the BGC. The use of this technique is usually technically more difficult for mid- to distal thrombus since navigation of the BGC is usually limited due to frequent tortuosity of the cervical segment of the internal carotid artery and higher risk for dissection at that level. Therefore the larger available stent retriever (6 mm) associated with balloon inflation and aspiration through the BCG is used for those thrombus located in tortuous cervical segments of the internal carotid artery as well as for distal cervical and petrous/cavernous locations (Fig. 7.2).

It has been our preference for thrombectomy of intracranial clots to position the BGC as distal as possible allowing for better support and control as well as more effective aspiration. It is important to understand that the ideal position of the BGC in the parent vessel is limited by its tortuosity (Figs. 7.3 and 7.4); therefore, in cases where the cervical segment of the parent vessel is fairly straight, the BGC can be safely navigated and positioned in the distal cervical segment.

The effectiveness of stent retriever thrombectomy has been proven by multiple RCTs in a recent past [3], including extended windows up to 24 h after onset as demonstrated by DAWN and DEFUSE trials [1, 2]. These types of devices work primarily by self-expanding inside occluded vessel and integrating the thrombotic

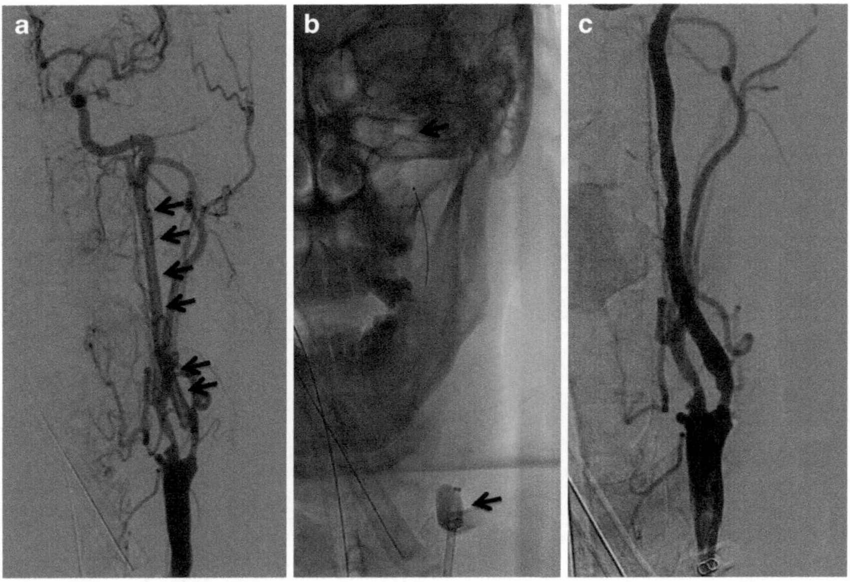

Fig. 7.2 Case demonstrating presence of a long clot affecting the entire cervical extension of the left ICA (**a** arrows). Thrombectomy was successfully performed using a combination of BGC at the left ICA origin for flow arrest and aspiration and a large 6 mm × 30 mm stent retriever (**b** arrows) resulting in complete recanalization (**c**) and no distal embolization

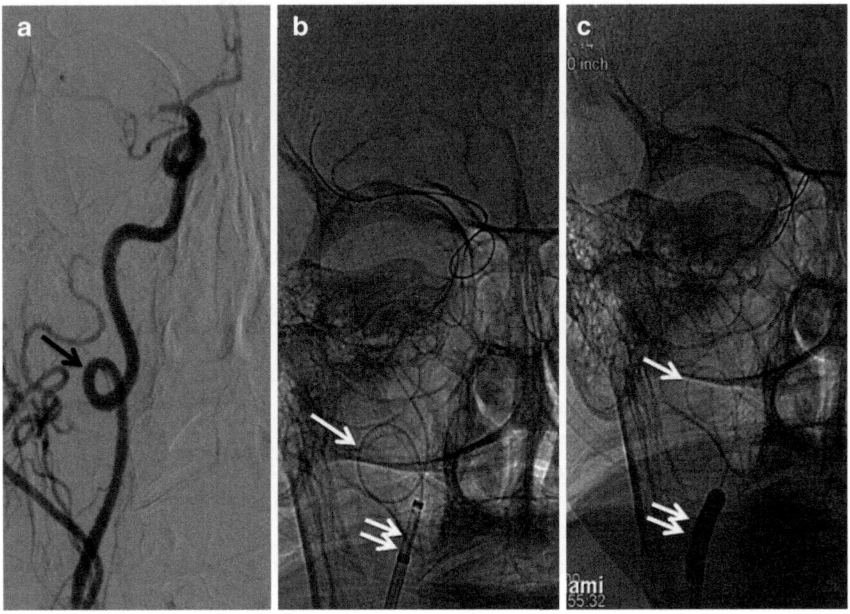

Fig. 7.3 A patient presenting with right M1 occlusion with a vascular loop in the cervical right ICA (**a**). It is our preference in these cases to keep the BGC immediately below the loop where the balloon can be safely inflated and thrombectomy performed, decreasing the risk of vascular injury and dissection (**b**, **c**)

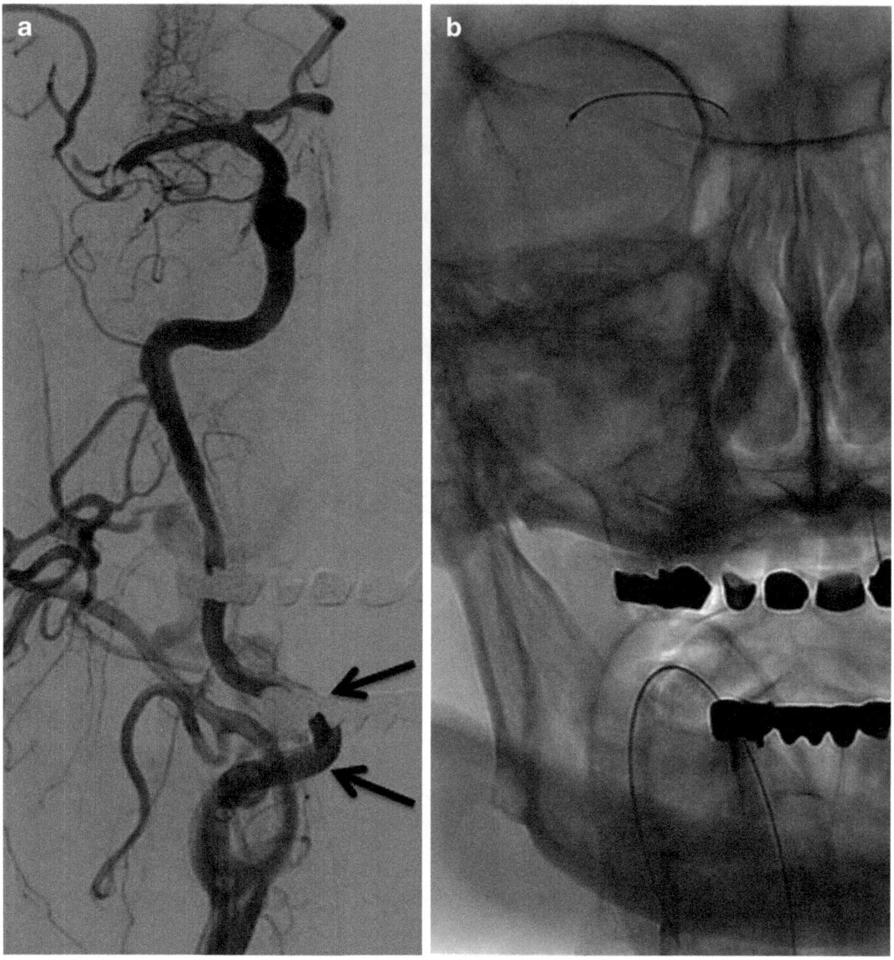

Fig. 7.4 Another example of vascular tortuosity in the cervical right ICA in a patient with distal right M1 occlusion (**a** arrows). Figure (**b**) demonstrating the position of the BGC immediately below the tortuosity and the stent retriever positioned for thrombectomy (**b**)

material into the stent's struts after waiting between 1 and 5 minutes. Additionally the stent retriever applies a radial force compressing the thrombus against the vessel wall partially restoring blood flow within the ischemic penumbra [13]. Successful positioning of a stent retriever across the thrombus is frequently influenced by the support provided from the balloon guide catheter to the delivering microcatheter with or without an intermediate catheter.

Once successful positioning of the stent retriever is achieved within the occluded segment, a time period is needed to allow thrombus integration within the stent retriever. In our experience, this is accomplished waiting from 2 to 5 minutes with

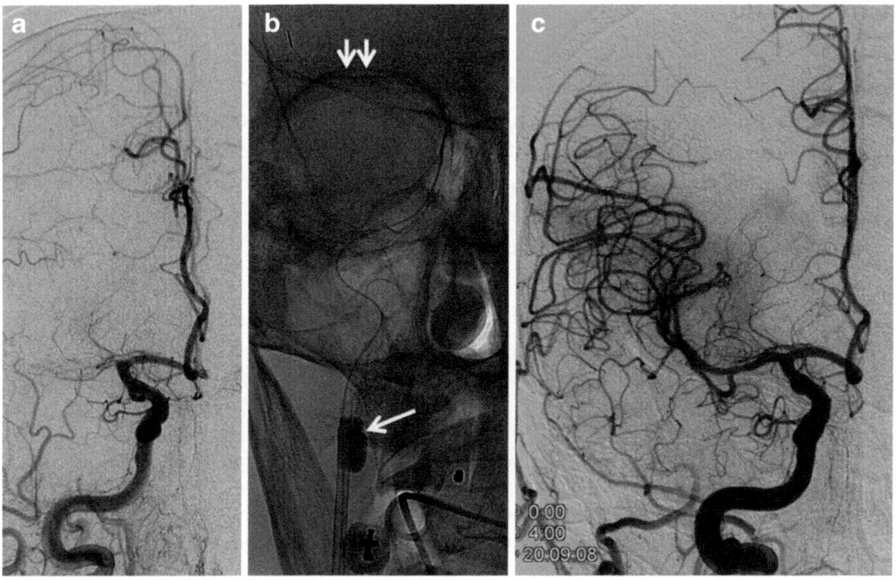

Fig. 7.5 A case demonstrating our usual technique for thrombectomy using BGC and stent retriever in a patient who presented with a right M1 occlusion (**a**). As usual, the BGC is advanced as distal as safely possible; the microcatheter is advanced over the microwire to cross the occluded segment; a small amount of contrast is gently injected through the microcatheter to confirm intraluminal position; the stent retriever is then advanced and deployed covering the occluded segment where the clot is located. After 2 to 5 minutes, the balloon is inflated and the stent retriever (**b**) withdrawn under continuous vigorous aspiration through the BGC. Angiography is then repeated to assess recanalization (**c**)

the stent retriever in place. Immediately prior to pulling the stent retriever, the balloon of the BGC is inflated, preferably within cervical segment of the parent artery (Fig. 7.5). Blood flow arrest with vigorous continuous aspiration within the parent artery facilitates retrieving the stent retriever with the integrated thrombus under negative pressures, theoretically decreasing the risk of distal embolization of thrombus fragments and better recanalization results. During the maneuver to pull the stent retriever, it is important to monitor the tip of the BGC as it can migrate distally increasing the risk of vasospasm or dissection within the parent vessel. After retrieving the stent retriever with the thrombus, the balloon is deflated during continuous aspiration. Further manual aspiration from the BGC is recommended for removal of residual thrombus. After any residual thrombus is cleared from the lumen of the BGC, recanalization status is determined by repeating a cerebral angiography. Before completion of the procedure, a cervical angiography is advisable to check for the presence of focal dissection secondary to the BGC manipulation. The balloon guide catheter is finally removed and the puncture site is closed with the standard devices.

Conclusion

Balloon guide catheter is a valuable tool in the neuro-interventionalist armamentarium. Its use is safe and technically easy with no need for advanced maneuvers. Understanding its advantages and disadvantages may increase the chances of obtaining an effective recanalization. The use of stent retriever in association with BGC seems beneficial to the patients when compared to use of stent retrievers with conventional large-bore guide catheters.

References

1. Albers GW, Marks MP, Kemp S, Christensen S, Tsai JP, Ortega-Gutierrez S, et al. Thrombectomy for stroke at 6 to 16 hours with selection by perfusion imaging. N Engl J Med. 2018;378(8):708–18.
2. Nogueira RG, Jadhav AP, Haussen DC, Bonafe A, Budzik RF, Bhuva P, et al. Thrombectomy 6 to 24 hours after stroke with a mismatch between deficit and infarct. N Engl J Med. 2018;378(1):11–21.
3. Goyal M, Menon BK, van Zwam WH, Dippel DW, Mitchell PJ, Demchuk AM, Dávalos A, Majoie CB, van der Lugt A, de Miquel MA, Donnan GA, Roos YB, Bonafe A, Jahan R, Diener HC, van den Berg LA, Levy EI, Berkhemer OA, Pereira VM, Rempel J, Millán M, Davis SM, Roy D, Thornton J, Román LS, Ribó M, Beumer D, Stouch B, Brown S, Campbell BC, van Oostenbrugge RJ, Saver JL, Hill MD, Jovin TG, HERMES collaborators. Endovascular thrombectomy after large-vessel ischaemic stroke: a meta-analysis of individual patient data from five randomised trials. Lancet. 2016;387(10029):1723–31.
4. Malisch TW, Zaidat OO, Castonguay AC, Marden FA, Gupta R, Sun CJ, et al. Clinical and angiographic outcomes with the combined local aspiration and retriever in the North American solitaire stent-retriever acute stroke (NASA) registry. Interv Neurol. 2018;7(1-2):26–35.
5. Brinjikji W, Starke RM, Murad MH, Fiorella D, Pereira VM, Goyal M, et al. Impact of balloon guide catheter on technical and clinical outcomes: a systematic review and meta-analysis. J Neurointerv Surg. 2018;10(4):335–9.
6. Lee DH, Sung JH, Kim SU, Yi HJ, Hong JT, Lee SW. Effective use of balloon guide catheters in reducing incidence of mechanical thrombectomy related distal embolization. Acta Neurochir. 2017;159(9):1671–7.
7. Zaidat OO, Castonguay AC, Nogueira RG, Haussen DC, English JD, Satti SR, et al. TREVO stent-retriever mechanical thrombectomy for acute ischemic stroke secondary to large vessel occlusion registry. J Neurointerv Surg. 2018;10(6):516–24.
8. Linfante I, Starosciak AK, Walker GR, Dabus G, Castonguay AC, Gupta R, et al. Predictors of poor outcome despite recanalization: a multiple regression analysis of the NASA registry. J Neurointerv Surg. 2016;8(3):224–9.
9. Zaidat OO, Castonguay AC, Linfante I, Gupta R, Martin CO, Holloway WE, et al. First pass effect: a new measure for stroke thrombectomy devices. Stroke. 2018;49(3):660–6.
10. Nguyen TN, Castonguay AC, Nogueira RG, Haussen DC, English JD, Satti SR, Chen J, Farid H, Borders C, Veznedaroglu E, Binning MJ, Puri AS, Vora NA, Budzik RF, Dabus G, Linfante I, Janardhan V, Alshekhlee A, Abraham MG, Edgell RC, Taqi MA, El Khoury R, Mokin M, Majjhoo AQ, Kabbani MR, Froehler MT, Finch I, Ansari SA, Novakovic R, Abdalkader M, Zaidat OO. Effect of balloon guide catheter on clinical outcomes and reperfusion in Trevo thrombectomy. J Neurointerv Surg. 2019; https://doi.org/10.1136/neurintsurg-2018-014452. [Epub ahead of print].

11. Okamura A, Kuroki K, Shinagawa K, Yamada N. Simple aspiration with balloon catheter technique (simple ABC technique) against proximal internal carotid artery occlusion in cases of cardiogenic cerebral embolism. Interv Neuroradiol: journal of peritherapeutic neuroradiology, surgical procedures and related neurosciences. 2018;24(3):317–21.
12. Haussen DC, Bouslama M, Grossberg JA, Nogueira RG. Remote aspiration thrombectomy in large vessel acute ischemic stroke. J Neurointerv Surg. 2017;9(3):250–2.
13. Chartrain AG, Awad AJ, Mascitelli JR, Shoirah H, Oxley TJ, Feng R, et al. Novel and emerging technologies for endovascular thrombectomy. Neurosurg Focus. 2017;42(4):E12.

Chapter 8
Direct Aspiration Thrombectomy for Acute Stroke: Evolution of Technique and Evidence

Sami Al Kasab and Alejandro M. Spiotta

Introduction

Mechanical thrombectomy (MT) is the standard of care for patients presenting with large vessel occlusion and salvageable brain tissue [1–3]. Most MT trials predominantly used stentriever devices as the first-line device [3–5]. Over the past few years, multiple large-scale studies and most recently two randomized trials have established non-inferiority of direct aspiration thrombectomy as first-line thrombectomy technique compared to stentriever [6–11]. Herein we review the key technological advances and design modifications that have allowed for navigation around the ophthalmic turn for more distal delivery of larger-bore catheters providing more aspiration force directly applied at the thrombus interface.

Direct Aspiration Origins: The Penumbra 054 Aspiration Catheter

The Penumbra aspiration system was first introduced in 2008. It involved maceration of the thrombus with a separator which was repeatedly introduced and withdrawn from the thrombus under direct aspiration to prevent distal embolization [12, 13]. While its market competitor at the time, the Merci system [14, 15], relied primarily on delivery of a microcatheter (the 18 L; Stryker, Kalamazoo, Michigan, USA) to the site of occlusion, the Penumbra aspiration system relied on the delivery

S. Al Kasab (✉) · A. M. Spiotta
Department of Neurosurgery, Medical University of South Carolina, Charleston, SC, USA
e-mail: alkasab@musc.edu

F. K. Hui et al. (eds.), *12 Strokes*, https://doi.org/10.1007/978-3-030-56857-3_8

of a much larger-bore catheter to the thrombus (up to effectively a 5 F device) [16]. The introduction of highly flexible lubricious polymers with good hoop strength allowed for safe placement of large intermediate-class catheters directly into the large intracranial vessels. The development of large-bore flexible catheters was essential to the function of the Penumbra system [7, 9, 17].

The original iteration of the Penumbra reperfusion catheter system included several different-sized catheters (internal diameter 0.026″, 0.032″, and 0.041″) and accompanying separators to maximize clot interaction and force of aspiration in vessels of differing diameters (internal carotid artery terminus, M1, M2, M3) to address both proximal and distal embolization [9, 17]. The largest catheter at the time of first launch had a lumen diameter of 0.041 inch, yet it tracked sub-optimally around the carotid siphon and required a median of 45 min to achieve acceptable recanalization [18]. The 054 reperfusion catheter became available in 2009; the large bore of this catheter has significantly improved the aspiration efficiency to a median 20 min by providing an estimated 4× aspiration force over the next smaller catheter, the 041 [19, 20].

Although a larger catheter lumen provides higher suction and more rapid removal of thrombus, a drawback of its larger size was that the 054 catheter often required the use of a coaxial technique to facilitate navigation to the middle cerebral artery. When navigated over a 0.014-inch microwire alone, a significant ledge would get held up at the origin of the ophthalmic artery. To overcome this obstacle to the target lesion, access with the 054 catheter could be optimized with a coaxial technique (Fig. 8.1). The smaller 032 and 026 reperfusion catheters could be delivered simply over either a 0.014- or 0.016-inch wire and the larger 054 delivered over those. One of the major advantages of the Penumbra aspiration system was that, once the catheter system was delivered to the target vessel, separator clot maceration could be performed without having to re-access (additional “passes”), as was the case for the Merci device.

Despite these advances in catheter technology, navigating past the carotid siphon was still a relative challenge during thrombectomy cases. In patients with very acute angulation in the ophthalmic segment, adjunctive techniques could be performed to obtain the necessary distal access. One approach used the Merci retriever system as an adjunct to improve the trackability of the 054 reperfusion catheter by altering the angle with which the catheter engages the ophthalmic segment and M1 origin. By deploying an appropriately sized Merci Retriever (Concentric Medical), such as a V.2.0 or V.2.5 soft, in the mid-M1 segment through either the 032 catheter or an 18-L microcatheter and then applying gentle traction on the Merci Retriever, the course of the wire straightens, approximating the inner curve of the vasculature, pulling the catheter complex away from the ledge of the vessel origins (“grappling hook” technique) [21], an approach now used routinely using stentrievers and intermediate catheters. The 054 catheter can then be more readily advanced into the target vessel. Once the 054 reperfusion catheter is in place, the retriever is resheathed into the 18-L microcatheter and then removed prior to separator placement and aspiration.

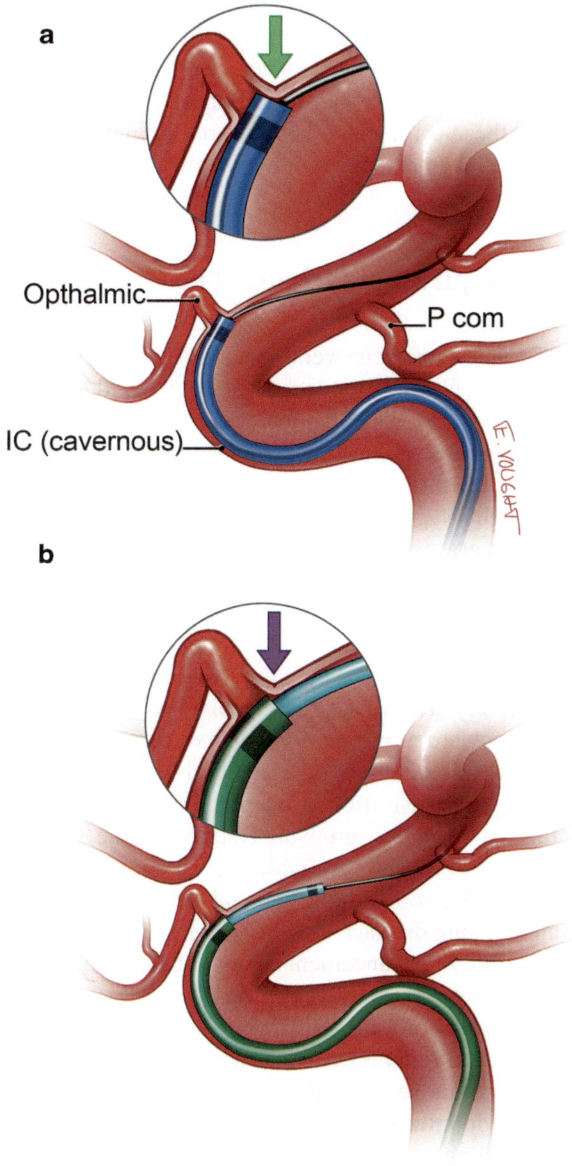

Fig. 8.1 (**a**) While a larger catheter lumen provides higher suction and more rapid removal of thrombus, it results in a larger catheter profile and "ledge effect" which renders navigation past the ophthalmic artery origin challenging. (**b**) To overcome this obstacle, access with an intermediate catheter is optimized with a coaxial technique resulting in a more tapered construct that minimizes the "ledge effect"

The most recent generation of the Penumbra aspiration catheters is called the "MAX" series. This was introduced in 2012 and also intended to be used with separators of varying sizes [22, 23]. The MAX series catheters included larger inner diameters at the distal end as well as the proximal end to increase the aspiration power. The larger proximal lumen reduces resistance to flow and therefore increases aspiration force at the catheter tip. Improvements in polymer and braid and ring reinforcement provide more catheter tip flexibility and an increased number of transition zones to improve trackability while maintaining hoop strength. The newly introduced intermediate catheters were named 5MAX, 4MAX, and 3MAX. An increased number of transition zones in the catheter design and manufacturing allowed these catheters to be delivered primarily over either a 0.014- or 0.016-inch microwire, even past the ophthalmic origin.

Direct Aspiration Origins: The Distal Access Catheter

In 2004 the Merci Retriever (Concentric Medical, Mountain View, California, USA) became the first mechanical thrombectomy device cleared for human use in the USA by the FDA [24]. The Merci device primarily works by engaging the thrombus with a "corkscrew" distal wire and suture tip deployed from within the clot and then removing the thrombus en bloc to achieve recanalization. The device was employed using a balloon guide catheter that was positioned at the carotid bifurcation or internal carotid artery to cause temporary flow reversal, allowing the Merci to be retrieved into the guide catheter while mitigating the possibility of emboli showering to distal territories. However, clot retrieval into the guide catheter still required a long distance to be traveled while maintaining purchase on the thrombus, most commonly from the M1 segment of the middle cerebral artery to the proximal cervical internal carotid artery. The vector force applied while pulling on the thrombus was suboptimal (downward along the long axis of the cervical carotid artery, not horizontally along the axis of the middle cerebral artery). This caused considerable torquing, stretching, and distortion of the parent vessel and presented a biomechanical disadvantage to thrombus removal. Traction on the vasculature resulted in pain for the patient. To avoid the inevitable movement induced, many operators chose to perform thrombectomy under general anesthesia. In addition, the Merci technique required a long distance to be traveled while remaining engaged with the thrombus.

A landmark advancement came in 2010 with the approval of the Outreach distal access catheter (DAC, Concentric Medical), which would have repercussions for the application of the Merci device and also for future iterations of thrombectomy approaches [17]. The DAC was designed for the purpose of buttressing access for the Merci thrombectomy device, affording stable access to the target vessel. Use of the DAC optimized the vectors at play during pulling of the device. With further understanding of clot fragmentation and distal embolization, the DAC was used as an intermediate aspiration device which aided in preventing showering of distal emboli during clot retrieval and increased the aspiration power applied directly to the thrombus [9, 17]. The development of large-bore flexible catheters that could be delivered into the intracranial circulation represented a major advancement in thrombectomy technology and also in intermediate catheter technology. The DAC has a flexible distal shaft with increased proximal shaft strength and axial load-bearing characteristics as well as good hoop strength, allowing it to be delivered to the intracranial circulation around the ophthalmic bend when navigated over a coaxial catheter system. A major drawback to the Merci retrieval system was that it necessitated navigating past the ophthalmic bend with every pass, decreasing the efficiency of the system and adding to procedure times.

Current-Generation Aspiration: "Solumbra" Technique

Another key milestone in the evolution of thrombectomy technique was developed in the early stages of widespread stentriever (SR) incorporation, the combined stentriever-Penumbra ("Solumbra") technique, which laid the foundation for direct aspiration alone (without the need for an SR) [25]. To minimize the distance, the SR must travel while engaging the thrombus, especially into larger-caliber vasculature such as the internal carotid artery from the middle cerebral artery, and mitigating the possibility of losing purchase of the clot, variations to the SR technique have been employed with incorporation of Penumbra reperfusion catheters. For example, a 5MAX catheter can be advanced over a 025 microcatheter and microwire up to the site of occlusion and left at the face of the thrombus. The SR is then deployed and the microcatheter is removed, leaving the SR in place. The SR is then pulled directly into the 5MAX while maintaining aspiration (so-called Solumbra technique since it combines a stentriever (Solitaire) with a Penumbra aspiration catheter), and both are removed together (Fig. 8.2), much in the same way as the Merci retriever device was removed with a DAC. However, traction is minimized as compared with the Merci system since the force vectors are horizontal in orientation from the aperture of the aspiration catheter in parallel to the M1. This eliminated the painful stimulus that patients were formerly experiencing. Thus, in addition to representing a more effective technique, the now painless procedure had the added advantage of reintroducing the concept of the awake thrombectomy, with many operators now electing to perform the procedure with minimal conscious sedation. Advantages included the ability to examine the patient's neurological status throughout the procedure, shorter CT-to-groin-stick times, and avoiding the imminent risk of systemic hypotension from induction of general anesthesia.

SR technology was employed exclusively in the ESCAPE, EXTEND-IA, SWIFT PRIME and REVASCAT trials [5, 26–28]. While the MR CLEAN trial did not dictate which thrombectomy device was to be utilized, the majority of cases were also SR based [4]. Given that SR were used in the overwhelming majority of patients enrolled in the positive trials, they have often been referred to as the "stentriever trials," which is reflected in the updated American Heart Association/American Stroke Association guidelines recommending thrombectomy to be performed with an SR [29]. However, thrombectomy techniques evolved even while those trials were enrolling, setting the stage for the next-generation strategy as detailed below.

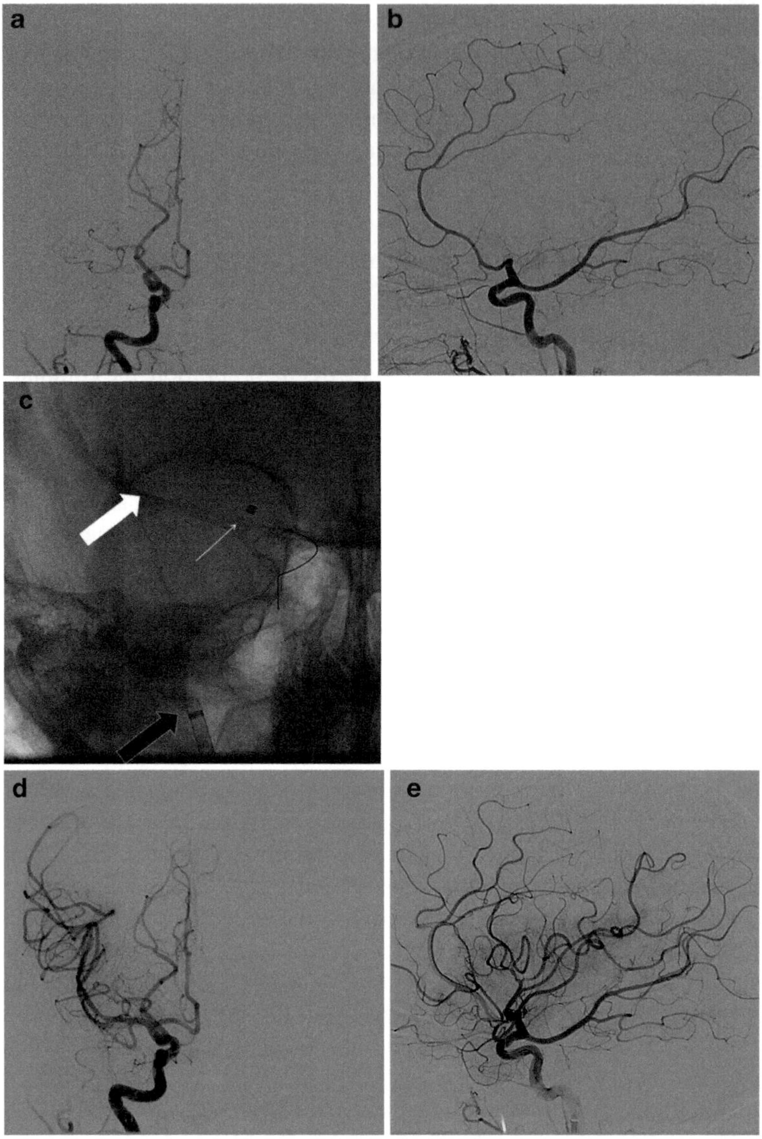

Fig. 8.2 "Solumbra" (Solitaire and Penumbra) technique. (**a**) Anteroposterior (AP) and (**b**) lateral digital subtraction angiography (DSA) demonstrates an M1 occlusion. (**c**) A Solitaire stentriever (SR) is deployed across the M1 segment occlusion (large white arrow), with the aspiration catheter in the proximal M1 segment (small white arrow) and the guide catheter in the distal cervical internal carotid artery (black arrow). The SR is then withdrawn back into the aspiration catheter under direct aspiration applied locally at the M1. Operator may choose to withdraw the SR entirely into the aspiration catheter, or to partially withdraw and then pull both the SR and the aspiration catheter together back to the guide catheter. Aspiration can also be applied at the guide catheter. Some may choose to perform this technique with a balloon guide catheter to affect flow reversal for added protection against distal emboli in the event of thrombus fragmentation. (**d**, **e**) AP and lateral DSA demonstrates recanalization of the M1 occlusion (TICI 2B) with showering of distal fragments and small vessel occlusions

Next Generation: Direct Aspiration

Direct aspiration has become possible due to advances in catheter technology that allow large-caliber aspiration catheters to be advanced intracranially to the thrombus [8, 22]. In general, the largest-sized aspiration catheter that the vessel can accommodate should be utilized. In the first iteration, this was most commonly a Penumbra 5MAX reperfusion catheter (Penumbra, Oakland, CA) for M1 or carotid terminus occlusions. The 5MAX can be advanced to the level of the thrombus over any microcatheter and microwire the operator chooses, but most commonly a Velocity microcatheter (Penumbra, Oakland, CA) over a 0.016-inch Fathom wire (Boston Scientific Corp, Natick, MA). The microcatheter and wire are removed and aspiration is applied by either a 20- or 60-cc syringe or use of the Penumbra aspiration pump that is part of the Penumbra thrombectomy/aspiration system [6, 8, 9]. Inability to draw back blood on aspiration confirms optimal position of the 5MAX catheter abutting the thrombus. The next iteration involved advancing the catheter slightly to ensure firm engagement with the thrombus. The 5MAX catheter is then slowly withdrawn while maintaining aspiration. Aspiration is also applied to the sideport of the guide catheter to prevent dislodging the thrombus from the 5MAX aperture as it is withdrawn into the sheath. Clots are typically removed en bloc, minimizing the risk of downstream emboli (Fig. 8.3). When this technique is successful, it eliminates the need to introduce stentriever or Penumbra separator devices, leading to an overall much lower procedure device cost[57,58]. Thus, we have found the initial application of this technique to provide the highest cost-effective value in acute stroke treatment.

This approach was facilitated by the development of the Penumbra MAX aspiration catheter technology which significantly increased the ease and speed of navigation of a large-bore catheter into the intracranial circulation. The direct aspiration technique differs from prior thrombectomy methods, as it focuses on engaging and removing the clot in its entirety rather than the use of the separator that was designed to macerate the thrombus and clear the tip of the aspiration catheter [6]. Historically, due to the challenges with tracking an aspiration catheter into the intracranial circulation, catheters had to be telescoped with other catheters together or other tricks employed to advance through the siphon. However, the superior trackability of the Penumbra MAX catheters has given operators the confidence to attempt direct aspiration alone without the fear that it will be a significant time and danger impediment to the patient if intracranial access is lost. The second iteration of the aspiration catheter, the 5MAX ACE, has an increased inner diameter of 0.060 at the distal 30 cm, while housing a 0.068 proximal end for larger aspiration forces. Advances in catheter technology would soon follow, allowing for even larger-bore catheters to be safely delivered to the intracranial circulation. With the introduction of the ACE 064 and the ACE 068 and later the 072 Jet 7 (Penumbra, Oakland, CA), the direct aspiration technique was refined further. Owing to the larger aperture of these catheters, rather than placing the catheter at the proximal extent of the thrombus and relying on the aspiration force to draw in the thrombus into the catheter, the aspiration catheter can now be advanced over the thrombus, to "ingest" the thrombus. Once

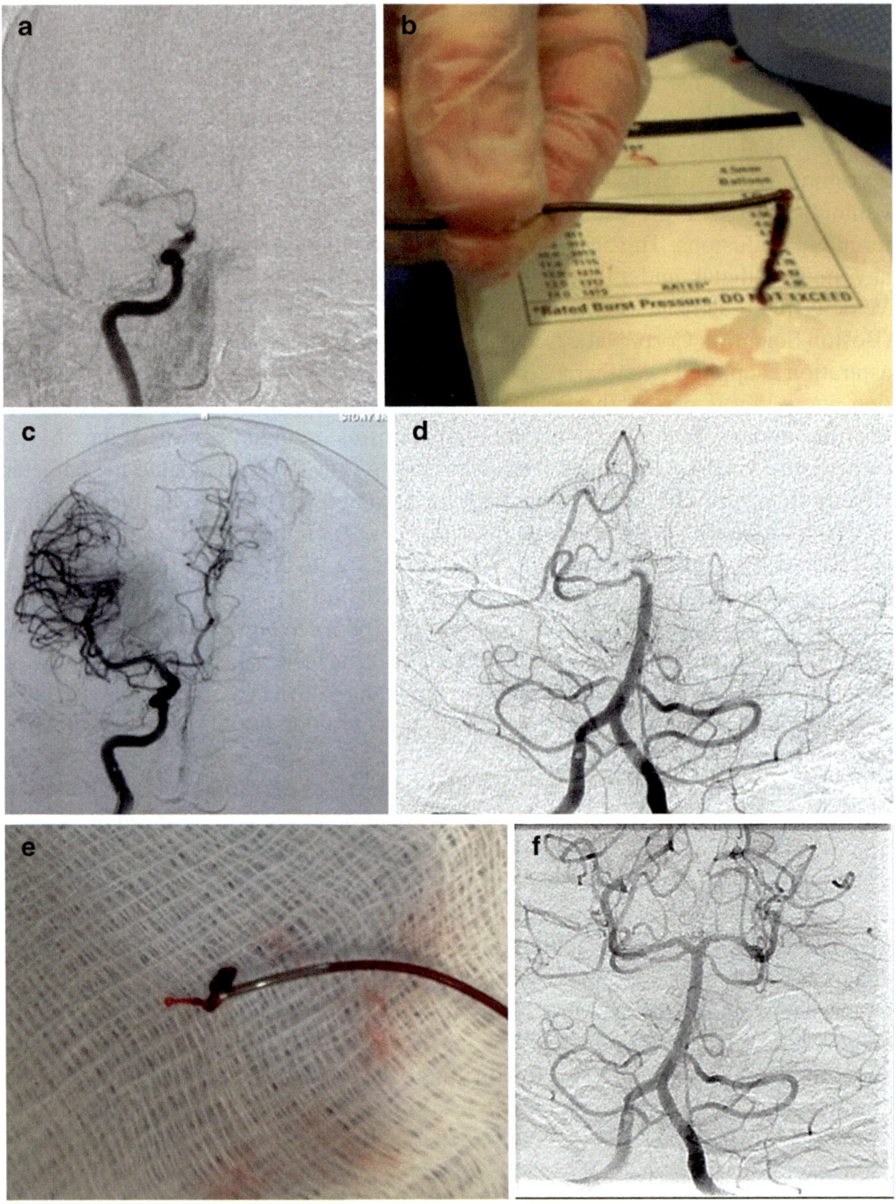

Fig. 8.3 ADAPT illustrations. Direct aspiration typically removed the thrombus en bloc, minimizing the risk of distal emboli. The largest-bore aspiration catheter that the occluded vessel will accommodate is advanced to the level of the thrombus. Aspiration is applied to engage the thrombus, which is then removed as demonstrated in the illustrations. (**a–c**) Carotid terminus occlusion recanalized in 15 minutes from groin puncture with direct aspiration thrombectomy in a single pass. (**d–f**) Basilar apex occlusion recanalized in 10 minutes with two passes of direct aspiration thrombectomy. (**g–i**) MCA bifurcation occlusion recanalized in 12 minutes with a single-pass direct aspiration. (**j–l**) MCA bifurcation occlusion recanalized in 7 minutes with a single-pass direct aspiration

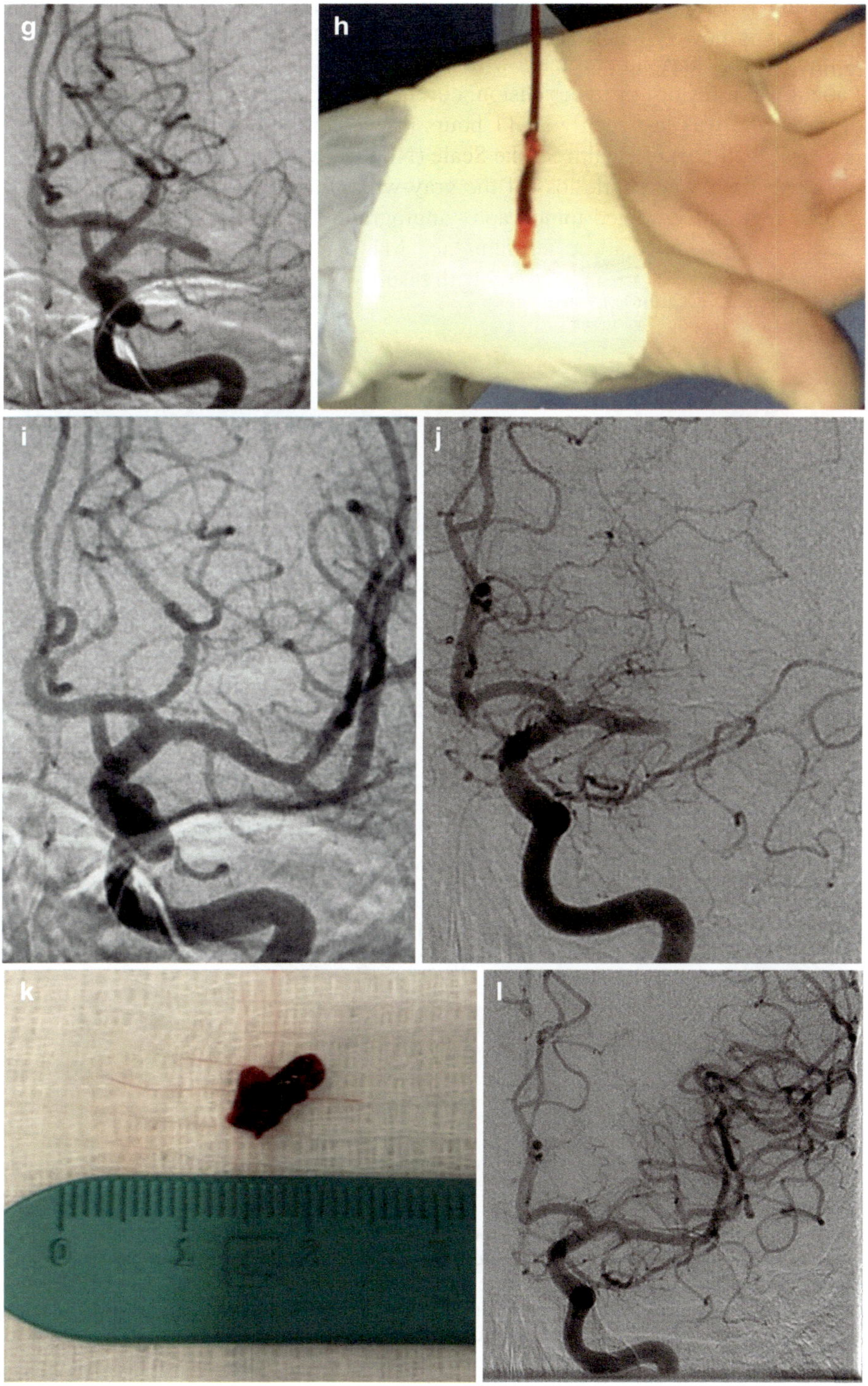

Fig. 8.3 (continued)

ingestion is achieved, aspiration then clears the lumen of the catheter, and the thrombus is now typically aspirated directly into the catheter without having to remove it (Fig. 8.4).

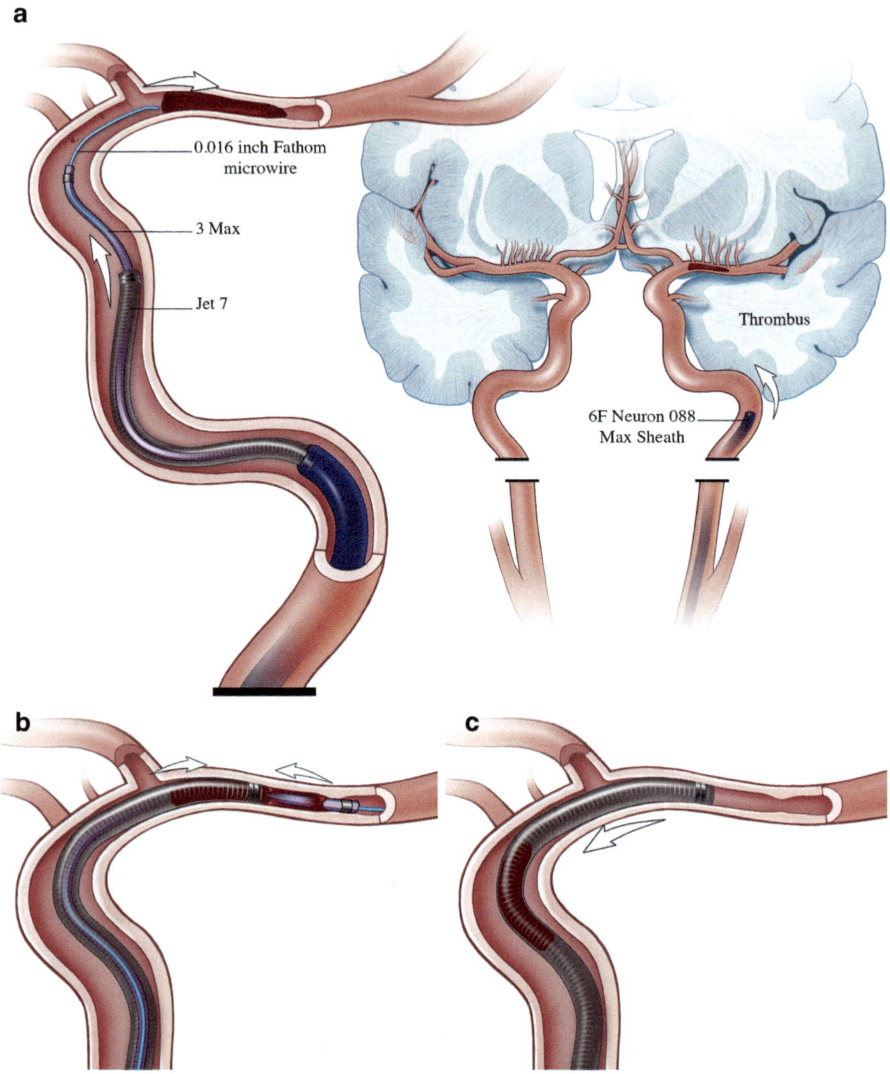

Fig. 8.4 Aspiration catheter technology has rapidly advanced. With the introduction of the ACE 068 and later 072 Jet 7 (Penumbra, Oakland, CA), the direct aspiration technique has been refined further (**a**, **b**). Owing to the larger aperture of these catheters, the aspiration catheter can now be advanced directly over the thrombus to "ingest" the thrombus under aspiration (**c**). The thrombus is now typically aspirated directly into the catheter aspiration tubing without having to remove it

Another advantage of this approach is that if aspiration alone is not successful at achieving revascularization of the occluded vessel, the Penumbra aspiration catheter can also function as a distal conduit for other devices such as a smaller 3MAX catheter for direct aspiration in more distal branches (e.g., M2, P2, or P3), stentrievers, balloons, or stents. This forms the basis of "ADAPT" (A Direct Aspiration First-Pass Technique) which is gaining in popularity. If direct aspiration attempts are unsuccessful, other attempts including SR thrombectomy can then be performed.

To date, two randomized controlled trials have compared the efficacy and adverse events using ADAPT compared to stentriever as a first-line thrombectomy technique [10, 11]. The first trial was the Contact Aspiration Versus Stentriever for Successful Revascularization (ASTER) trial [11]. This trial was done in Europe. ASTER was a randomized, open-label, blinded end-point clinical trial. Patients were randomly assigned to first-line aspiration or first-line stentriever. Total of 381 patients were randomized (174 women, mean age 69.9 years). Successful revascularization was achieved in 164 (85.4%) in the aspiration group compared to 157 (83.1%) in the stentriever group (OR 1.2 [95% CI, 0.68–2.10], $p = 0.53$). Similarly, there was no difference in adverse events, time to revascularization, or long-term functional outcome between the two groups. The second randomized trial was the Aspiration Thrombectomy Versus Stentriever Thrombectomy as First-Line Approach for Large Vessel Occlusion (COMPASS): a multicenter, randomized, open-label, blinded outcome, non-inferiority trial [10]. In COMPASS, 270 patients were enrolled (125 men, mean age 71 years). Patients who presented with anterior circulation large vessel occlusion within 6 hours of symptom onset, with a non-contrast computed tomography (CT) Alberta Stroke Program Early CT Score (ASPECTS) of 6 or more, were randomized to either direct aspiration first-pass technique ($n = 134$) or stentriever first-line thrombectomy ($n = 136$). A good functional outcome of modified Rankin Scale (mRS) of 0–2 at 90 days was achieved in 52% in the aspiration group and 67% in the stentriever group ($p = 0.0014$ for non-inferiority). While the recanalization rates were similar between the two modalities, ADAPT resulted in faster recanalization times (11 minutes). An important finding of COMPASS was a cost-benefit to direct aspiration. A pre-specified cost analysis showed that the use of aspiration first-line technique was associated with lower cost of approximately 4541 USD compared to stentriever.

The newest iteration of direct aspiration involves its application in more distal vasculature. In smaller caliber vessels, the technique can be employed with either a 4MAX or 3MAX reperfusion catheter (Penumbra Inc., Oakland, CA). In principle, the largest-bore catheter that the occluded vessel can accommodate is selected for aspiration (Fig. 8.5), with effective (TICI 2B 97.1%) and fast recanalization (mean 35.7 min) achieved safely. In addition, newer-generation catheters (Sofia 070 Microvention, Vecta 071 Stryker, Jet 7 072 Penumbra) are being introduced with potential benefits including the promise of higher first-pass success and shorter procedure times.

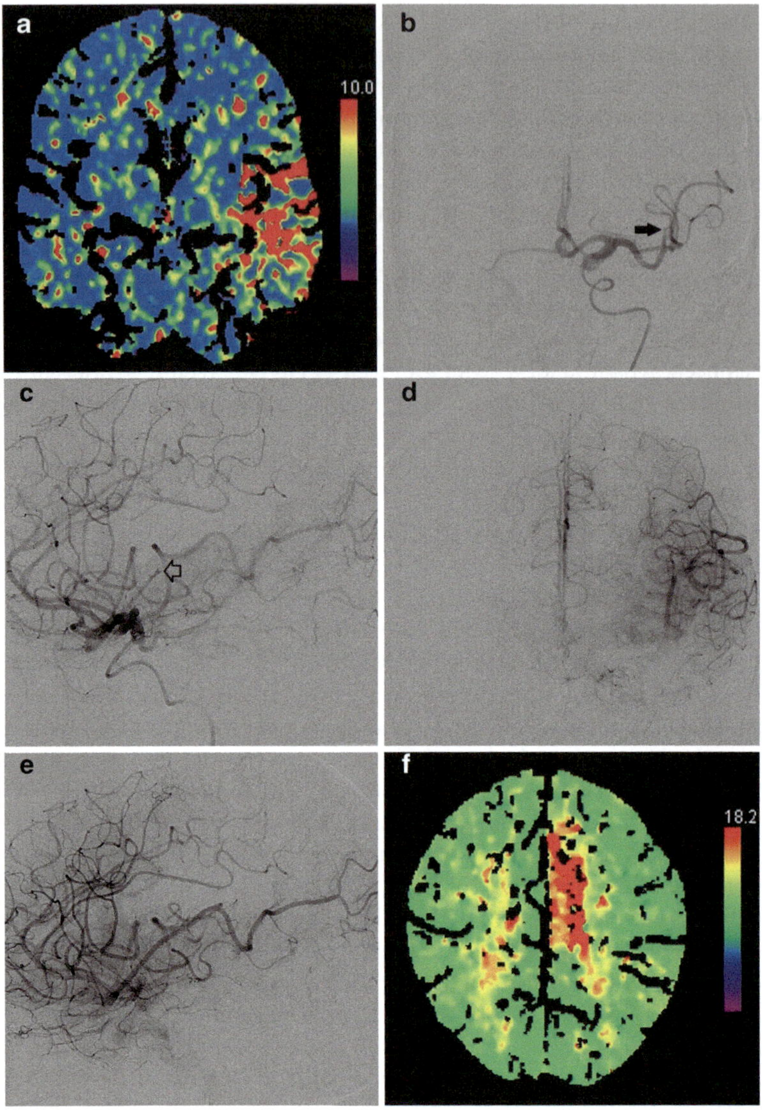

Fig. 8.5 (**a**) CT perfusion imaging demonstrating elevated mean transit time in the left frontal lobe consistent with a left M2 occlusion. (**b**) AP and (**c**) lateral projection cerebral angiogram during a left internal carotid injection demonstrating a distal M2 occlusion with no flow past the site of thrombus (arrows). (**d**) AP and (**f**) lateral projection cerebral angiogram during a left internal carotid injection following thrombectomy demonstrating resolution of M2 occlusion and opacification of distal branches. (**e**) CT perfusion imaging demonstrating elevated mean transit time consistent with a left A2 occlusion. (**f**) Lateral projection cerebral angiogram demonstrating A2 occlusion (arrow). (**g**) Post-thrombectomy lateral projection cerebral angiogram with resolution of A2 occlusion and complete opacification of distal branches. (**h**) CT perfusion imaging demonstrating elevated mean transit time in the right occipital lobe consistent with right P2 ischemia. (**i**) Cerebral angiogram with AP projection from a left vertebral artery injection demonstrating right P2 occlusion and no opacification distal to the thrombus (arrow). (**j**) Post-thrombectomy cerebral angiogram with AP projection from a left vertebral artery injection demonstrating resolution of the thrombus with opacification of the distal PCA branches (**k**)

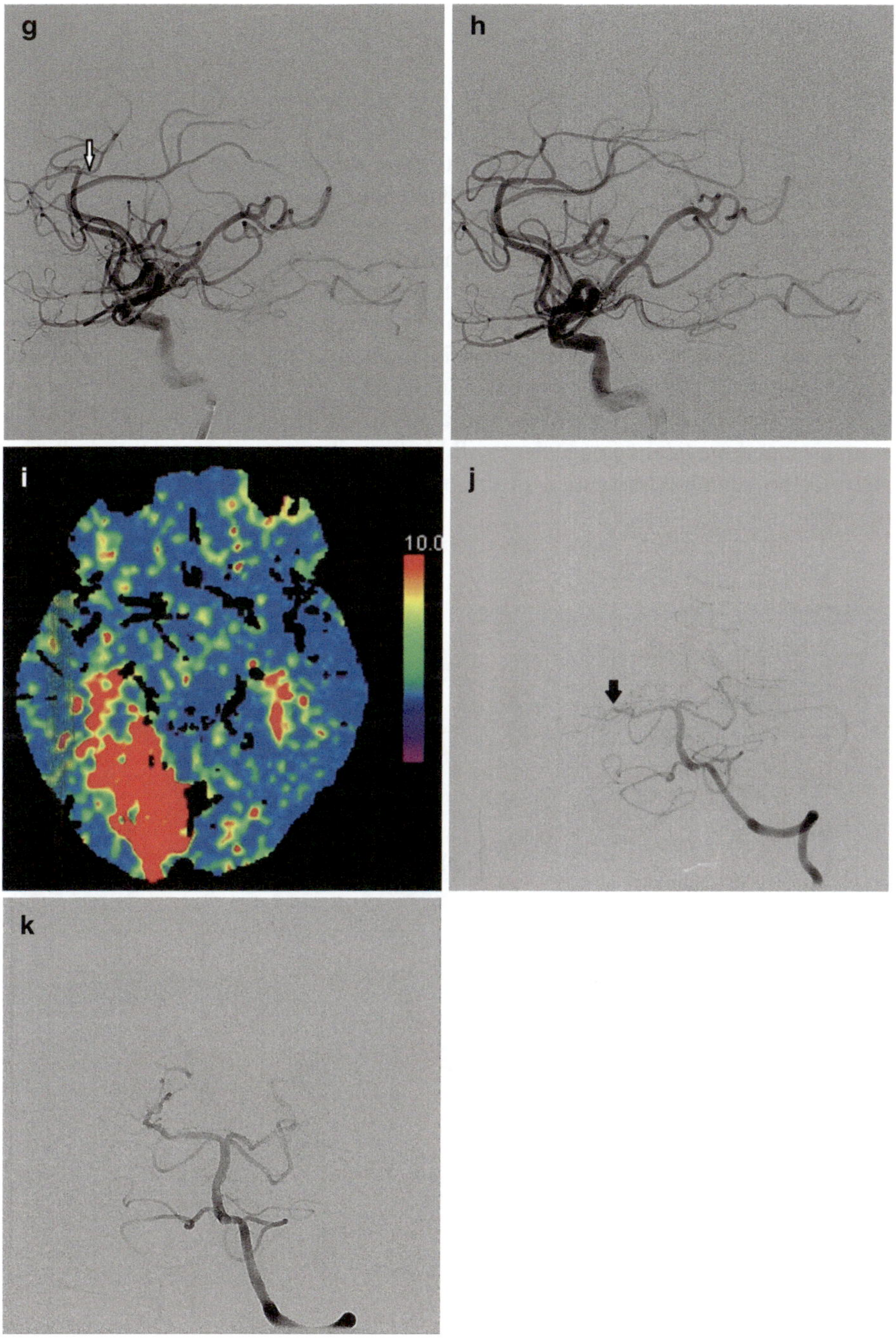

Fig. 8.5 (continued)

Conclusions

There have been rapid advances in thrombectomy devices and approaches over the past decade, from rudimentary mechanical disruption, followed by intra-arterial thrombolytic infusions, to increasingly effective thrombectomy devices (Fig. 8.6). Ongoing improvements in the devices and techniques are yielding improved angiographic and clinical outcomes, allowing patients to enjoy the best outcomes following LVO in recorded history. Direct aspiration, once considered the next-generation thrombectomy approach, is now an established methodology with two randomized controlled trials supporting its use as a frontline modality. Direct aspiration has also undergone considerable evolution and refinement, not only with the introduction of larger, more trackable catheters but also in the technique of ingesting the thrombus with the catheter prior to applying aspiration force. Device technology, selection strategies, and medical management will likely evolve in tandem, and we look forward to the continued evolution of thrombectomy approaches for acute stroke in the future.

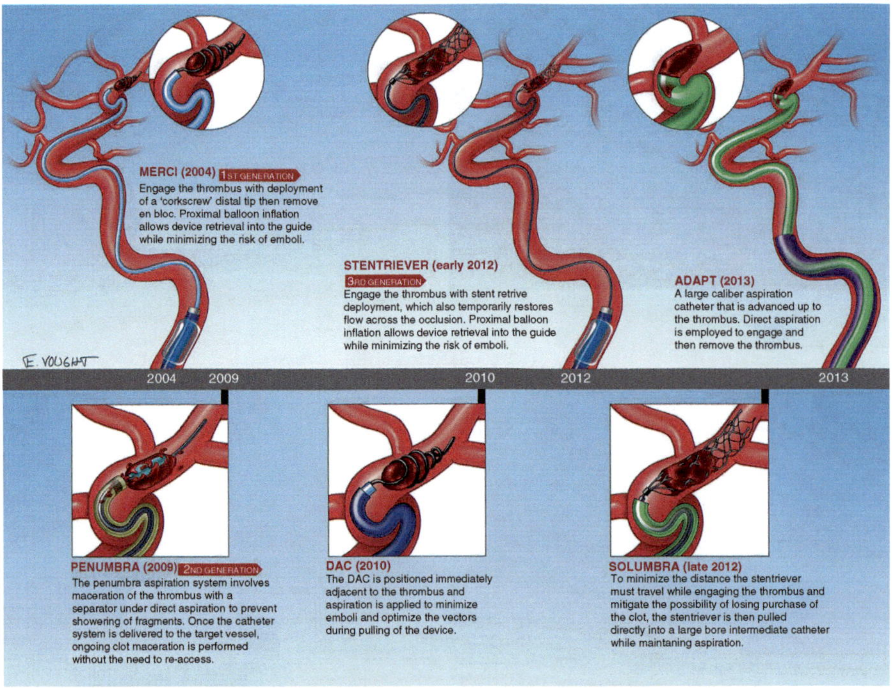

Fig. 8.6 Illustration depicting the major steps in evolution of thrombectomy devices, beginning from the first-generation concept to state-of-the-art approaches

References

1. Albers GW, et al. Thrombectomy for stroke at 6 to 16 hours with selection by perfusion imaging. N Engl J Med. 2018;378(8):708–18.
2. Nogueira RG, et al. Thrombectomy 6 to 24 hours after stroke with a mismatch between deficit and infarct. N Engl J Med. 2018;378(1):11–21.
3. Goyal M, et al. Endovascular thrombectomy after large-vessel ischaemic stroke: a meta-analysis of individual patient data from five randomised trials. Lancet. 2016;387(10029):1723–31.
4. Fransen PS, et al. MR CLEAN, a multicenter randomized clinical trial of endovascular treatment for acute ischemic stroke in the Netherlands: study protocol for a randomized controlled trial. Trials. 2014;15:343.
5. Saver JL, et al. Solitaire with the intention for thrombectomy as primary endovascular treatment for acute ischemic stroke (SWIFT PRIME) trial: protocol for a randomized, controlled, multicenter study comparing the solitaire revascularization device with IV tPA with IV tPA alone in acute ischemic stroke. Int J Stroke. 2015;10(3):439–48.
6. Turk AS, et al. Initial clinical experience with the ADAPT technique: a direct aspiration first pass technique for stroke thrombectomy. J Neurointerv Surg. 2013;6:231.
7. Alawieh A, et al. Lessons learned over more than 500 stroke thrombectomies using ADAPT with increasing aspiration catheter size. Neurosurgery. 2018;86:61.
8. Vargas J, et al. Long term experience using the ADAPT technique for the treatment of acute ischemic stroke. J Neurointerv Surg. 2017;9(5):437–41.
9. Vargas J, et al. Experience with A Direct Aspiration First Pass Technique (ADAPT) for thrombectomy in distal cerebral artery occlusions causing acute ischemic stroke. World Neurosurg. 2017;99:31–6.
10. Turk AS 3rd, et al. Aspiration thrombectomy versus stent retriever thrombectomy as first-line approach for large vessel occlusion (COMPASS): a multicentre, randomised, open label, blinded outcome, non-inferiority trial. Lancet. 2019;393(10175):998–1008.
11. Lapergue B, et al. Effect of endovascular contact aspiration vs stent retriever on revascularization in patients with acute ischemic stroke and large vessel occlusion: the ASTER randomized clinical trial. JAMA. 2017;318(5):443–52.
12. Bose A, et al. The Penumbra system: a mechanical device for the treatment of acute stroke due to thromboembolism. AJNR Am J Neuroradiol. 2008;29(7):1409–13.
13. Nogueira RG, et al. Trevo versus Merci retrievers for thrombectomy revascularisation of large vessel occlusions in acute ischaemic stroke (TREVO 2): a randomised trial. Lancet. 2012;380(9849):1231–40.
14. Tenser MS, Amar AP, Mack WJ. Mechanical thrombectomy for acute ischemic stroke using the MERCI retriever and Penumbra aspiration systems. World Neurosurg. 2011;76(6 Suppl):S16–23.
15. Smith WS. Safety of mechanical thrombectomy and intravenous tissue plasminogen activator in acute ischemic stroke. Results of the multi Mechanical Embolus Removal in Cerebral Ischemia (MERCI) trial, part I. AJNR Am J Neuroradiol. 2006;27(6):1177–82.
16. Yoo AJ, et al. The penumbra stroke system: a technical review. J Neurointerv Surg. 2012;4(3):199–205.
17. Spiotta AM, et al. The versatile distal access catheter: the Cleveland Clinic experience. Neurosurgery. 2011;68(6):1677–86; discussion 1686.
18. Turk AS 3rd, et al. An investigation of the cost and benefit of mechanical thrombectomy for endovascular treatment of acute ischemic stroke. J Neurointerv Surg. 2014;6(1):77–80.
19. Turk AS, et al. Initial clinical experience with the ADAPT technique: a direct aspiration first pass technique for stroke thrombectomy. J Neurointerv Surg. 2018;10(Suppl 1):i20–5.
20. Frei D, et al. The SPEED study: initial clinical evaluation of the Penumbra novel 054 Reperfusion Catheter. J Neurointerv Surg. 2013;5(Suppl 1):i74–6.
21. Hui FK, et al. Merci retrievers as access adjuncts for reperfusion catheters: the grappling hook technique. Neurosurgery. 2012;70(2):456–60; discussion 460.

22. Turk A, et al. Initial experience with distal guide catheter placement in the treatment of cerebrovascular disease: clinical safety and efficacy. J Neurointerv Surg. 2012;5:247.
23. Turk AS, et al. ADAPT FAST study: a direct aspiration first pass technique for acute stroke thrombectomy. J Neurointerv Surg. 2014;6(4):260–4.
24. Devlin TG, et al. The Merci retrieval system for acute stroke: the Southeast Regional Stroke Center experience. Neurocrit Care. 2007;6(1):11–21.
25. Delgado Almandoz JE, et al. Comparison of clinical outcomes in patients with acute ischemic strokes treated with mechanical thrombectomy using either Solumbra or ADAPT techniques. J Neurointerv Surg. 2016;8(11):1123–8.
26. Jovin TG, et al. Diffusion-weighted imaging or computerized tomography perfusion assessment with clinical mismatch in the triage of wake up and late presenting strokes undergoing neurointervention with Trevo (DAWN) trial methods. Int J Stroke. 2017;12(6):641–52.
27. Campbell BC, et al. Endovascular therapy for ischemic stroke with perfusion-imaging selection. N Engl J Med. 2015;372(11):1009–18.
28. Jovin TG, et al. Thrombectomy within 8 hours after symptom onset in ischemic stroke. N Engl J Med. 2015;372(24):2296–306.
29. Powers WJ, et al. 2018 guidelines for the early management of patients with acute ischemic stroke: a guideline for healthcare professionals from the American Heart Association/American Stroke Association. Stroke. 2018;49(3):e46–e110.

Chapter 9
The Stentriever-Mediated Aspiration Thrombectomy (SMAT) Technique

Benjamin Zussman, Ashutosh Jadhav, and Tudor G. Jovin

Clinical Case Vignette

A 42-year-old male with a mechanical mitral heart valve awoke with left-sided facial droop, dysarthria, left hemiparesis, and a right gaze preference. He was last seen well the night before. His NIH Stroke Scale (NIHSS) was found to be 14. His international normalized ratio (INR) was found to be sub-therapeutic at 1.2 (goal 2.5–3.5). A CT of the head did not show any hemorrhage and the Alberta Stroke Program Early CT Score (ASPECTS) was nine. A CT angiogram showed a right middle cerebral artery (MCA) M2 segment occlusion. Based on the presence of substantial mismatch between the clinical exam and radiographic imaging, he was transferred urgently from the emergency department to the neuroendovascular surgery suite for endovascular thrombectomy. Door-to-groin puncture time was 35 minutes.

Description

Radial expansion of a stent retriever device within a clot pushes thrombus circumferentially against the vessel wall and creates a functional vessel lumen that restores anterograde blood flow. The trapped thrombus becomes entangled in the stent retriever struts and removal of the stent retriever may drag the clot along with it. Aggressive suction aspiration during removal of the stent retriever performed with

B. Zussman (✉)
Wellstar Health System, Atlanta, GA, USA
e-mail: Benjamin.Zussman@wellstar.org

A. Jadhav
Barrow Neurological Institute, Phoenix, AZ, USA

T. G. Jovin
Cooper University Health Care, Camden, NJ, USA
e-mail: jovin-tudor@cooperhealth.edu

F. K. Hui et al. (eds.), *12 Strokes*, https://doi.org/10.1007/978-3-030-56857-3_9

a 60-cc syringe attached to a large-bore aspiration catheter positioned at the face of the clot facilitates thrombus capture and reduces the risk of distal embolization.

Key Principles

Rapid thrombectomy that achieves effective reperfusion requires robust catheter support, precise stent retriever deployment, and aggressive suction aspiration.

Indications

Primary treatment of acute large vessel occlusion of the proximal intracranial arteries in patients with suspected salvageable brain, second-line treatment after failure of primary stent retriever thrombectomy, primary manual aspiration, and primary pump aspiration to achieve satisfactory reperfusion.

Contraindications

Lack of salvageable brain distal to the occluded vessel. Occlusion of small, distal intracranial arteries that – in the judgment of the operator – cannot withstand the mechanical and shearing forces of stent retriever deployment and aggressive suction aspiration.

Special Considerations

There are myriad technical permutations for performing intracranial thrombectomy. The SMAT technique described herein utilizes a stent retriever, a large-bore aspiration catheter, and manual syringe suction aspiration. This technique does not use a balloon guide catheter or pump suction. There remains significant controversy regarding optimal aspiration methods. We feel that manual syringe aspiration may be more effective than pump aspiration and it is less expensive [1].

A key element of this technique relates to the diameter of the aspiration catheter. In general, the larger the catheter, the more effective the reperfusion results. For carotid terminus and proximal MCA occlusions, we attempt to use a 0.070-inch range size catheter (e.g., 0.072″ Navien, Medtronic; 0.070″ Sofia, Microvention; 0.068″ ACE, Penumbra), while for distal MCA M1 and M2 segments, we prefer a 0.060-inch range (e.g., 0.064″ or 0.060″ ACE, Penumbra; 0.060″ AXS Catalyst 6, Stryker). For smaller branches, we prefer smaller-diameter catheters (e.g., 0.050″ Sofia, Microvention; 0.054″ 5MAX and 0.041″ 4MAX, Penumbra; 0.044″ DAC, Concentric Medical).

No published, prospective randomized trials compare SMAT to other thrombectomy techniques, although the ASTER trial [2] – which showed equivalence between first-line contact aspiration and first-line stent retriever with balloon guide catheter – comments that evaluating stent retriever with local aspiration in combination versus aspiration alone versus stent retriever alone in a randomized trial is a potential area of future study. Nevertheless, the SMAT technique is probably the most effective first-line strategy to achieve reperfusion [3]. When it is used as a first-line strategy, non-randomized trials suggest it may be associated with increased likelihood of patient functional independence [4]. And, based on studies utilizing first-generation aspiration catheters only, SMAT is associated with faster access-to-reperfusion times than manual aspiration thrombectomy alone [5].

Special Instructions, Positioning, and Anesthesia

If possible, no sedation or conscious sedation should be used instead of general anesthesia. The patient's blood pressure should not be lowered unless it is greater than 200–220 mm Hg systolic, in order to support collateral flow to the ischemic penumbra. Once reperfusion is achieved, especially when reperfusion is complete or near complete (i.e., mTICI 2B or 3), the systolic blood pressure may be capped at 140 mm Hg for 12–24 hours to prevent any reperfusion injury or perioperative intracranial hemorrhage.

Step-By-Step Description of the Technique

- Obtain access using a transfemoral or transradial artery approach.
- Advance a 6 Fr or larger base (support) catheter to the aortic arch under road-map guidance.
- Advance a 5 Fr diagnostic catheter and guidewire into the target supra-aortic artery and then, typically over a glidewire, serially track the base catheter to the cervical internal carotid or distal vertebral V2 segment.
- Remove the diagnostic catheter and guidewire. Perform an angiographic run through the base catheter (Fig. 9.1) to confirm persistence of a large vessel occlusion and to delineate the relevant arterial anatomy.
- Advance a coaxial system consisting of an aspiration catheter, a microcatheter, and a microwire through the base catheter up to the cavernous internal carotid or vertebral V4 segment under road-map guidance
- Serially track the base catheter as distal as possible, typically up to the petrous or proximal cavernous internal carotid or proximal vertebral V3 segment.
- Advance the microcatheter and microwire across the clot and then gently remove the microwire.
- Aspirate blood through the microcatheter and optionally perform an angiographic run through the microcatheter to confirm that the microcatheter position is both within the vessel lumen and distal to the clot.

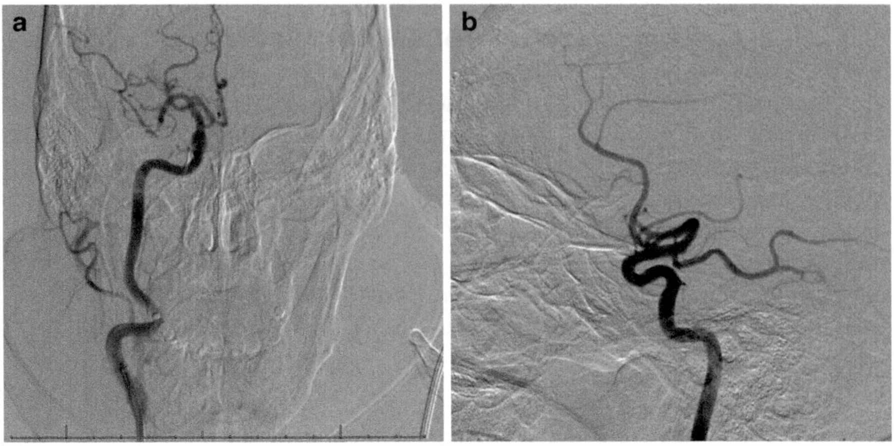

Fig. 9.1 Anteroposterior (**a**) and lateral (**b**) runs through the base catheter placed in the proximal right ICA confirm the right MCA large vessel occlusion

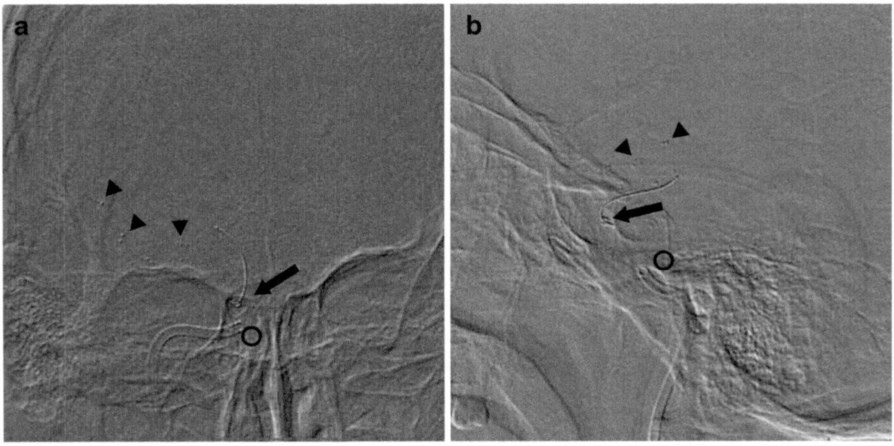

Fig. 9.2 AP (**a**) and lateral (**b**) views show the unsheathed stent retriever (*arrow heads*) in the occluded right MCA M2 division. The aspiration catheter (*arrows*) is parked proximal to the occlusion in the cavernous segment. The base catheter (*circle*) has been tracked as distally as possible in the petrous segment

- Advance the stent retriever device through the microcatheter up to its tip and then slowly unsheathe the stent retriever by withdrawing the microcatheter. During this maneuver, the aspiration catheter should remain proximal to the occlusion, generally in the cavernous internal carotid or proximal vertebral V3 segment (Fig. 9.2).
- Wait 2 minutes with the stent retriever deployed and perform a run through the aspiration catheter to assess for flow restoration.
- Advance the aspiration catheter toward the clot.
- Once the aspiration catheter reaches the proximal aspect of the clot, remove the microcatheter from the body and subsequently steadily withdraw the stent retriever into the base catheter followed by removal of the stent retriever from the body while applying continuous suction at the level of the aspiration catheter.

- Steadily withdraw the aspiration catheter while applying continuous syringe suction and assess for captured thrombus.
- Perform additional aspiration from the base catheter prior to performing a post-pass angiographic run.
- Perform additional passes until satisfactory reperfusion is achieved or until the risk of further attempts outweighs the benefit. Be certain to thoroughly flush the coaxial system and clean the stent retriever of debris before re-inserting it into the body.
- Remove the coaxial system and withdraw the base catheter to the common carotid or vertebral V2 segment. Perform control angiography (Fig. 9.3).
- Remove the base catheter and achieve hemostasis with a closure device or manual pressure.

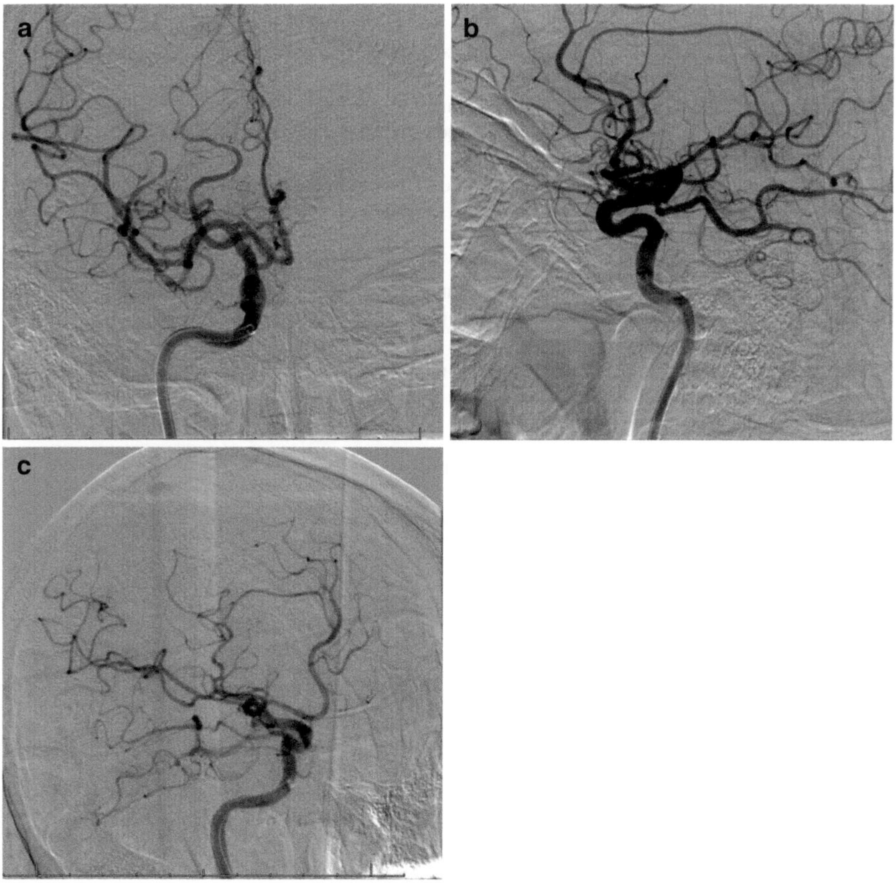

Fig. 9.3 AP (**a**), lateral (**b**), and oblique (**c**) post-thrombectomy control runs through the base catheter show revascularization of the occluded branch and modified treatment in cerebral ischemia (TICI) 2C reperfusion

Tips, Pearls, and Lessons Learned

- Advancement of the aspiration catheter to the clot face is facilitated by traction on the deployed stent retriever that functions as an anchor for the system.
- Following stent retriever removal, clot is often "corked" at the tip of the aspiration catheter, and swift, vacuum force applied using a 60-cc syringe transforms the aspiration catheter into a suction grasper that is then removed from the body while manual suction is maintained.

References

1. Gross BA, Jadhav AP, Jovin TG, Jankowitz BT. Dump the pump: manual aspiration thrombectomy (MAT) with a syringe is technically effective, expeditious, and cost-efficient. J Neurointerv Surg. 2018;10:354–7.
2. Lapergue B, et al. Effect of endovascular contact aspiration vs stent retriever on revascularization in patients with acute ischemic stroke and large vessel occlusion: the ASTER randomized clinical trial. JAMA. 2017;318:443–52.
3. Hesse AC, et al. Comparing different thrombectomy techniques in five large-volume centers: a 'real world' observational study. J. Neurointerv Surg. neurintsurg-2017-013394. 2017; https://doi.org/10.1136/neurintsurg-2017-013394.
4. Saber H, Rajah GB, Kherallah RY, Jadhav AP, Narayanan S. Comparison of the efficacy and safety of thrombectomy devices in acute stroke : a network meta-analysis of randomized trials. J Neurointerv Surg. neurintsurg-2017-013544. 2017; https://doi.org/10.1136/neurintsurg-2017-013544.
5. Jadhav AP, et al. Stent retriever-mediated manual aspiration thrombectomy for acute ischemic stroke. Interv Neurol. 2017;6:16–24.

Chapter 10
Transradial Approach for Stroke

Stephanie H. Chen, Robert M. Starke, Dileep R. Yavagal, and Eric C. Peterson

Introduction

Mechanical thrombectomy has become the standard of care for acute large vessel occlusion ischemic strokes, with time to reperfusion being the critical factor in determining outcomes [1]. Complex aortic arch and carotid arterial anatomy is associated with increased technical difficulty and thus prolonged procedural times and complication rates [1–3]. In particular for mechanical thrombectomy, patients with complex aortic arch anatomy and ICA tortuosity are associated with significant increases in puncture-to-reperfusion times [4]. A transradial approach (TRA) from the right subclavian artery offers a technically favorable trajectory in folded over arches and tortuosity (Fig. 10.1). Furthermore, as compared to TFA, TRA is associated with a greater than 60% reduction in vascular complications, overwhelming patient preference, and reduced post-procedure nursing care, hospital stay, and cost, although this is primarily from the coronary literature [5–10]. In this chapter, we review the TRA technique for mechanical thrombectomy.

Patient Selection

There are currently no formal guidelines for TRA vs. TFA approach in mechanical thrombectomy. A primary transradial approach is used for posterior circulation strokes. Due to the short, direct catheterization of the vertebral artery from the subclavian artery,

S. H. Chen (✉) · R. M. Starke · E. C. Peterson
Department of Neurosurgery, University of Miami, Miami, FL, USA
e-mail: stephanie.chen@jhsmiami.org

D. R. Yavagal
Department of Neurology, University of Miami, Miami, FL, USA

F. K. Hui et al. (eds.), *12 Strokes*, https://doi.org/10.1007/978-3-030-56857-3_10

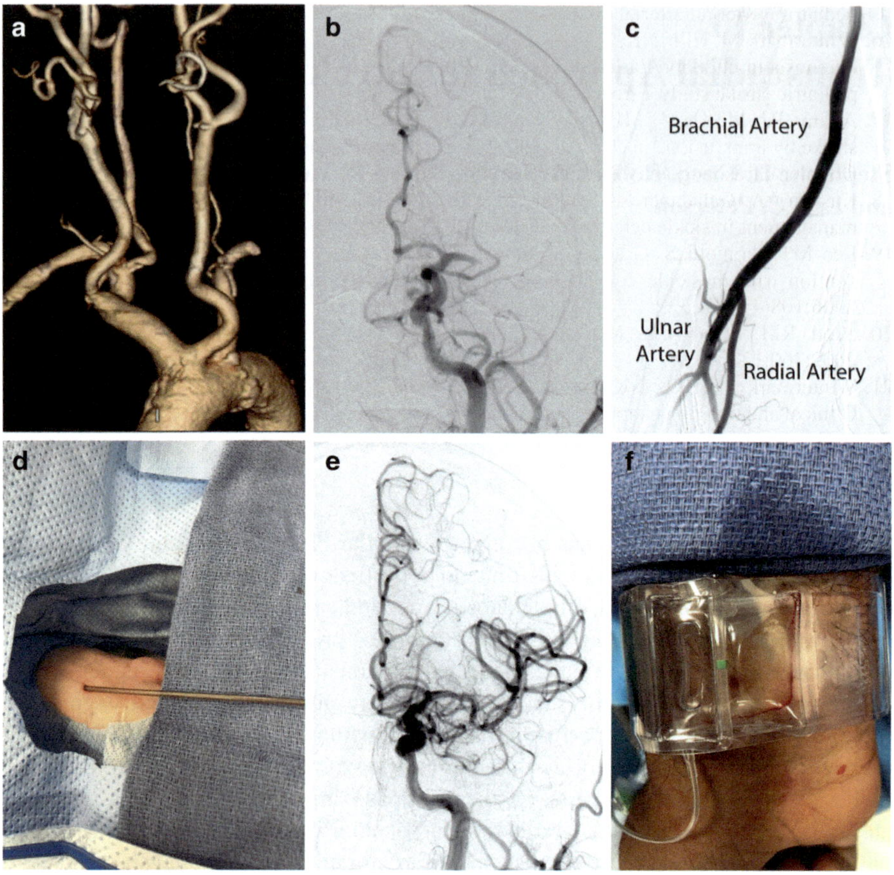

Fig. 10.1 A transradial approach (TRA) from the right subclavian artery. (**a**) CTA reconstruction revealing bovine arch more favorable for TRA. (**b**) DSA of left ICA demonstrating acute left M1 occlusion. (**c**) Right radial artery angiogram demonstrating a normal brachial bifurcation. (**d**) TRA with 0.088″ guide catheter inserted sheathless in the radial artery. (**e**) DSA s/p first pass with aspiration alone, TICI 3 recanalization. (**f**) Closure of radial artery arteriotomy with TR band

it has been shown that the transradial approach is associated with significantly shorter puncture-to-recanalization time in posterior circulation strokes (29.2 ± 17.6 min in the transradial group vs. 63.9 ± 56.7 min in the transfemoral group) [11]. For anterior circulation strokes, we evaluate the pre-procedural CTA of the head and neck including the aortic arch that is obtained in all acute stroke patients. In cases of a bovine arch variant, aortic arch type II, or aortic arch type III, an initial transradial approach is preferred. In our initial experience, we found equipoise between TRA and TFA undergoing MT with challenging vascular anatomy [12]. However, with more experience, efficiency, and equipment improvements, we anticipate improved outcomes and a transition to default radial akin to interventional cardiology. Finally, we also consider primary TRA in patients with large body habitus, previous iliac stenting or bypass, or femoral occlusion or on antiplatelets and anticoagulation.

Procedure Details

Radial Artery Access

The right radial artery is used for MT of the anterior circulation or for posterior circulation LVOS from the right vertebral artery. The left radial artery is used in cases of posterior circulation LVOS with a left dominant vertebral artery. The patient is placed supine with an extension arm board under the patient. For right radial access, the arm is positioned tightly against the hip of the patient and the palm supinated approximately 45 degrees. Towels are placed under the arm and caudal to the hand to elevate it to the level of the hip, thus creating a flat surface for the catheters to lie on. A pulse oximeter is attached to the ipsilateral hand and the radial artery area is prepped and draped in usual surgical fashion. If the patient is awake, the periarterial tissue is infiltrated with 1 cc of lidocaine (± nitroglycerin). Under ultrasound guidance, the RA is cannulated using a 20 gauge needle. A 6 or 7 French (F) transradial introducer sheath (Glidesheath Slender, Terumo, Somerset, New Jersey) is placed and a radial angiogram obtained. Prophylactic spasmolytic agents (2.5 mg verapamil, 200 μg nitroglycerin) are diluted in saline or blood and given intra-arterially through the sheath. For TRA MT, prophylactic intravenous heparin to prevent radial artery occlusion is not given, due to the potentially devastating risks of hemorrhagic conversion after stroke as compared to clinically insignificant and low radial artery occlusion rates (4%) [13].

Catheter Selection

Our preferred technique for mechanical thrombectomy is to use a 0.088″ Infinity guide catheter (Stryker Neurovascular, Kalamazoo, Michigan, USA) which is placed into the radial artery without a sheath. After access is obtained, the 7 Fr Glidesheath Slender (Terumo, Somerset, New Jersey, USA) is exchanged over a 0.035″ guidewire for the 0.088″ Infinity guide catheter with the stylet. The catheter is advanced over the wire into the subclavian artery, and the stylet and wire are then removed. A 125 cm Simmons 2 Select catheter (Penumbra, Alameda, California, USA) is navigated over a guidewire into the target ICA. A 125 cm Berenstein Select catheter is used for VA catheterization from the subclavian artery. The guide catheter is tracked over the Select catheter and thrombectomy is performed with either "Solumbra" technique or first-pass aspiration alone with the operator's aspiration catheter of preference (0.068″ or 0.071″).

Although that is our preferred approach, various other systems have been employed. In patients with posterior circulation occlusions and/or small radial arteries, a 6 F Benchmark (Penumbra, Alameda, California, USA) or Envoy DA guide catheter (Codman Neuro, Raynham, Massachusetts, USA) can be coaxially navigated into distal ICA/VA over a 125 cm Simmons 2/Berenstein Select diagnostic catheter (Penumbra, Alameda, California, USA). The stent retriever is then deployed using standard procedure and retrieved with manual aspiration of the guide catheter. For balloon guide plus stent retriever techniques, a 5 F Simmons 2 catheter is introduced into a 6 or 7 F sheath and used to navigate to the target ICA. Over an exchange-length guidewire, the sheath and catheter are removed, and a 6 or 7 F Cello balloon guide (Medtronic, Irvine, California, USA) is brought into the ICA or VA. However, this can be time-consuming and cumbersome and is thus not preferred.

At this time catheter and device selection for mechanical thrombectomy is limited for the transradial approach. A 6F and 7F system limits use of larger balloon guide catheters. Additionally, access catheters and guide systems have been designed for TFA primarily and there are no commercially available systems designed specifically for navigating the cervical and cranial vasculature via TRA at this time. Furthermore, with our preferred approach of using a 0.088″ guide catheter sheathless in the radial artery, the lack of hydrophilic coating can increase risk of severe radial artery spasm prohibiting completion of the procedure. With the advent of newer devices and technology, there is great potential for taking better advantage of the anatomical configuration of the great vessels approached via the right or left subclavian artery. Finally, it should be noted that there is a significant learning curve to the transradial approach, which should be traversed in non-emergent procedures, to prevent unnecessary prolongation of TRA MT.

Closure

Radial artery arteriotomy closure with patent hemostasis decreases risk of RAO. While RAO is rare and almost always clinically silent, RAO can preclude any future use of the radial artery for procedures or grafting. Patent hemostasis describes holding the bare amount of pressure needed to prevent bleeding. A radial armband is snugly secured 1–2 cm proximal to the point of the arteriotomy and inflated 10–15 cc. The guide catheter or sheath is removed with the band inflated. Then the band is slowly deflated until oozing is seen from the puncture site, at which time 1–2 cc of air is reintroduced to the band to achieve hemostasis. A reverse Barbeau test wherein the ulnar artery is compressed manually and the pulse oximetry wave is monitored for radial artery patency can be performed. If the RA does not appear to be patent, compression of the ulnar artery can be continued. The band is slowly deflated after 30 minutes and removed if there is no evidence of bleeding.

Case Example A. CTA reconstruction revealing bovine arch more favorable for TRA. B. DSA of left ICA demonstrating acute left M1 occlusion. C. Right radial artery angiogram demonstrating a normal brachial bifurcation. D. TRA with 0.088″ guide catheter inserted sheathless in the radial artery. E. DSA s/p first pass with aspiration alone, TICI 3 recanalization. F. Closure of radial artery arteriotomy with TR band.

*CTA = computed tomography angiogram, TRA = transradial approach, DSA = digital subtraction angiography

References

1. Goyal M, et al. Endovascular thrombectomy after large-vessel ischaemic stroke: a meta-analysis of individual patient data from five randomised trials. Lancet. 2016;387(10029):1723–31.
2. Togay-Isikay C, et al. Carotid artery tortuosity, kinking, coiling: stroke risk factor, marker, or curiosity? Acta Neurol Belg. 2005;105(2):68–72.
3. Maus V, et al. Maximizing first-pass complete reperfusion with SAVE. Clin Neuroradiol. 2018;28(3):327–38.
4. Snelling BM, et al. Unfavorable vascular anatomy is associated with increased revascularization time and worse outcome in anterior circulation thrombectomy. World Neurosurg. 2018;120:e976–83.
5. Jolly SS, et al. Radial versus femoral access for coronary angiography or intervention and the impact on major bleeding and ischemic events: a systematic review and meta-analysis of randomized trials. Am Heart J. 2009;157(1):132–40.
6. Jolly SS, et al. Radial versus femoral access for coronary angiography and intervention in patients with acute coronary syndromes (RIVAL): a randomised, parallel group, multicentre trial. Lancet. 2011;377(9775):1409–20.
7. Khanna O, et al. Radial artery catheterization for neuroendovascular procedures. Stroke. 2019;50(9):2587–90.
8. Kok MM, et al. Patient preference for radial versus femoral vascular access for elective coronary procedures: the PREVAS study. Catheter Cardiovasc Interv. 2018;91(1):17–24.
9. Kolkailah AA, et al. Transradial versus transfemoral approach for diagnostic coronary angiography and percutaneous coronary intervention in people with coronary artery disease. Cochrane Database Syst Rev. 2018;4:CD012318.
10. Mamas MA, et al. Health economic analysis of access site practice in England during changes in practice: insights from the British Cardiovascular Interventional Society. Circ Cardiovasc Qual Outcomes. 2018;11(5):e004482.
11. Maud A, et al. Transradial access results in faster skin puncture to reperfusion time than transfemoral access in posterior circulation mechanical thrombectomy. J Vasc Interv Neurol. 2019;10(3):53–7.
12. Chen SH, et al. Transradial versus transfemoral access for anterior circulation mechanical thrombectomy: comparison of technical and clinical outcomes. J Neurointerv Surg. 2019;11:874.
13. Pancholy SB, et al. Prevention of radial artery occlusion after transradial catheterization: the PROPHET-II randomized trial. JACC Cardiovasc Interv. 2016;9(19):1992–9.

Chapter 11
Thrombectomy Techniques: Remote Aspiration

David Dornbos III, Tarek Abuelem, David J. Fiorella, and Adam S. Arthur

Case Presentation

An otherwise healthy 90-year-old female presented with sudden-onset right-sided hemiplegia, right facial droop, and dysarthria, 4 hours following stroke onset. On presentation to the hospital, her National Institutes of Health Stroke Scale (NIHSS) score was 10. A non-contrast CT was unremarkable, while CT angiography revealed a left proximal supraclinoid ICA occlusion. CT-perfusion imaging identified a large penumbra and no ischemic core within the left MCA territory (Fig. 11.1). Given the compelling clinical history and radiographic findings, the patient was taken for intervention.

Angiography revealed an occlusion of the left supraclinoid ICA (Fig. 11.2). Utilizing an 8F FlowGate2 balloon-guide catheter (BGC), proximal flow was arrested and aspiration was employed with the use of a large-volume locking hand syringe in an attempt to reverse flow through and deliver the thrombus into the BGC (Fig. 11.3). Following aspiration, clot material was noted within the suction tubing, followed by arrest of backflow. Shortly thereafter, backflow resumed within the aspiration tubing. The BGC was deflated and control angiography revealed TICI 3 revascularization (Fig. 11.4). The patient had no neurological deficits after the procedure and was discharged home after a short hospital stay.

D. Dornbos III · A. S. Arthur (✉)
Department of Neurosurgery, University of Tennessee Health Sciences Center and Semmes-Murphey Clinic, Memphis, TN, USA
e-mail: aarthur@semmes-murphey.com

T. Abuelem
Department of Neurosurgery, St. Vincent Arkansas Neuroscience Institute, Little Rock, AR, USA

D. J. Fiorella
Department of Neurosurgery, Stony Brook University, Stony Brook, NY, USA

F. K. Hui et al. (eds.), *12 Strokes*, https://doi.org/10.1007/978-3-030-56857-3_11

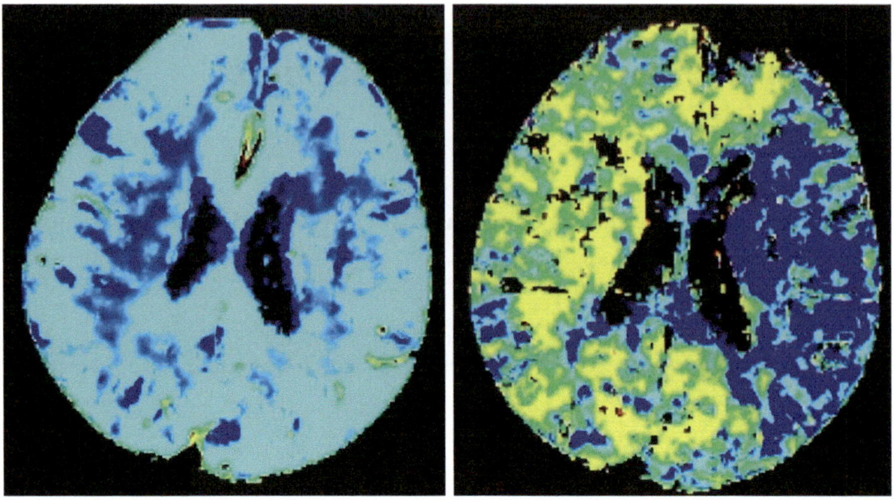

Fig. 11.1 CT perfusion imaging revealing a large area of penumbra with no ischemic core

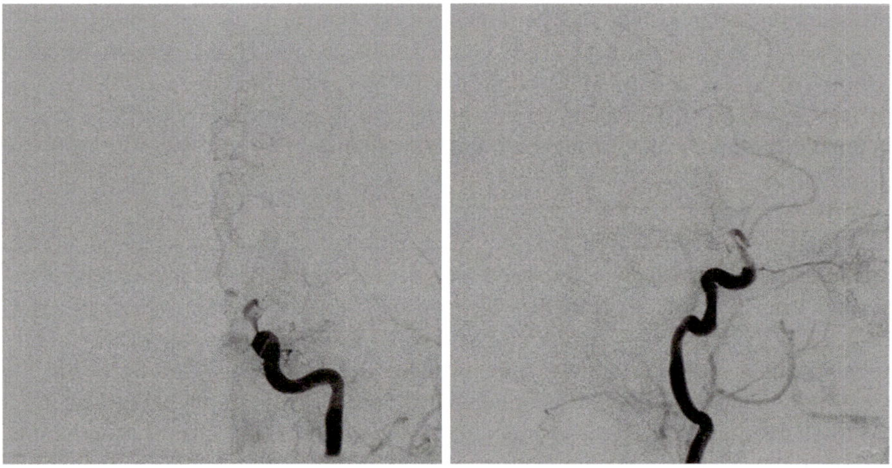

Fig. 11.2 Initial control angiography (A/P and lateral) identifying an occlusion of the supraclinoid internal carotid artery

Introduction

While the benefits of endovascular intervention for ELVO have been well established over the past several years, the optimal method of mechanical thrombectomy (MT) is largely dependent on various patient factors. Stentrievers (S-R), heavily utilized in the trials establishing the efficacy of MT, have been shown to provide excellent recanalization [1–4], either used alone or in combination with distal aspiration [5].

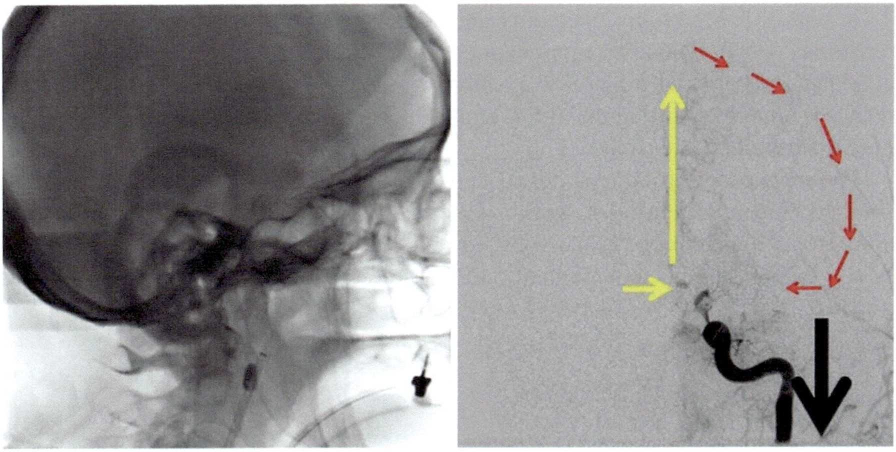

Fig. 11.3 Fluoroscopic imaging (lateral) of the inflated balloon-guide catheter and theoretical flow diagram depicting flow reversal following proximal balloon occlusion and remote aspiration

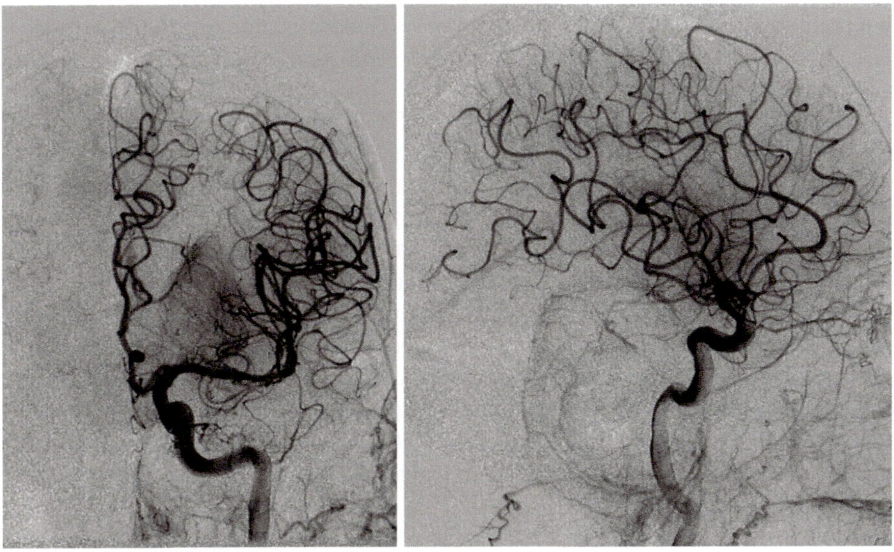

Fig. 11.4 Final control angiography (A/P and lateral) revealing TICI 3 revascularization following successful aspiration thrombectomy

Direct aspiration alone has also proven to be a highly effective and efficient means by which to achieve revascularization. In two prospective randomized controlled trials (ASTER and COMPASS), investigators found no difference in patient outcomes between the two techniques. The ADAPT technique proved to be slightly faster in both studies [6, 7]. Moreover, the direct aspiration first-pass technique (ADAPT) provided a more cost-effective method of revascularization when compared to S-R-based thrombectomy [8, 9].

In both S-R-based thrombectomy and ADAPT, the risk of embolization to new territories (ENT) remains a significant concern. With S-R thrombectomy, the available data indicate that the use of a balloon-guide catheter decreases this risk. Less data is available regarding the utility of a BGC within the context of ADAPT and its potential role in decreasing ENT.

The increasingly routine application of BGCs during thrombectomy procedures provides the opportunity to assess the potential for extraction of remote intracranial clots through aspiration on the BGC located within the proximal cervical carotid artery. We discuss this technique of remote aspiration and its application in clinical practice.

Balloon-Guide Catheters

While nearly 90% of patients experience successful recanalization following MT in most published series, less than 50% will achieve functional independence in long-term follow-up studies. The reasons underlying this discrepancy are multifactorial, but premorbid functional status, delayed time to recanalization, incomplete revascularization, showering of distal thromboemboli, and other factors likely contribute in some capacity.

Embolization of clot into a new territory (ENT) represents a major limitation of both major thrombectomy techniques. ENT is particularly detrimental as it not only results in new, previously uninvolved, vascular territory strokes, but it can also result in the occlusion of collaterals that are imperative for maintaining perfusion of the penumbra, thus worsening the extent of the presenting infarct [3, 10, 11]. Several studies have revealed new occlusions of the anterior cerebral artery in greater than 10% of patients following M1 thrombectomy, demonstrating the significant rate at which ENT occurs during these procedures [10, 11]. Furthermore, among patients with ENT, 70% experienced clinical deterioration with a mortality rate that was double that of the remainder of patients without new post-procedural emboli [11]. While these studies predominantly evaluated radiographically visible occlusions, other studies have also revealed thousands of microemboli being released during MT [12].

Balloon-guide catheters (BGCs) were brought into use in MT to ameliorate some of this secondary injury, given their ability to arrest ipsilateral flow during MT whether using stentrievers, distal aspiration, or a combination of these methods. The combination of BGCs and aspiration can potentially reverse flow in the ipsilateral vasculature. Previous in vitro studies have identified that BGCs are particularly useful to prevent fragmentation of small elastic thromboemboli during MT [13] and can decrease embolic events when used in conjunction with distal devices [14]. Furthermore, the use of BGCs has been shown to increase suction effectiveness during distal aspiration, leading to a decrease in distal thromboemboli and improved thrombectomy efficiency [12, 15–17].

Given these beneficial effects of BGCs, their use has clinically been associated with improved rates of recanalization compared to MT without a BGC [15, 18]. Utilizing BGCs and distal aspiration as adjunctive applications to stentriever thrombectomy is both safe and effective and limits new occlusions following the procedure [13, 19, 20]. BGCs have also been shown to decrease the number of thrombectomy attempts, adjunctive treatment modalities, and overall procedural times [15, 18]. Most importantly, the use of BGCs during thrombectomy has been shown to be an independent predictor of good clinical outcome [18]. While BGCs carry theoretical risks of local vascular injury and increased procedural costs, these have not been demonstrated clinically nor studied systematically.

Remote Aspiration

In addition to arresting antegrade flow during MT and subsequently reducing new distal thromboemboli in previously affected (or unaffected) vascular territories, BGCs have also been used as a standalone vehicle for primary aspiration of proximal large vessel occlusions. Following flow arrest with BGC inflation, subsequent aspiration through a large-bore BGC theoretically generates flow reversal and provides an avenue for subsequent clot retrieval. This form of remote aspiration was initially described as an adjunctive treatment to decrease overall thrombus burden prior to distal thrombectomy modalities [21].

Remote aspiration is particularly useful in cases with extensive clot burden in the proximal internal carotid artery (ICA), although consideration can be given to distal ICA and proximal anterior cerebral and middle cerebral artery occlusions, depending on collateral vasculature. Proximal aspiration through an inflated BGC for such cases has been shown to decrease overall procedural times, and it improves revascularization rates with subsequent distal MT procedures when used as an augmentation procedure for proximal anterior circulation thrombectomies [21].

More recently, remote aspiration has been used with success without the need for subsequent treatment measures. Principally used for proximal petrous to supraclinoid ICA occlusions, aspiration through a BGC can eliminate the need for intracranial catheterization [22, 23]. Remote aspiration in such a manner has proven to be especially useful for occlusive thrombi originating from a cardiogenic etiology and with a high degree of clot burden [23]. This particular technique relies on flow reversal, not just flow arrest, for clot retrieval.

Utilization of remote aspiration yields faster time to reperfusion than other thrombectomy techniques with reported mean times from puncture to reperfusion of 14 minutes [22, 23]. These faster reperfusion times are observed in spite of the additional time required to prepare the BGC prior to use. In instances where this technique is not successful, the operator simply proceeds with conventional intracranial thrombectomy techniques, using the BGC as the guiding catheter [24].

Theoretical Considerations

Remote aspiration provides a technically straightforward, fast, effective, and safe technique, which can be readily transitioned to other treatment modalities if needed. Another substantial benefit to this technique is that catheter manipulation remains entirely extracranial, eliminating potential injury posed by distal intracranial thrombectomy modalities. While the risks remain relatively small, distal thrombectomy with microwires, microcatheters, and stentrievers carries standard risks of vessel perforation, dissection, and vasospasm, all of which are minimized with the sole use of proximal aspiration on a BGC.

Patent collateral circulation is helpful in promoting reversal of flow during remote aspiration. Depending on the precise location of the occlusion, flow reversal within the carotid system can be augmented by leptomeningeal collateral support, which provides a pressure head against the distal aspect of the in situ thrombus. This phenomenon may actually assist in delivering the thrombus into the BGC. Unfortunately, robust direct collateral flow through a large posterior communicating artery or the ophthalmic artery may diminish suction effectiveness, particularly if a large component of the clot burden is distal to these vessels. In contrast, the efficacy of remote aspiration on a thrombus entirely proximal to the posterior communicating artery is likely aided by robust flow reversal with a large collateral vessel.

Methodology

A variety of devices are currently commercially available for use with the remote BGC aspiration technique. Typically, operators have used 8F (FlowGate2, Stryker, Minneapolis, MN) or 9F (Concentric, Stryker, Minneapolis, MN; Cello, Medtronic, Irvine, CA) BGCs through similarly sized femoral sheaths. The BGC is placed as distally as technically feasible and safe within the cervical segment of the carotid artery ipsilateral to the anterior circulation occlusion. Once in position and initial control angiography is performed, the operator can arrest antegrade flow by inflating the balloon on the guide catheter. Next, aspiration is applied to the BGC in order to reverse flow. This can be achieved with either a large-volume locking hand syringe or one of the commercially available aspiration pumps (e.g., Pump MAX aspiration pump, Penumbra, Alameda, California). Please note that the use of commercially available aspiration pumps for this purpose represents an off-label use.

At the point of connection to the aspiration pump, several phenomena can be observed. First, a column of blood is typically aspirated into the tubing. Observation of the tubing for obvious clot material provides an indication that thrombus is being evacuated successfully. In this setting, the operator simply monitors the tubing until a continuous free backflow of blood (without clot material) is noted. The balloon is then deflated under continuous aspiration. Once fully deflated, aspiration may be halted, and angiography can be performed to assess efficacy.

Second, after initial backflow of blood, the column becomes arrested within the tubing. This likely indicates that either thrombus has occluded the tip of the BGC or that the vessel has collapsed around the outside of the BGC. In this scenario, the balloon can be deflated under continuous aspiration. If there is thrombus at the tip of the BGC, it will remain occluded and flow within the tubing will remain arrested. In this scenario, with aspiration still connected, the BGC can be removed from the cervical target artery and withdrawn through the femoral sheath. The operator then must re-access the cervical artery with a diagnostic catheter for control angiography. This technique often yields voluminous clot material extraction and typically results in complete or substantial target artery revascularization.

On the other hand, if the BGC is deflated and flow is immediately restored through the system, this indicates that aspiration resulted in collapse of the parent artery around the orifice of the BGC. This collapse of the vessel negates the transmission of the full vacuum to the intracranial circulation, and the procedure is not successful in yielding thrombus. The operator at that point can decide to reposition the BGC (more distal position is often helpful) and attempt the maneuver again or can abandon the technique and proceed with a conventional distal aspiration or S-R-based thrombectomy procedure.

Conclusion

Numerous studies have demonstrated the ability of BGCs to increase the efficiency and extent of revascularization during traditional intracranial thrombectomy procedures. With the described technique, remote aspiration through a cervical BGC is sometimes able to not only arrest flow but also to reverse it within the affected vasculature, facilitating delivery of the thrombus into the BGC. In some circumstances, this provides a safe, efficient, and efficacious means of MT, particularly in distal cervical or proximal intracranial ICA occlusions. Furthermore, in instances where this thrombectomy modality is insufficient, the BGC provides an excellent platform for subsequent attempts. Preliminary, retrospective series have demonstrated this technique to be feasible and successful in some cases. A prospective study will be required to better define the success rate of the procedure.

References

1. Nogueira RG, Lutsep HL, Gupta R, Jovin TG, Albers GW, Walker GA, et al. Trevo versus Merci retrievers for thrombectomy revascularisation of large vessel occlusions in acute ischaemic stroke (TREVO 2): a randomised trial. Lancet. 2012;380(9849):1231–40.
2. Saver JL, Jahan R, Levy EI, Jovin TG, Baxter B, Nogueira RG, et al. Solitaire flow restoration device versus the Merci Retriever in patients with acute ischaemic stroke (SWIFT): a randomised, parallel-group, non-inferiority trial. Lancet. 2012;380(9849):1241–9.

3. Berkhemer OA, Fransen PS, Beumer D, van den Berg LA, Lingsma HF, Yoo AJ, et al. A randomized trial of intraarterial treatment for acute ischemic stroke. N Engl J Med. 2015;372(1):11–20.
4. Nogueira RG, Jadhav AP, Haussen DC, Bonafe A, Budzik RF, Bhuva P, et al. Thrombectomy 6 to 24 hours after stroke with a mismatch between deficit and infarct. N Engl J Med. 2018;378(1):11–21.
5. Humphries W, Hoit D, Doss VT, Elijovich L, Frei D, Loy D, et al. Distal aspiration with retrievable stent assisted thrombectomy for the treatment of acute ischemic stroke. J Neurointerv Surg. 2015;7(2):90–4.
6. Turk AS, Siddiqui AH, Mocco J. A comparison of direct aspiration versus stent retriever as a first approach ('COMPASS'): protocol. J Neurointerv Surg. 2018;10(10):953–7.
7. Lapergue B, Blanc R, Gory B, Labreuche J, Duhamel A, Marnat G, et al. Effect of endovascular contact aspiration vs stent retriever on revascularization in patients with acute ischemic stroke and large vessel occlusion: the ASTER randomized clinical trial. JAMA. 2017;318(5):443–52.
8. Turk AS, Frei D, Fiorella D, Mocco J, Baxter B, Siddiqui A, et al. ADAPT FAST study: a direct aspiration first pass technique for acute stroke thrombectomy. J Neurointerv Surg. 2014;6(4):260–4.
9. Turk AS, Spiotta A, Frei D, Mocco J, Baxter B, Fiorella D, et al. Initial clinical experience with the ADAPT technique: a direct aspiration first pass technique for stroke thrombectomy. J Neurointerv Surg. 2014;6(3):231–7.
10. Kurre W, Vorlaender K, Aguilar-Perez M, Schmid E, Bazner H, Henkes H. Frequency and relevance of anterior cerebral artery embolism caused by mechanical thrombectomy of middle cerebral artery occlusion. AJNR Am J Neuroradiol. 2013;34(8):1606–11.
11. Gascou G, Lobotesis K, Machi P, Maldonado I, Vendrell JF, Riquelme C, et al. Stent retrievers in acute ischemic stroke: complications and failures during the perioperative period. AJNR Am J Neuroradiol. 2014;35(4):734–40.
12. Chueh JY, Kuhn AL, Puri AS, Wilson SD, Wakhloo AK, Gounis MJ. Reduction in distal emboli with proximal flow control during mechanical thrombectomy: a quantitative in vitro study. Stroke. 2013;44(5):1396–401.
13. Chueh JY, Puri AS, Wakhloo AK, Gounis MJ. Risk of distal embolization with stent retriever thrombectomy and ADAPT. J Neurointerv Surg. 2016;8(2):197–202.
14. Gralla J, Schroth G, Remonda L, Nedeltchev K, Slotboom J, Brekenfeld C. Mechanical thrombectomy for acute ischemic stroke: thrombus-device interaction, efficiency, and complications in vivo. Stroke. 2006;37(12):3019–24.
15. Velasco A, Buerke B, Stracke CP, Berkemeyer S, Mosimann PJ, Schwindt W, et al. Comparison of a balloon guide catheter and a non-balloon guide catheter for mechanical thrombectomy. Radiology. 2016;280(1):169–76.
16. Ansel GM, Hopkins LN, Jaff MR, Rubino P, Bacharach JM, Scheinert D, et al. Safety and effectiveness of the INVATEC MO.MA proximal cerebral protection device during carotid artery stenting: results from the ARMOUR pivotal trial. Catheter Cardiovasc Interv. 2010;76(1):1–8.
17. Chartrain AG, Awad AJ, Mascitelli JR, Shoirah H, Oxley TJ, Feng R, et al. Novel and emerging technologies for endovascular thrombectomy. Neurosurg Focus. 2017;42(4):E12.
18. Nguyen TN, Malisch T, Castonguay AC, Gupta R, Sun CH, Martin CO, et al. Balloon guide catheter improves revascularization and clinical outcomes with the Solitaire device: analysis of the North American Solitaire Acute Stroke Registry. Stroke. 2014;45(1):141–5.
19. Matsumoto H, Nishiyama H, Tetsuo Y, Takemoto H, Nakao N. Initial clinical experience using the two-stage aspiration technique (TSAT) with proximal flow arrest by a balloon guiding catheter for acute ischemic stroke of the anterior circulation. J Neurointerv Surg. 2017;9(12):1160–5.
20. Stampfl S, Pfaff J, Herweh C, Pham M, Schieber S, Ringleb PA, et al. Combined proximal balloon occlusion and distal aspiration: a new approach to prevent distal embolization during neurothrombectomy. J Neurointerv Surg. 2017;9(4):346–51.

21. Kim YW, Kang DH, Hwang YH, Park J, Kim YS. Efficacy of proximal aspiration thrombectomy for using balloon-tipped guide catheter in acute intracranial internal carotid artery occlusion. J Korean Neurosurg Soc. 2016;59(4):379–84.
22. Haussen DC, Bouslama M, Grossberg JA, Nogueira RG. Remote aspiration thrombectomy in large vessel acute ischemic stroke. J Neurointerv Surg. 2017;9(3):250–2.
23. Okamura A, Kuroki K, Shinagawa K, Yamada N. Simple aspiration with balloon catheter technique (simple ABC technique) against proximal internal carotid artery occlusion in cases of cardiogenic cerebral embolism. Interv Neuroradiol. 2018;24(3):317–21.
24. Demerath T, Reinhard M, Elsheikh S, Keuler A, Urbach H, Meckel S. Balloon guide catheter in complex anterior circulation mechanical thrombectomy: beyond proximal occlusion and flow reversal. Clin Neuroradiol. 2016;26(3):369–73.

Part III
Core

Chapter 12
Endovascular Therapy for Middle Cerebral Artery Occlusions

Ansaar T. Rai

Introduction

The middle cerebral artery is the most common large vessel occlusion presenting with acute ischemic stroke. Traditionally the MCA segments are numerically labeled from its origin to its first-, second-, and third-order branches. This numerical classification is based on anatomical landmarks primarily for microsurgical planning. From a neurological perspective, the more proximal the occlusion, the larger the deficit. However, due to variations in anatomy, it is possible that an MCA branch is functionally dominant affecting a large part of the brain demonstrable by cerebral perfusion and the severity of the clinical deficit.

The mean length and diameter of the M1 segment (from the origin to branching) was measured as 22.5 ± 8 mm (95% CI 20.9–24.1) and 3.1 ± 0.4 mm (95% CI 3–3.1) in one study using CT angiography and a vascular post-processing software. The study also found that the MCA diameter marginally increased with age (>60 versus 40–60). This information can be pertinent when positioning large-bore catheters in the MCA. It is important to know not only the inner but also the outer diameter of a catheter that may be placed in a small blood vessel. Typically, these sizes are listed on the packaging. The units in which these diameters are reported can be in French, millimeters, or inches. One French equals exactly 1/3 mm or 0.013 inches. Conversely 1 mm is equal to 3F. So, for example, an intermediate catheter with an inner diameter of 5.5F (0.072 inches or 1.83 mm) may have an outer diameter of 6.5F (0.085 inches or 2.17 mm). A 3-mm MCA can potentially accommodate a 9F (outer diameter) catheter; obviously at this size it will be approaching the lumen diameter and can be dangerous. Navigation of such a large catheter may also

A. T. Rai (✉)
Department of Neuroradiology, West Virginia University School of Medicine, Morgantown, WV, USA

F. K. Hui et al. (eds.), *12 Strokes*, https://doi.org/10.1007/978-3-030-56857-3_12

be challenging. However, as the quest to develop large-bore catheters for boosting aspiration increases, we will likely see and use catheters with outer diameter up to or slightly larger than 8F (0.1 inches or 2.67 mm) – which will be just under the average lumen diameter of the middle cerebral artery. It is important to note that an occluded MCA with a thrombus may be less receptive to the larger catheters and diseased vessels with less compliance may be less tolerant to stretching, increasing the risk of vessel injury.

The critical component in treatment planning for a stroke intervention is access. Stable and distal access can make the difference between a speedy recanalization versus a prolonged frustrating procedure. Vascular imaging from the aortic arch to the cranial vertex outlays the roadmap and helps plan access, for example, multi-axial catheter constructs in tortuous access.

The current mechanical thrombectomy techniques generally involve retrieval devices, aspiration catheter, or increasingly a combination of both. In clinical trials no one technique has been shown to be clearly superior to another. The use of balloon guide catheters has been associated with improved recanalization and outcomes presumably by reducing clot fragmentation and distal emboli. The general current consensus is that some form of flow arrest and flow reversal aids in recanalization with or without a retrieval device.

Over the past decade, refinement in devices, access catheters, and techniques has steadily improved recanalization rates. With high recanalization rates reported in clinical trials, the current and future goals of measuring the efficacy of a technique are not only procedural recanalization but complete recanalization in the first pass. As such technical factors such as stable access, flow reversal, and ability to capture and retain the clot are important determinants of efficient recanalization. Peri-procedural factors such as general anesthesia have been the topic of much debate, and some studies have shown them to have a negative impact on outcomes; however, others show no effect. Generally, if there is maintenance of blood pressure parameters and efficiency in administering intubation, then the negative effects are mitigated. Like in other aspects of intervention planning, a case-by-case approach over a dogmatic paradigm will give the most tailored patient care.

Case – 1 (Primary Aspiration of an M1 Occlusion)

Presentation

A 56-year-old man presented 9 hours after onset of acute left-sided hemiplegia with an NIHSS of 24. The patient had a history of uncontrolled atrial fibrillation, hyperlipidemia, and previous history of congestive heart failure. CT imaging (Fig. 12.1) confirmed a right MCA occlusion at the M1 origin. The non-contrast head CT did not show any significant early ischemic changes with an ASPECTS of 9. The perfusion parameters showed an elevated mean transit time (MTT) and time to peak (TTP) involving the right hemisphere in the MCA distribution. Interestingly, the

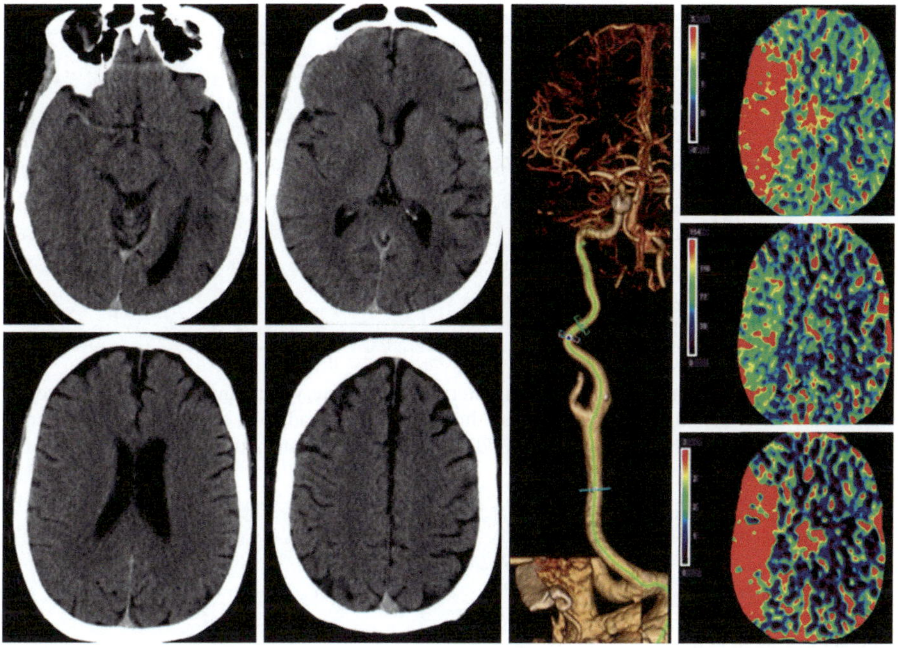

Fig. 12.1 The non-contrast component of the CT examination shows a favorable ASPECTS of 9. The volume-rendered 3D image in the center shows a mid-right M1 occlusion. The last column shows from top to bottom: MTT, CBF, and CBV. Notice the elevated CBV in this case

cerebral blood flow (CBF) and cerebral blood volume (CBV) were elevated which, in the absence of any non-contrast CT ischemic changes, are likely related to robust cerebral autoregulation and good collaterals.

Intervention and Outcome

The procedure was performed under conscious sedation. Access was via an 8F sheath in the right common femoral artery. A 90-cm Infinity guide catheter was advanced to the mid-cervical ICA on the right. An angiogram confirmed the right M1 occlusion and also showed good pial collaterals from the right anterior cerebral artery reaching the proximal M2 branches in a retrograde fashion (Fig. 12.2). A 6F (0.079 inches, 2 mm) intermediate catheter with an inner diameter of 4.6F (0.06, 1.53 mm) was advanced through the guide catheter over a 0.027″ microcatheter and a 0.014″ microwire into the proximal MCA. The microwire and microcatheter were removed. Manual aspiration through the intermediate catheter was performed with a 60-cc syringe which did not yield any aspirate (Fig. 12.3). The syringe was locked in aspiration and gently withdrawn out. The catheter was flushed on the table yielding clot material. Angiogram following aspiration

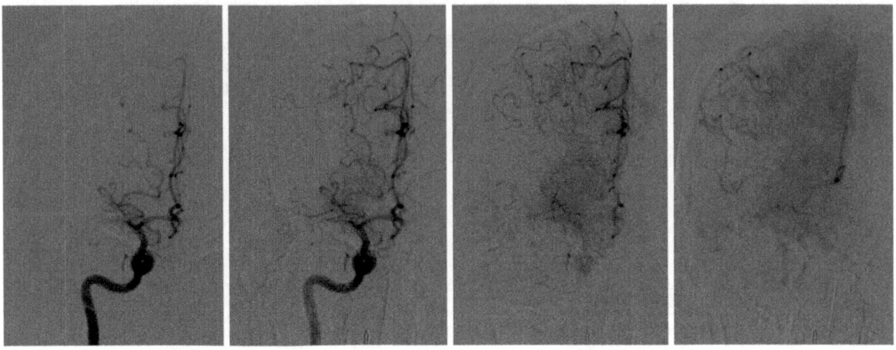

Fig. 12.2 A selective injection of the right internal carotid artery with an anteroposterior projection in early arterial and late capillary phase shows good retrograde pial collaterals from the anterior cerebral artery reaching the Sylvian middle cerebral artery distribution

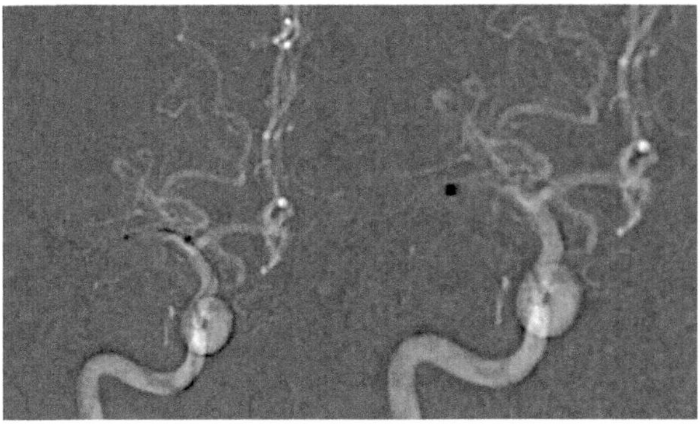

Fig. 12.3 The first picture shows placement of the microcatheter in the mid-M1 segment followed by the intermediate catheter as shown in the second picture

showed recanalization of the M1 segment and the M2 divisions. A prefrontal branch of the inferior division demonstrated persistent occlusion; however, because of the small size of the blood vessel and relatively distal occlusion, this was not treated (Fig. 12.4). There was good capillary perfusion over the right hemisphere (Fig. 12.5). A non-contrast CT scan performed at 48 hours showed small patchy infarcts in the right inferior division but no major vascular territory infarction. The patient had significant clinical improvement (NIHSS returning to 6) over the 72 hours post-procedure.

Discussion

Even though this patient presented fairly late after symptom onset, his imaging especially the CT perfusion was interesting in that it showed an elevated cerebral blood volume and blood flow compared to the normal side. In this patient this was likely related to good collaterals and robust cerebral vascular autoregulation without

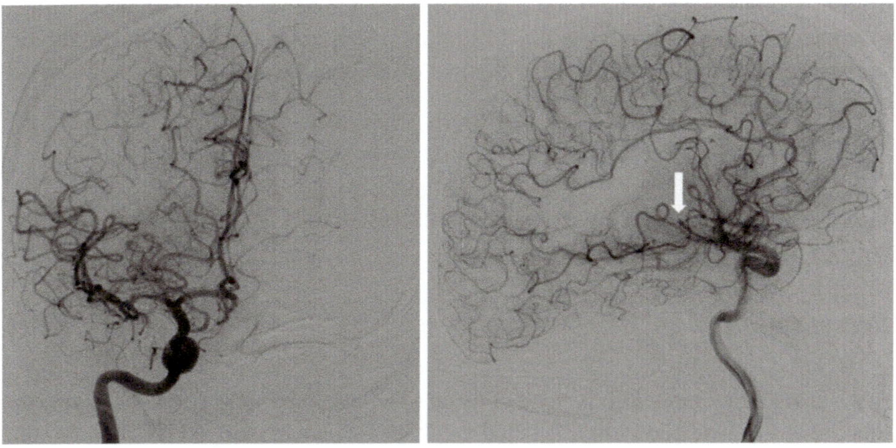

Fig. 12.4 An AP and lateral projection from a right internal carotid injection shows recanalization of the right middle cerebral artery. Persistent occlusion of a prefrontal branch is demonstrated by an arrow on the lateral projection

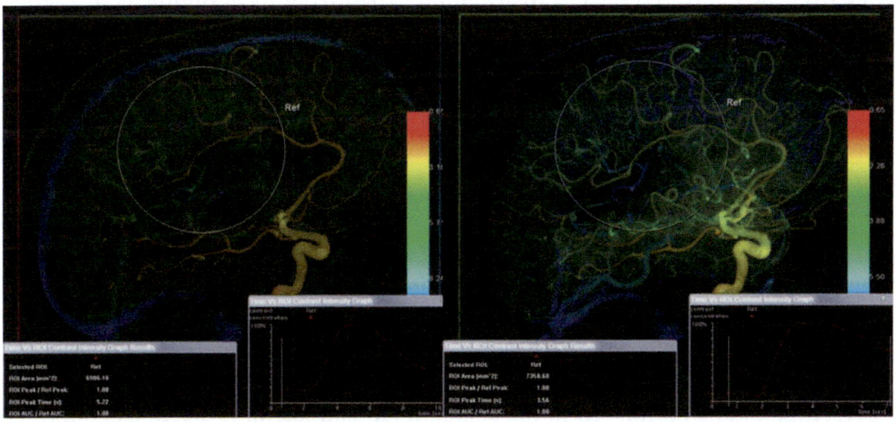

Fig. 12.5 Pre- and post-parenchymal perfusion maps created from the lateral angiogram show significantly improved perfusion in the right middle cerebral artery distribution

any ischemic changes on the non-contrast brain CT. The second discussion point is whether the small prefrontal branch arising from the inferior division should have been recanalized. Treatment options would have been placement of a stent retriever or a small-bore aspiration catheter. The concern with stent retrievers in the small branch at an angulation would be vessel injury or spasm and proximal migration of the clot potentially occluding the inferior division or even the MCA. A small-bore aspiration catheter and clot ingestion could be a safer option possibly with less risk of proximal clot migration. A third option would be the administration of local intra-arterial thrombolytics such as r-tPA through a microcatheter. The typical dose used in a small artery is between 2 and 6 mg administered in 2-ml aliquots diluted in saline and administered over 10–15 minutes. Availability of newer thrombolytics such as tenecteplase may increase the use of adjunct thrombolytics when considered safe.

Case – 2 (Stent Retriever and Intermediate Catheter for a Low NIHSS M1 Occlusion)

Presentation

A 77-year-old woman with history of atrial fibrillation, hypertension, and hyperlipidemia was transferred with left-sided weakness. She had stopped her anticoagulation (apixaban) for 3 months. At arrival, the patient was 9 hours after symptom onset and had an NIHSS of 5. Imaging work-up confirmed a right M1 occlusion (Fig. 12.6). Time-resolved CT angiography showed good collaterals to the MCA distribution. Perfusion parameters showed increased time to peak and mean transit time over the entire right MCA distribution. Apart from focal diminished cerebral blood volume at the right basal ganglia, there was no core infarct on CBV. Due to the large tissue at risk, it was decided to intervene despite the patient's relatively low NIHSS.

Intervention and Outcome

The procedure was performed under conscious sedation. An 8F sheath was placed in the right common femoral artery and an 8F (0.088″) guide catheter was navigated over a diagnostic catheter into the right proximal cervical internal carotid artery. The guide catheter was positioned just proximal to a loop in the cervical ICA. Angiograms performed in the standard AP and lateral projections confirmed the right M1 occlusion at the origin with good pial collaterals from the anterior cerebral artery up to the proximal MCA branches in the Sylvian fissure (Fig. 12.7). A construct of a 125-cm 6.3F (OD 0.083″, ID 0.070″) intermediate catheter and a 150-cm 2.9F (OD 0.038″, ID 0.027″) microcatheter was navigated over a 0.014 microwire through the guide catheter into the cervical and intracranial internal carotid artery in a tandem fashion. The microwire was advanced beyond the occluded MCA into the inferior division; this was followed by the microcatheter. The position of the microcatheter was confirmed by a very gently puff of contrast. A 6x25-mm stent retriever was advanced through the microcatheter and deployed from the proximal inferior division to the internal carotid artery terminus centering

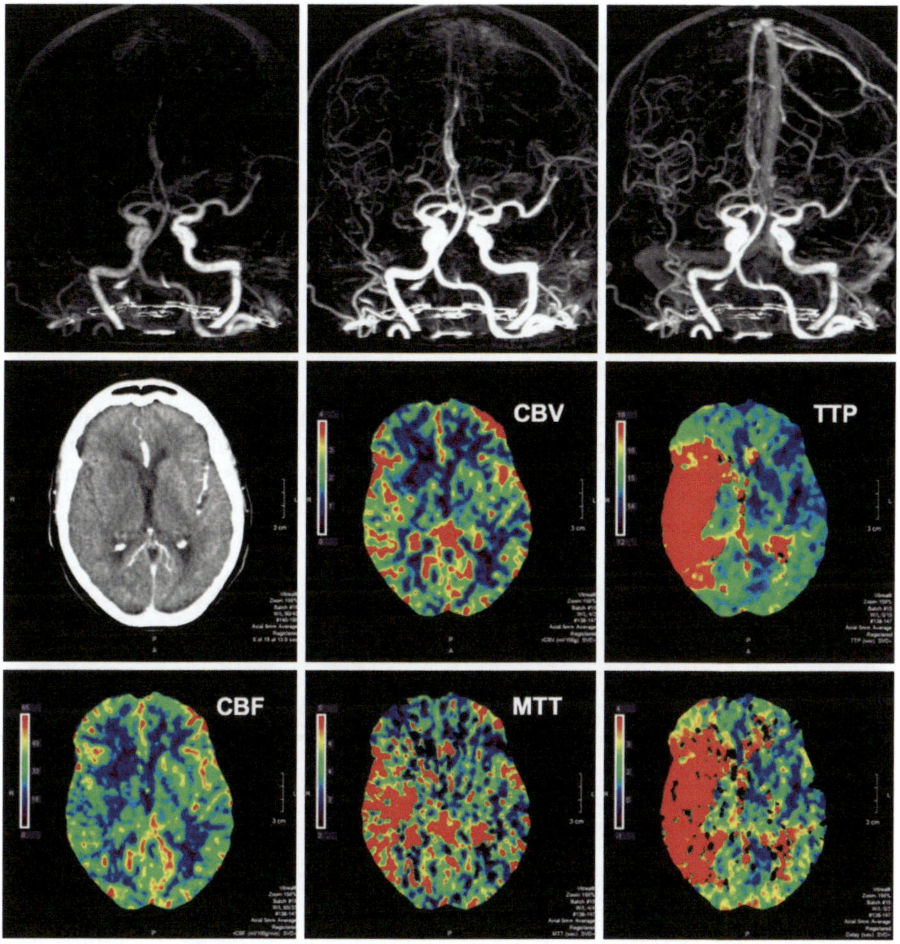

Fig. 12.6 Top row shows images from time-resolved CTA with a right M1 occlusion at the origin. The bottom two rows show elevated TTP and MTT with slightly reduced CBF but mostly preserved CBV

the device over the occluded MCA (Fig. 12.8). An injection performed through the intermediate catheter showed some recanalization through the deployed stent retriever with flow past the occlusion into the inferior division branches. Keeping the stent retriever in place, the microcatheter was carefully removed leaving the stent retriever inside the intermediate catheter which was advanced up to the ICA terminus and connected to pump aspiration. The stent retriever was then slowly withdrawn toward the intermediate catheter under constant aspiration. About

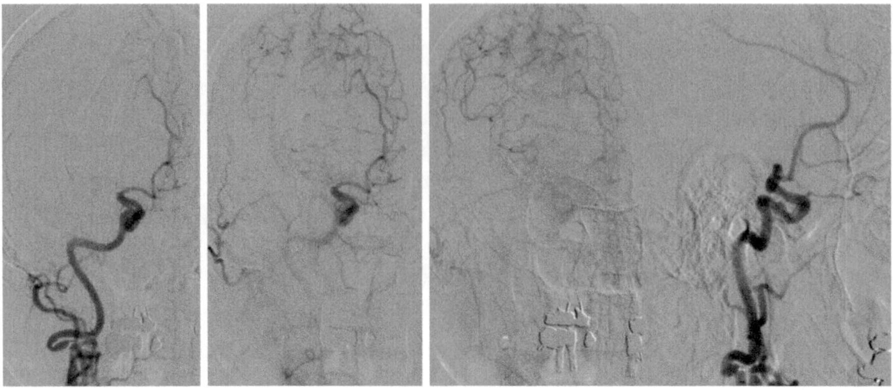

Fig. 12.7 The first three images are from a right internal carotid artery injection showing an M1 occlusion at the origin with good pial collaterals from the anterior cerebral artery. The last image is a lateral projection showing the M1 occlusion in the early arterial phase. Notice position of the guide catheter proximal to a bend in the cervical ICA

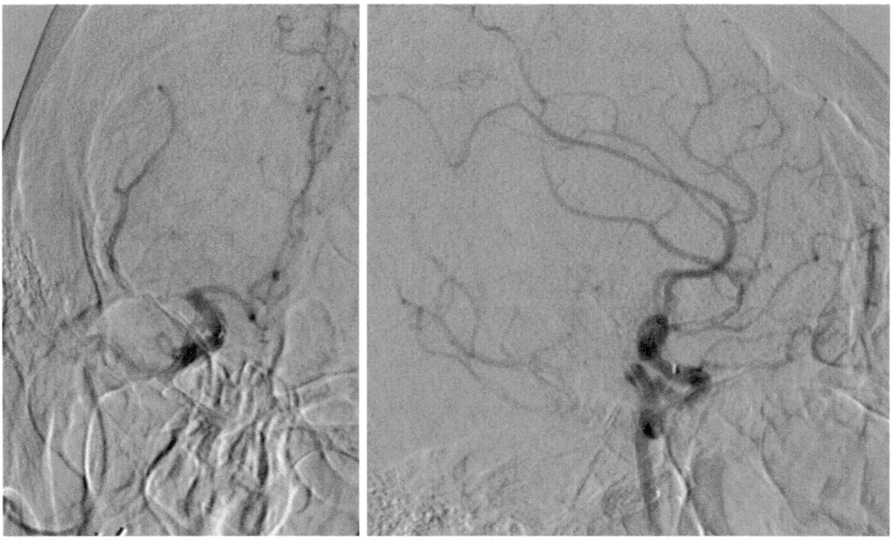

Fig. 12.8 The AP and lateral angiograms show recanalization of the middle cerebral artery with the stent retriever in place. The intermediate catheter is in the communicating segment of the internal carotid artery and the microcatheter has been removed

one-third of the device was withdrawn into the intermediate catheter with cessation of aspirate; at this time these were removed in tandem. An angiogram performed through the 8F guide catheter showed complete recanalization of the middle cerebral artery and its branches (Fig. 12.9).

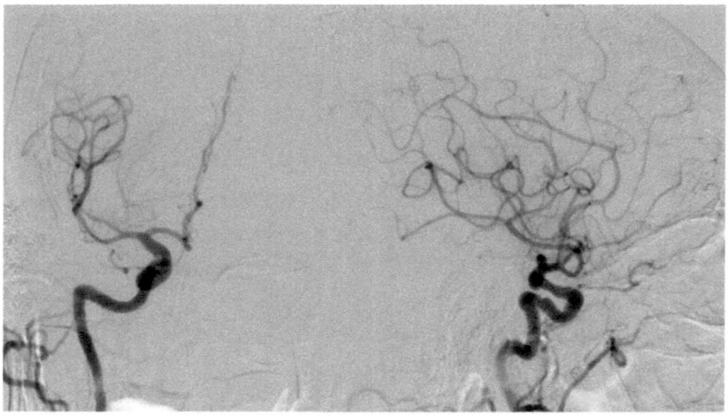

Fig. 12.9 Post-thrombectomy AP and lateral angiogram shows complete recanalization

Discussion

The interesting feature of the case is the late presentation combined with the low NIHSS. The decision to treat was not based on one factor but a combination of her functional and independent status prior to the stroke and the large tissue at risk on parametric perfusion imaging. The patient had good collaterals explaining her minor neurological symptoms and low NIHSS despite a completely occluded middle cerebral artery and a large perfusion deficit. The patient had arrived late in the evening and there was concern of neurological worsening with any hypotensive episode in the middle of the night. In cases such as these, the trend is moving toward earlier intervention than relying on medical management to sustain and preserve the collateral circulation.

Case – 3 (Stent Retriever and Intermediate Catheter for M1 Occlusion in Tortuous Cervical ICA)

Presentation

An 88-year-old woman with atrial fibrillation and hypertension but not on anticoagulation fell in the bathroom and was found by her son. She presented with profound right hemiplegia and aphasia with an NIHSS of 28. Prior to this presentation, she lived independently performing all her activities of daily living. She presented about 3 and a half hours after symptom onset and was given intravenous r-tPA on arrival. Imaging at presentation showed a left M1 occlusion with favorable parameters on perfusion and non-contrast CT (Figs. 12.10 and 12.11). The patient was taken for endovascular treatment.

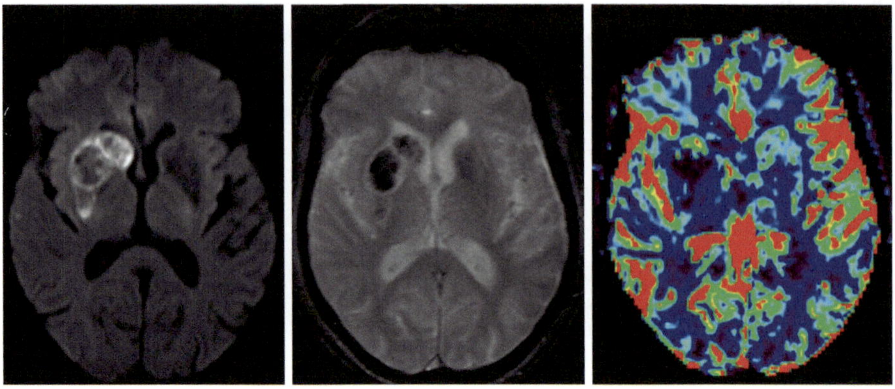

Fig. 12.10 The 24-hour MRI shows focal basal ganglia infarct (first image – diffusion-weighted image) with petechial hemorrhage (second image – gradient echo) corresponding to the pre-procedure focal CBV core. The last image shows normalization of the CBF

Intervention and Outcome

The procedure was performed under conscious sedation. Femoral access was established with an 8F sheath. A 90-cm 8F (0.88″) guide catheter was advanced over a 5F diagnostic catheter into the left common carotid artery just proximal to its bifurcation. Angiography performed through the guide catheter confirmed the left MCA occlusion with good pial collateral (Fig. 12.12).

Because of the cervical ICA tortuosity observed on the CT angiography, a 6F (OD 0.079″, ID 0.060″) was advanced over a 150-cm 2.9F (OD 0.038″, ID 0.027″) microcatheter and a 0.014″ microwire through the cervical ICA into the intracranial circulation. The 8F guide catheter was then advanced over this construct into the proximal cervical ICA past the carotid bulb. The microcatheter over the wire was then advanced into the left inferior division and the position was confirmed with small puff of contrast. A 6 × 25-mm stent retriever was then deployed through the microcatheter with a push and pull technique from the inferior M2 division to proximal to the M1 origin. With the stent retriever in place, the microcatheter was removed allowing the intermediate catheter to advance up to the M1 origin. Angiography through the intermediate catheter showed recanalization through the stent retriever (Fig. 12.13).

Under vigorous manual aspiration from the intermediate catheter with a 60-cc syringe, the stent retriever was gently partially withdrawn into the intermediate catheter. Once there was loss of aspiration, the syringe suction was locked in place using a one-way valve switch. The partially withdrawn stent retriever and the intermediate catheter were then removed in tandem through the guide catheter. Post-first-pass angiography showed minimal recanalization through the occluded MCA (Fig. 12.14).

The procedure was repeated a second time without the intermediate catheter with just the microcatheter which was navigated over a 0.014 microwire through the 8F guide catheter past the occluded MCA. However, this time the wire was advanced

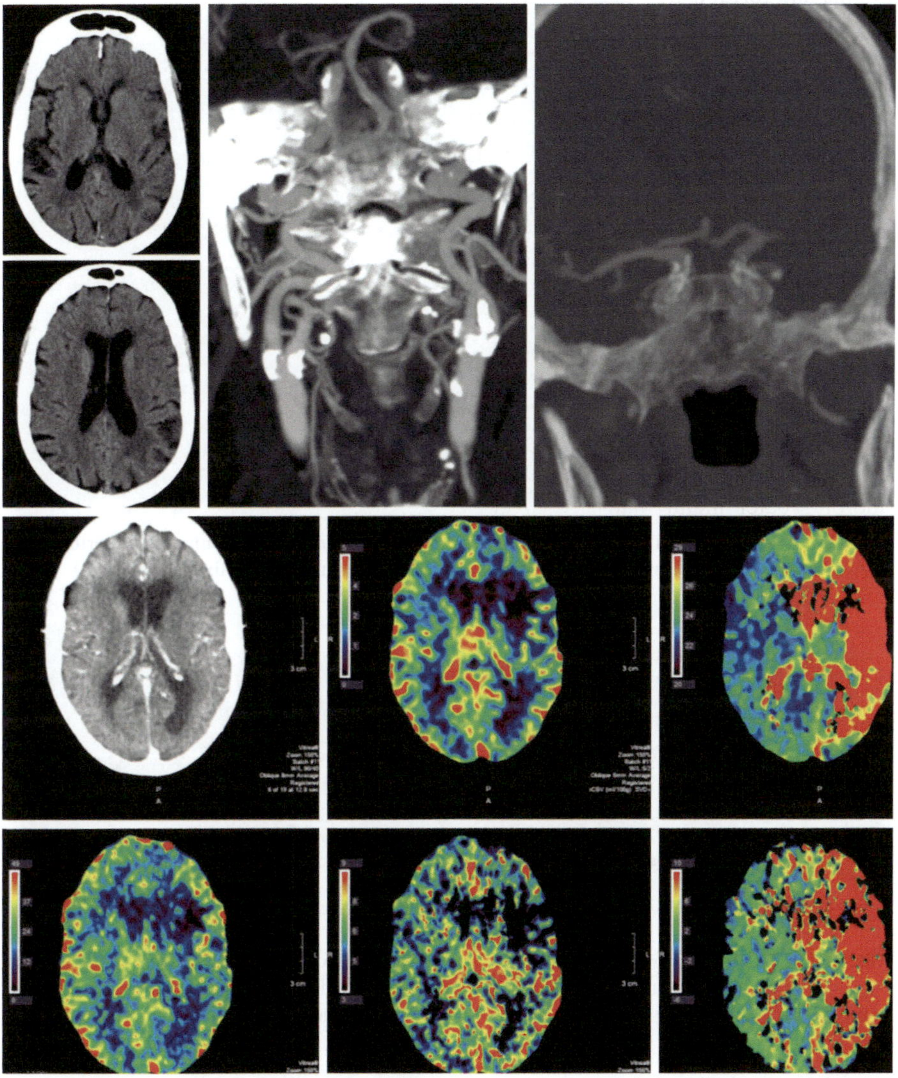

Fig. 12.11 The top half shows NCCT in the first column without significant early ischemic change. The middle column which is a coronal multiple intensity projection image of the CTA shows significant tortuosity in the cervical internal carotid arteries bilaterally, and the last column shows complete abrupt occlusion of the left M1 at its origin

into the superior division followed by the microcatheter with position confirmed through gentle microcatheter injection. The same stent retriever was then deployed from the superior division into proximal to the M1 origin in the ICA terminus. Recanalization through the deployed device was observed on angiography. The device was then gently withdrawn under vigorous aspiration from the guide catheter. Once the device reached the guide catheter and was partially withdrawn into it, there was loss of aspiration. In a similar fashion as the previous case, aspiration was

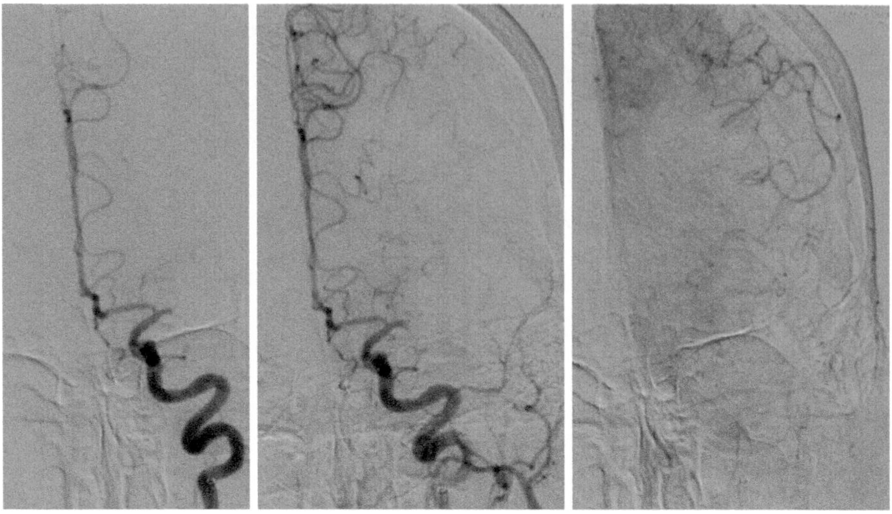

Fig. 12.12 AP projection from a left internal carotid artery angiogram confirms the tortuous left ICA with an M1 occlusion. The capillary phase shows good pial collaterals from the ACA

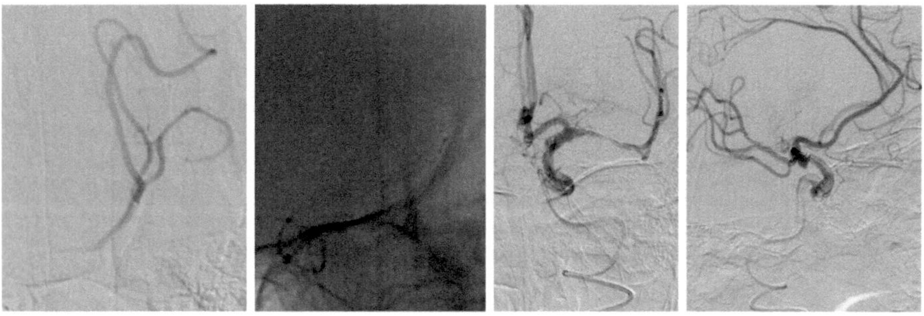

Fig. 12.13 The first image shows a gentle microcatheter injection in the M2 branch followed by deployment of the stent retriever in the second image. Intermediate catheter injection after removal of the microcatheter shows flow through the occluded M1 segment on the AP and lateral projections

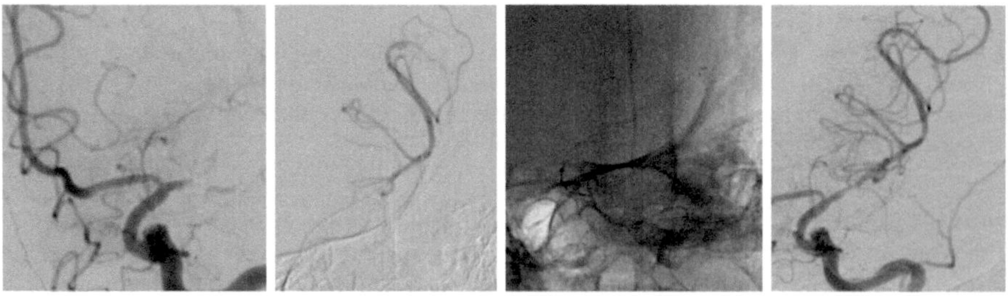

Fig. 12.14 The first image shows almost no recanalization following the first pass. The second image shows microcatheter placement in the superior division followed by deployment of the stent retriever in the third image. The fourth image confirms flow through the stent retriever in the occluded middle cerebral artery

locked at the 60-cc syringe and the guide catheter along with the microcatheter and the stent retriever were removed. Clot was observed on the microcatheter outside the body. The cervical ICA was accessed with the guide catheter for angiography which showed recanalization of the occluded left M1 segment with good distal perfusion (Fig. 12.15).

The patient had partial clinical recover post-operatively. Over the next 48 hours, she had persistent aphasia but improvement in the right hemiplegia. An MRI at 48 hours showed left basal ganglia and localized frontal opercular infarct and petechial hemorrhagic conversion in the basal ganglia without mass effect (Fig. 12.16).

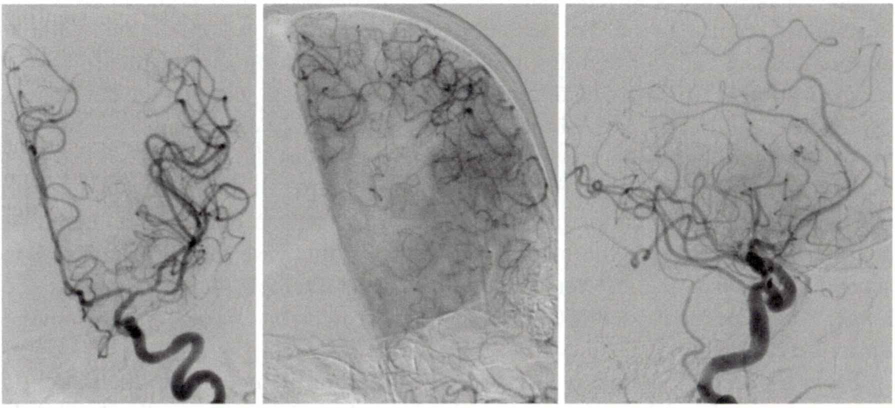

Fig. 12.15 There is complete recanalization following the second pass with good capillary perfusion

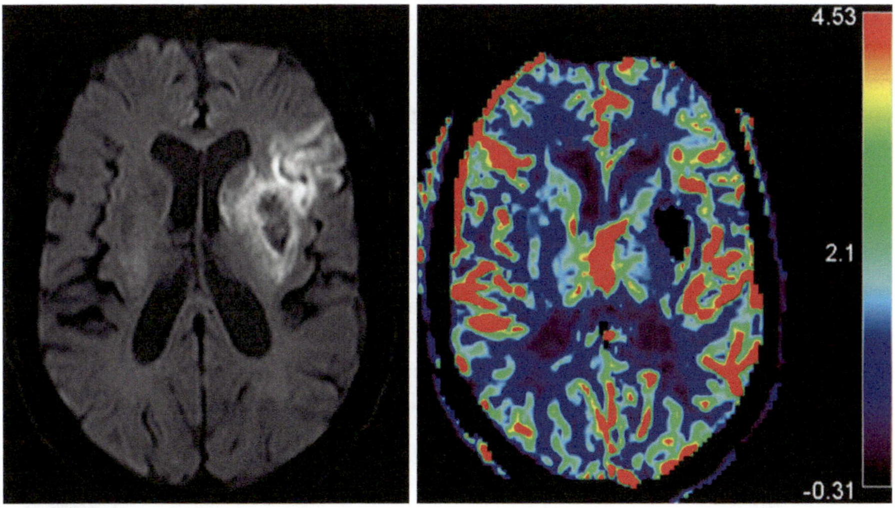

Fig. 12.16 An MRI at 24 hours shows localized left basal ganglia infarct and petechial hemorrhage with normalization of the CBF

She was discharged 6 days later to a rehabilitation unit and followed up at 3 months at which time other than mild upper extremity deficit she had recovered from her neurological acute stroke presentation.

Discussion

From a technical perspective, the discerning feature of the case is the cervical ICA tortuosity because of which an intermediate catheter was deployed. The first pass that was done with the intermediate catheter and the stent retriever did not result in meaningful recanalization. The second pass even though it was performed without an intermediate catheter and despite the cervical ICA tortuosity resulted in good recanalization (TICI 2B). The difference from the first pass was that the device was deployed in a different MCA branch than the first time, i.e., the superior division versus the inferior division. In vitro flow modeling studies show that an embolic clot to the MCA bifurcation often flips on itself with "limbs" of the clot extending into and occluding the bifurcation branches. Repeating the procedure after a failed first attempt by catheterizing the other M2 branch (in this case the superior division second time versus the inferior division in the first attempt) may help capture the longer "limb" of the flipped MCA clot and thus provide better traction in removing the entire clot.

From a clinical perspective, the relevant feature of the case is the patient's advanced age. The life expectancy at birth continues to increase in the developed world, and the life expectancy at age 65 is increasing at a much higher rate than life expectancy at birth. The incidence and prevalence of stroke is highest in patients ≥80 years of age. The randomized clinical trials did show a benefit in all age groups, although some recent studies have shown persistent challenges in achieving good outcomes in the elderly. A major factor in elderly patients undergoing any surgical or interventional procedure, other than the comorbidities, is the baseline functional and cognitive status. A well-developed social or family support structure can be very helpful in the recovery of an elderly patient. Depression is a significant independent risk factor for stroke and depression and social isolation is significantly associated with poor recovery following a stroke. Conversely, better cognitive and mental health correlates with improved physical function and pre-stroke physical activity is associated with good outcomes following a large vessel stroke. Thus, older age by itself should not be an exclusion to therapy; however, patient selection should be more rigorous including an assessment of the level of independence and functional status and the level of family support versus isolation.

Case – 4 (Stent Retriever with Balloon Guide Catheter)

A 77-year-old man presented 50 minutes after acute onset of left-sided weakness. His presentation NIHSS was 23. Imaging was consistent with a right MCA syndrome secondary to an M1 occlusion (Fig. 12.17). The patient was administered intravenous thrombolytics and taken to the neurointerventional suite.

Intervention and Outcome

The procedure was done under conscious sedation via a right transfemoral approach through an 8F sheath. An 8F balloon guide catheter was placed in the right common carotid artery; however, due to abdominal aortic tortuosity, this could not be advanced beyond the carotid bifurcation into the internal carotid artery. The femoral sheath was removed over the wire and the BGC was directly placed through the femoral artery increasing its workable length. It could now be advanced into the proximal internal carotid artery. An angiogram performed through the BGC

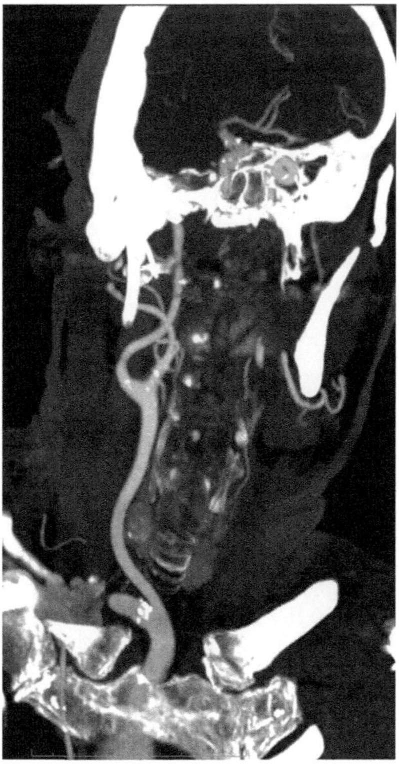

Fig. 12.17 Coronal CTA image shows an occlusion beginning at the ICA terminus extending into the right M1

confirmed the right M1 occlusion with pial collateralization from the anterior cerebral artery up to the proximal MCA branches (Fig. 12.18).

A 150-cm 2.9F (OD 0.038″, ID 0.027″) microcatheter and a 0.014″ microwire were navigated into the right internal carotid artery. The wire was manipulated across the occlusion through a very firm clot based on the tactile feedback. Attempts to advance the microcatheter over the wire were met with resistance at the clot face resulting in prolapse of the BGC. To stabilize the BGC, the balloon was inflated and "locked" in the cervical internal carotid which allowed the microcatheter to be advanced over the wire up to the mid-M1. A 6x25-mm stent retriever was then deployed from the distal M1 segment into the internal carotid artery in a standard unsheathing and push fashion to allow opening of the device (Fig. 12.19). A post-deployment angiogram showed good expansion of the device and flow through the MCA (Fig. 12.20). The microcatheter and device were then withdrawn under flow arrest and vigorous manual aspiration through the BGC using a 60-cc syringe. The

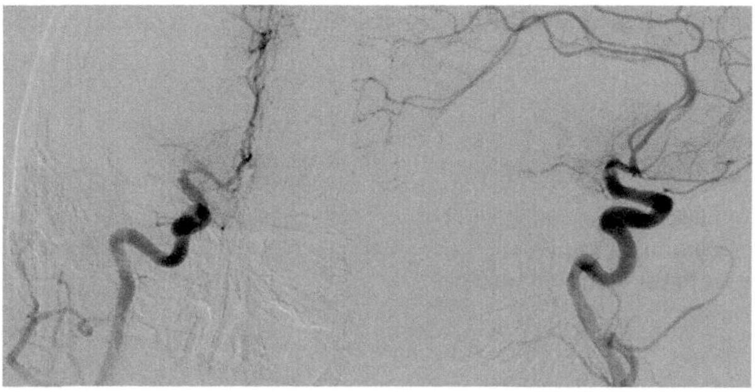

Fig. 12.18 AP and lateral projections from a right internal carotid artery angiogram confirm the occluded right M1 with occlusion slightly extending into the ICA terminus

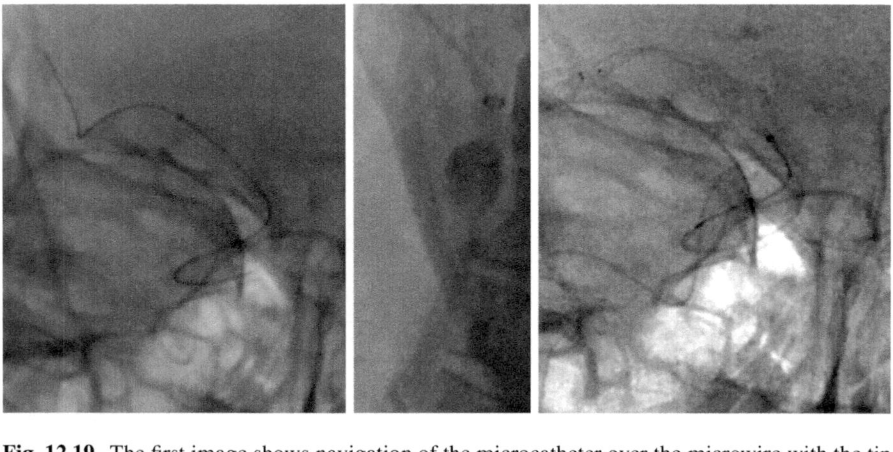

Fig. 12.19 The first image shows navigation of the microcatheter over the microwire with the tip of the microcatheter in the proximal M1. The second image shows balloon inflated at the guide catheter in the cervical ICA to help stabilize the guide catheter. The third image shows the deployed stent retriever

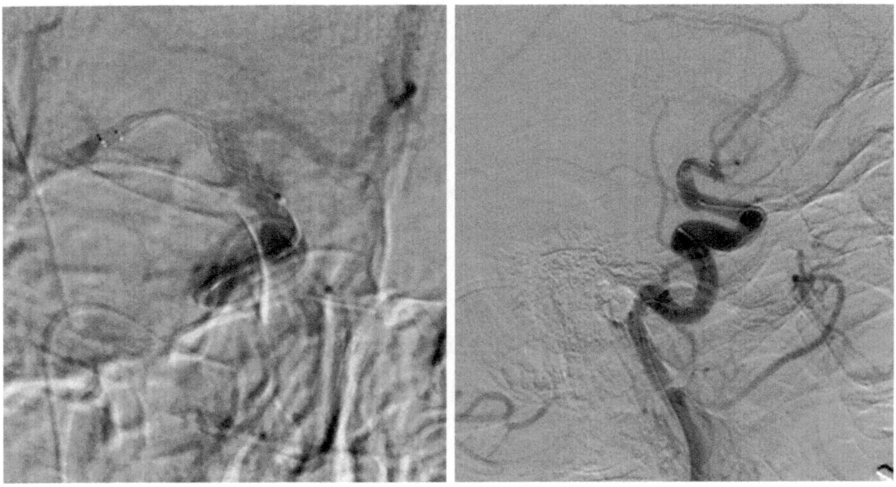

Fig. 12.20 Angiogram shows flow through the stent retriever in the occluded middle cerebral artery

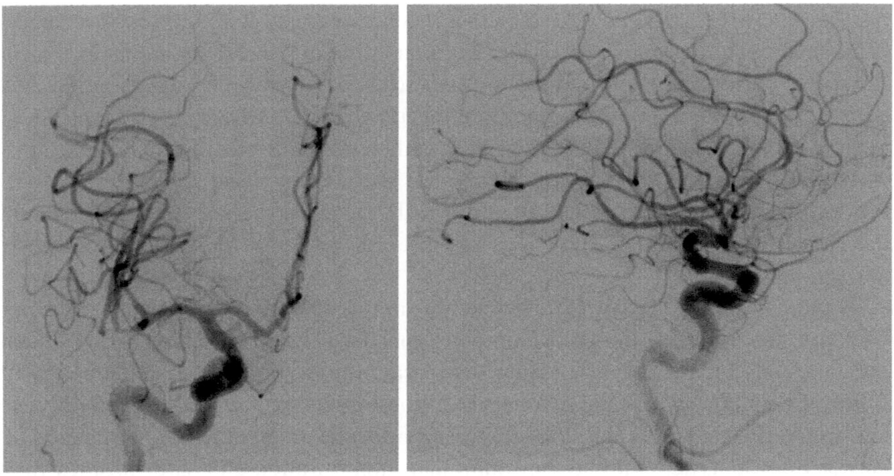

Fig. 12.21 Post-thrombectomy AP and lateral projections from a right ICA injection show complete recanalization

device was withdrawn into the BGC and removed. There was visible clot entangled with the stent retriever. Post-retrieval angiogram showed complete recanalization (Fig. 12.21). The puncture to closure time was 28 minutes.

The patient had steady recovery over the next 24 hours and was discharged to home after 6 days with a discharge NIHSS of 2. The patient's 24-hour MRI showed right basal ganglia and caudate infarct with petechial hemorrhage (Fig. 12.22).

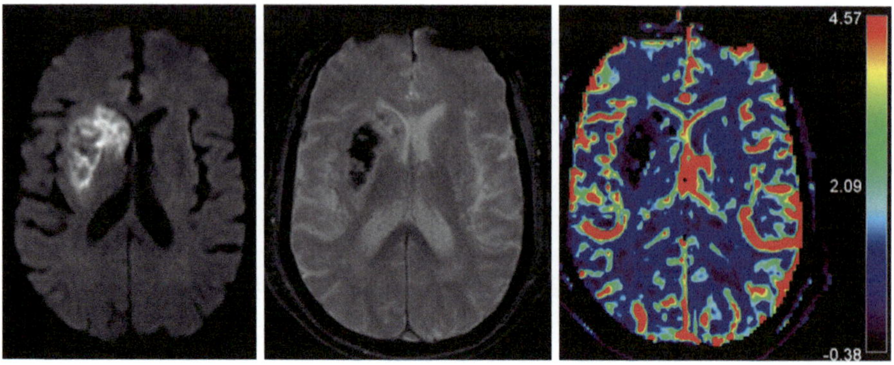

Fig. 12.22 The 24-hour MRI shows focal basal ganglia infarct (first image – diffusion-weighted image) with petechial hemorrhage (second image – gradient echo) corresponding to the pre-procedure focal CBV core. The last image shows normalization of the CBF

Discussion

This is a relatively straightforward case of mechanical thrombectomy with a stent retriever and BGC. The use of a BGC has been associated with improved recanalization and outcomes and reduced clot fragmentation in clinical studies as well as in in vitro experiments. However, randomized trials have shown relatively equal efficacy of stent retriever and aspiration thrombectomy. Advances in novel stent retriever designs and large-bore aspiration catheters are aiming to enhance recanalization rates, and the measure for procedural success for these newer devices will move to fast and complete recanalization with one pass. Inflation of the balloon in this case helped lock it in place and prevent prolapse during microcatheter advancement.

Administration of costly intravenous thrombolytics prior to mechanical thrombectomy has not been shown to improve procedural success or long-term clinical outcomes. As access to endovascular stroke care improves, it is possible that it will follow the trajectory of acute coronary syndromes where intravenous thrombolytics are reserved for cases when immediate endovascular intervention is not available. Newer thrombolytics with shorter administration duration and safer profiles may enhance the endovascular procedure. Similarly, clinical trials studying efficacy of neuroprotective agents may also show improved stroke outcomes with adjunctive use of these agents in endovascular stroke interventions.

Chapter 13
Thrombectomy for Basilar Occlusion: Approach and Strategy

Amin Aghaebrahim, Mohamad A. Asfour, John J. Entwistle, Manuel F. Granja, and Ricardo A. Hanel

Background

Posterior circulation strokes represent 20% of all ischemic strokes. Several different factors including onset of symptoms, location of the occlusion, infarct size, and management strategies constitute major challenges for the treating physicians [1]. Vertebrobasilar occlusion strokes (VBOS), also known as posterior circulation emergent large vessel occlusions (pc-ELVO), represent 1% of all ischemic strokes and 5% of all large vessel occlusion strokes. They are associated with a mortality rate of approximately 90% as well as severe neurological dysfunction in 65% of post-VBOS survivors [2, 3].

The basilar artery is the main vessel of the posterior circulation and supplies the majority of the brainstem, occipital lobes, and parts of the cerebellum and thalami. Because of the diversity and sensitivity of the areas that are supplied by this crucial vessel, patients with acute basilar artery occlusion can present symptoms that range from cranial nerve palsy or hemiparesis to locked-in syndrome or coma. Basilar artery occlusive disease most commonly presents as ischemia in the pons with the most extensive damage subjected to the midline.

Modern endovascular thrombectomy (ET) approaches have demonstrated superiority in reducing the mortality and disability in selected patients with anterior ischemic stroke (AIS) secondary to a large vessel occlusion [4]. However, none of the previous randomized trials included a population of patients with posterior

A. Aghaebrahim · M. F. Granja · R. A. Hanel (✉)
Baptist Medical Center, Baptist Neurological Institute, Jacksonville, FL, USA
e-mail: Ricardo.Hanel@bmcjax.com

M. A. Asfour
Baptist Medical Center, Lyerly Neurosurgey, Jacksonville, FL, USA

J. J. Entwistle
Department of Neurosurgery, Carilion Clinic, Roanoke, VA, USA

F. K. Hui et al. (eds.), *12 Strokes*, https://doi.org/10.1007/978-3-030-56857-3_13

circulation stroke [5–9]. Although the American Heart Association guidelines recommend ET for select patients with VBOS (class IIb, level of evidence C) [10], there have not been any definite randomized trials in this population to date [11]. There are however retrospective and prospective trials looking at this disease. BASIC, for example, was a prospective trial which analyzed 592 patients, of which 183 were treated with medical therapy, 121 received IV-tPA, and 288 received intra-arterial therapy. Overall, 68% of those studied had poor outcomes with no one treatment showing any statistically significant superiority over the others. The BEST trial [12] randomized 131 patients at 28 Chinese sites within 8 hours of stroke onset. Although slow recruitment and crossovers significantly fogged the results of the intention-to-treat analysis, the per-protocol and as-treated analysis both showed superiority of thrombectomy when compared with best medical management. The study's primary endpoint of a modified Rankin Scale (mRS) of 0–3 at 90 days after treatment was 44% in 63 patients who underwent thrombectomy and 26% in the 51 patients randomized to best medical therapy. This trial reached statistical significance unlike the BASIC trial. The progressive loss of equipoise for endovascular therapy for severe ELVO makes this data the best evidence available up to date. Due to the superiority in therapeutic effect of thrombectomy in anterior circulation strokes, it is unlikely that there will ever be a randomized trial comparing thrombectomy vs. medical management in VBOS attempted in the USA.

Anatomy

The Vertebrobasilar Arterial System (VBAS)

The vertebral arteries (VAs) originate from the right and left subclavian arteries. They run posterosuperiorly behind the anterior scalene muscle and travel through the foramina of the transverse processes of the sixth and seventh cervical vertebrae. From here, they traverse the transverse foramen at C6 and ascend vertically to C2 to finally reach the foramen magnum where they pierce the dura. The VAs are commonly divided in four classic anatomical segments described by Huber in 1979 (Table 13.1, Figs. 13.1, and 13.2).

Table 13.1 Segments of the vertebral artery

V1	Is the most proximal segment from the origin of the vertebral artery to the point of entry in the transverse foramen of C6
V2	Ascends along with vertebral veins and sympathetic nerves through the transverse foramina of C6 to C2
V3	From the exit of the transverse foramen of C2 to its entrance into the spinal canal and piercing of the posterior atlanto-occipital membrane
V4	Intracranial portion after entering the dura. It reaches the pontomedullary sulcus where it forms the basilar artery

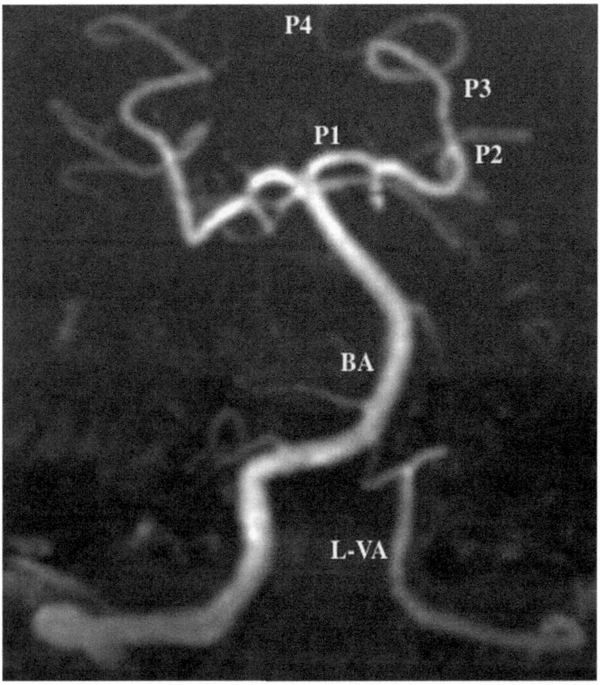

Fig. 13.1 Magnetic resonance angiography (MRA) showing an otherwise normal basilar artery (BA) with a left-sided deviation in the context of a hypoplastic left vertebral artery (L-VA). P1 to P4 segments of the posterior cerebral artery can also be identified (P1-P4)

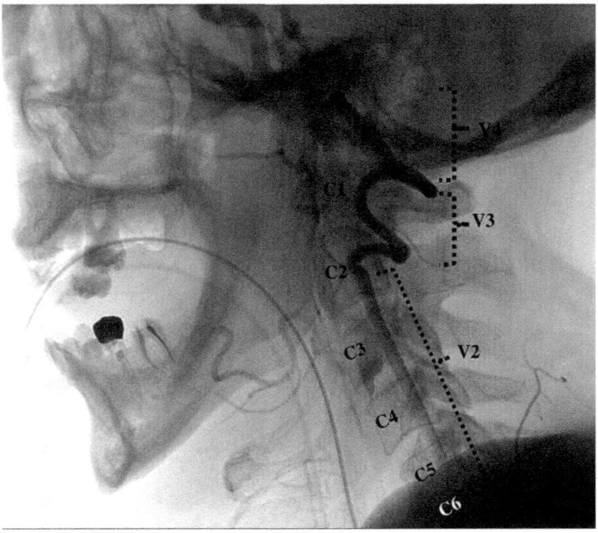

Fig. 13.2 Lateral angiogram showing the V2-V4 vertebral artery segments

The Basilar Artery (BA)

The VAs merge at the pontomedullary junction giving rise to the basilar artery (BA). This important vessel travels rostrally along the ventral medulla and basis pontis to bifurcate into the right and left posterior cerebral arteries at the ponto-mesencephalic junction. The BA is embryologically derived from the fusion of the longitudinal neural system and often deviates to one side, as its curvature usually tends toward the opposite side of the larger vertebral artery (Fig. 13.1). This may result from a congenital asymmetric blood flow to the vertebrobasilar junction with consequent asymmetric vessel wall tension and elongation of the BA. The stress may result in endothelial injury, thrombosis, and pre- and post-junctional infarctions. Pontine infarctions usually occur contralateral to the site of the BA displacement in 72% of patients, whereas PICA territory infarcts occurred ipsilateral to the hypoplastic vertebral artery in almost the same rate of patients [13, 14].

Common Anatomical Variations of the Vertebrobasilar System

The vertebrobasilar system and its major cerebellar arteries are characterized by a high degree of variability in comparison to the vascular anatomy of the ventral brainstem which is more constant and reliable. Viewing the arterial system of the brainstem and cerebellum as a natural extension of the segmental arrangement found in the spinal cord will facilitate the understanding of the myriad variations to which the basilar artery and its daughter vessels are subjected [15, 16].

- Asymmetric vertebral arteries (VAs) are present in up to two-thirds of individuals. Approximately 70% of people have a left dominant vertebral artery which is associated with pontine infarcts and posterior circulation strokes affecting the brainstem and cerebellum [17].
- An incomplete circle of Willis is another common anatomical variation that can be seen in up to 60% of the population and has no significant pathologic associations [18].
- The most common carotid-vertebrobasilar anastomosis is a persistent primitive trigeminal artery (PPTA). It is usually unilateral and can be observed in 0.1–0.6% of cerebral angiograms. PPTA usually arises from the junction between the petrous and cavernous internal carotid artery (ICA) segments (Figs. 13.3 and 13.4).
- Fenestration of the vertebrobasilar junction is present in 0.3–0.6% of the population and is usually associated with the formation of aneurysms of the posterior cerebral arteries [19].

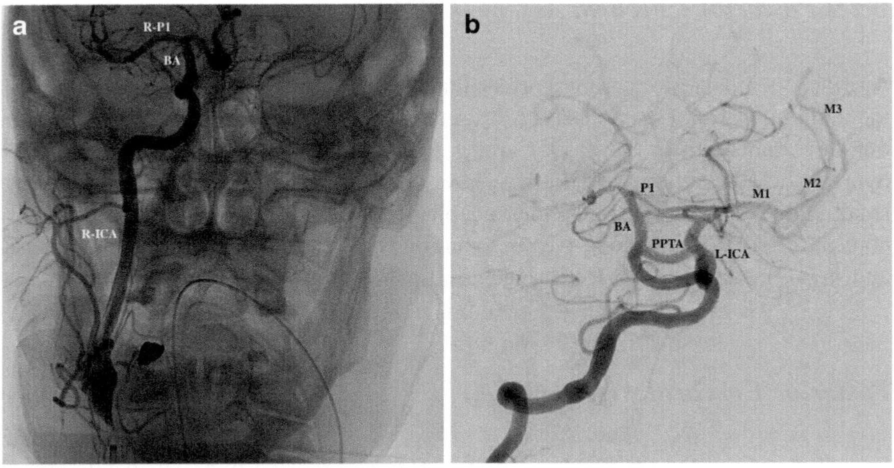

Fig. 13.3 Vertebral angiogram. (**a**) AP view and (**b**) lateral view of a persistent trigeminal artery (PPTA) that originates from the left internal carotid artery (L-ICA)

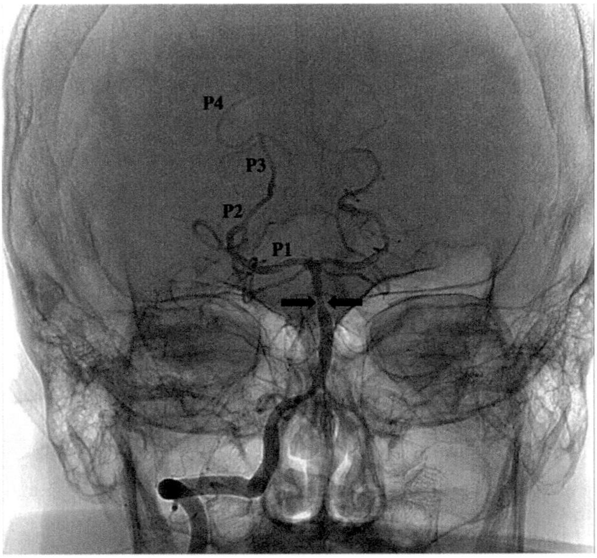

Fig. 13.4 Vertebral angiogram, AP view. The P1 to P4 segments of the posterior cerebral artery (PCA) can be identified along with mild vasospasm of the basilar artery (arrows)

The Artery of Percheron

The rostral mesencephalon and both paramedian thalami are supplied by the artery of Percheron that originates from P1, the most proximal segment of the posterior cerebral artery (PCA). Strokes in the aforementioned territories are often secondary to proximal embolisms of this well-known variant ending up with asymmetric thalamic involvement in approximately 66% of cases and midbrain infarction in almost 50% of the cases [20].

Fetal Posterior Cerebral Artery (fPCA)

An fPCA is a posterior cerebral artery that arises directly from an intracranial segment of the ICA. A complete fPCA originates from the internal carotid artery without any connection to the basilar artery. On the other hand, a partial fPCA has a hypoplastic connection with the BA. Every time that two fPCA coexist, there is a small-caliber BA because no mesencephalic, temporal, or occipital blood flow comes from it. There is no proven association between bilateral or unilateral fPCAs and stroke in any vascular territory [1, 21].

Posterior Cerebral Artery (PCA)

In the human embryo, the PCA originates as a branch of the ICA. The basilar artery divides into the two PCAs at the level of the interpeduncular fossa under the floor of the third ventricle. Hypertension and atherosclerosis can elongate this artery which bulges to the floor of the third ventricle. The posterior communicating artery (PComA) originates as a connection between the PCA and the ICA, but it can also regress creating an incomplete circle of Willis. The PCAs are classically divided into four anatomical segments described by Huber in 1979 (Fig. 13.5 and Table 13.2).

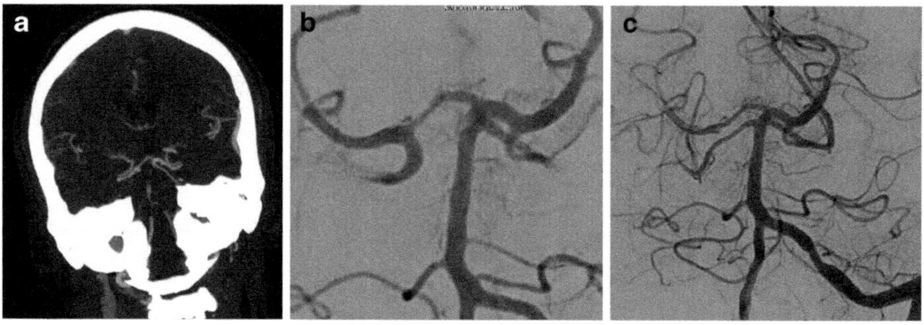

Fig. 13.5 Acute basilar tip occlusion. **(a)** Computed tomography angiography and coronal maximal intension projection demonstrating a total obstruction of the basilar artery in a patient with an NIHSS of 16. **(b)** Digital subtraction angiography left vertebral injection demonstrating subocclusive clot at the tip of the basilar and right P1 occlusion. **(c)** Post-thrombectomy angiography demonstrating complete revascularization of the basilar artery and P1 segment (TICI 3)

Table 13.2 Segments of the posterior cerebral artery

P1	From the origin at the basilar artery to the junction with the PComA
P2	Surrounds the midbrain
P3	Over the surface of the quadrigeminal plaque
P4	Give rise to parieto-occipital branches supplying the medial surface of the parietal lobe

Clinical Presentation of Posterior Circulation Stroke

Basilar occlusion is usually associated with a significant delay in primary presentation mostly due to its non-specific presentation. Gradual loss of consciousness, nausea, headache, dizziness, imbalance, gait disturbance, double vision, and unilateral weakness may suggest an ongoing posterior circulation stroke. There is significant variation in symptoms presentation according to the specific segment of the BA that is occluded.

- An occlusion of the proximal BA can result in "locked-in" syndrome with quadriplegia, bilateral facial plegia, anarthria, horizontal gaze paresis, and sparing of the vertical gaze movements and blinking. Reduced consciousness and several cranial nerve palsies may also be seen.
- A mid-basilar occlusion may result in lateral and mid-pontine syndrome with ipsilateral loss of facial sensation and ipsilateral ataxia.
- Distal BA artery occlusion also known as top of the basilar syndrome usually has an embolic etiology and may present as motor dysfunction, vivid hallucinations, and somnolence. This anatomical location can also present with decreased consciousness and oculomotor and pupillomotor dysfunction.

One of the major considerations in the clinical evaluation of patients with a stroke of the posterior circulation is the inherent limitation of the National Institutes of Health Stroke Scale (NIHSS). Its main focuses are on limb and speech impairment, specifically involving the more common left-dominant hemisphere with less emphasis on cranial nerve lesions. The NIHSS is not as accurate for posterior circulation stroke diagnosis. Even patients with a posterior circulation emergent large vessel occlusion can score 0 on the NIHSS with non-specific symptoms such as nausea, vertigo, or headache. Due to difficulty in timely recognition of the posterior circulation stroke, there may be significant delay in neurological evaluation and door to needle time for intravenous tPA or longer time from door to groin puncture in these patients that are considered candidates for endovascular thrombectomy (Figs. 13.6 and 13.7).

Role of Computed Tomography, Digital Subtraction Angiography, and Magnetic Resonance Imaging in Acute Occlusion of the Basilar Artery

Vascular imaging should always be included in the evaluation of any patient with clinical signs that suggest a pc-ELVO. Computed tomography angiography (CTA), digital subtraction angiography (DSA), and magnetic resonance angiography (MRA) are the primary imaging modalities to identify large vessel occlusion in a patient with a posterior circulation stroke. Non-contrast CT is usually the first-line imaging modality to exclude intracranial hemorrhage even though it may not be

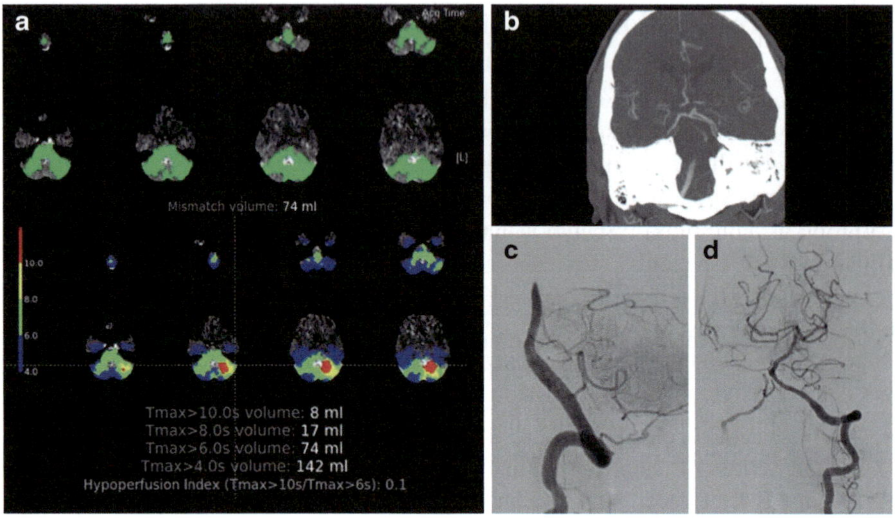

Fig. 13.6 Acute basilar tip occlusion in an 89-year-old female who presented with altered mental status and an NIHSS of 13. Patient last known well was 10 hours before presentation. (**a**) CT perfusion demonstrates a favorable mismatch volume as well as good collateralization with a hypoperfusion intensity ratio (hypoperfusion index) of 0.1. Pre-thrombectomy CT coronal MIP projections (**b**) and lateral angiography (**c**) demonstrating a basilar tip obstruction. Post-thrombectomy coronal angiography (**d**) after first pass with aspiration catheter only (TICI 3). Neuron MAX + ACE 68 aspiration only

very accurate to show early signs of ischemia in the posterior circulation. Up to 83% of patients with a partial or complete basilar artery occlusion can have a hyperdense basilar artery visible on a non-contrast CT scan [22]. CTA evaluation of patients with posterior circulation stroke also carries an important prognostic value. A hyperdense basilar artery has been identified as an independent predictor of a poor outcome at 6 months. A favorable posterior circulation collateral score and patency of the distal third of the basilar artery has been linked to a modified Rankin Score (mRS) of ≤ 3 at 90 days [22, 23]. Similarly, the presence of bilateral posterior communicating arteries in the pretreatment CTA was associated with a favorable outcome after endovascular treatment, whereas having a posterior circulation ASPECTS (pc-ASPECTS) < 8 has been linked with an increased risk of mortality [24–26]. Although initially described using CTA source images, pc-ASPECTS is frequently calculated using diffusion-weighted sequences (DWI). When scoring a pc-ASPECTS, one point is subtracted for any ischemic change in the right or left thalamus, cerebellum, or posterior cerebral artery territories, whereas two points are subtracted whenever an ischemic change is observed in the midbrain or pons [27]. Another important CTA-based scoring tool is the Basilar Artery on Computed Tomography Angiography (BATMAN) score. This score is a ten-point grading system that incorporates thrombus burden and the presence of collaterals. The BATMAN score allocates two points for each PCom or one point

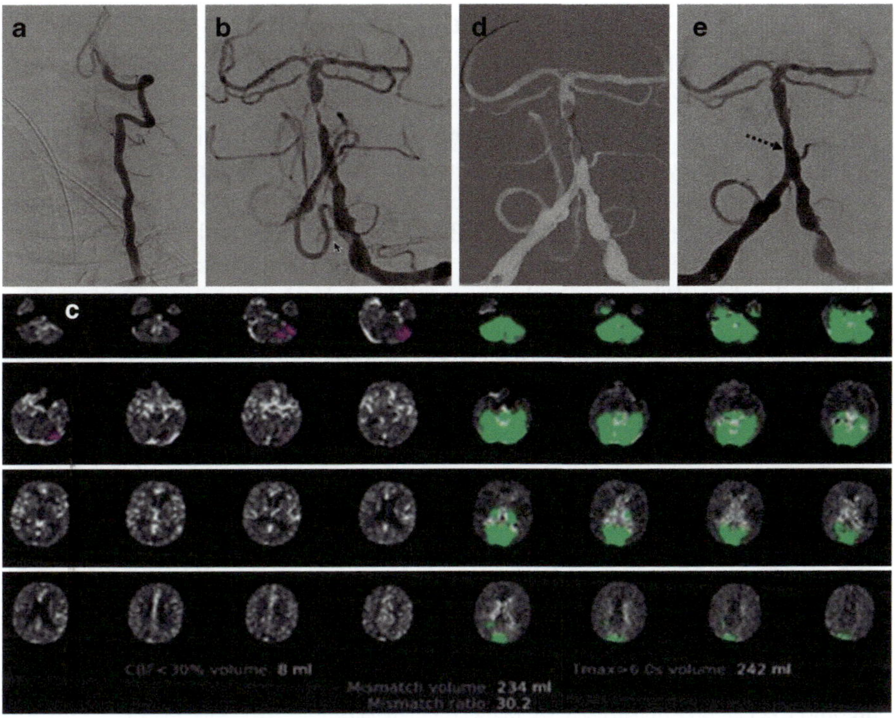

Fig. 13.7 Basilar tip occlusion in a 79-year-old male presenting with aphasia and global weakness. NIHSS of 20. Intravenous thrombolysis was given 2 h after symptoms onset. (**a**) Pre-thrombectomy lateral angiography demonstrating a mid-basilar obstruction (TICI 0). (**b**) Post-thrombectomy coronal angiography after manual aspiration. There is flow through the basilar artery (TICI 3); however, there is evidence of high-grade mid-basilar atherosclerotic stenosis. (**c**) CT perfusion demonstrates a favorable mismatch volume with an 8-mL infarct core. (**d**) Coronal angiography while performing balloon angioplasty, 2.75 × 15 mm. (**e**) Coronal angiography projection after successful (TICI 3) recanalization, balloon angioplasty, and Wingspan stent, 4x20 mm (arrow points to proximal stent marker)

for a hypoplastic PCom defined as being smaller than 1 mm. It also allocates one point if either intracranial vertebral artery is patent, one point for each open segment of the basilar artery (i.e., the proximal, middle, and distal basilar segments), and one point for each permeable P1 segment of the PCA for a total of ten points. When compared with the posterior circulation collateral score (PC-CS), BATMAN score was found to be more prognostically accurate than PC-CS in both ROC and logistic regression analysis with a higher interrater agreement for the BATMAN score [28]. DWI sequences are considered a powerful imaging tool, especially for late arrivals to exclude patients with a poor pc-ASPECTS or large core infarcts before they are taken to the angiosuite for further intervention (AHA class I, level of evidence c-LD).

Thrombectomy Techniques for the Treatment of Acute Basilar Artery Occlusion

Early recanalization is the standard of care for stroke. Interventions have included intravenous tissue-type plasminogen activator (IV-tPA), intra-arterial tissue-type plasminogen activator (IA-tPA), and mechanical thrombectomy. Randomized trials have shown the safety and efficacy of intravenous thrombolysis given within 4.5 hours, and more recently they have shown very good clinical outcomes after endovascular thrombectomy as it has been evidenced in both early and late window trials for strokes in the anterior circulation [29, 30]. The BASICS (Basilar Artery International Cooperation Study) registry [31] reported no benefit from intra-arterial treatment versus medical therapy alone. However, modern thrombectomy devices were not utilized during this prospective registry.

A more recent published registry, ENDOSTROKE, enrolled 148 patients with angiography-proven BAOs between January 2011 and June 2013. A total of 84% of patients were treated with a stent retriever either as the only device or in combination with others. Good clinical outcome (mRS = 0–2) was reached by 34% and moderate clinical outcome (mRS = 0–3) by 42%. In this cohort of patients, lower National Institutes of Health Stroke Scale (NIHSS) score, use of MRI, and better collateralization status independently predicted a good clinical outcome. Recanalization was achieved in 79% but was not found to be a predictor of good outcome [32].

Although mechanical thrombectomy has been validated through multiple international randomized controlled studies for anterior stroke [29], BAO patients have been commonly excluded from all of these papers except for one of them, the THRACE trial (**THR**ombectomie des **A**rtères **CE**rebrales) that only included few patients with acute BAO [33]. The exact relationship between reperfusion and outcome is not fully understood at this moment. However, recent studies have shown a full range of imaging and clinical predictors based on retrospective case series [12, 34, 35].

In general, patients who present with acute basilar artery occlusion are taken for thrombectomy if plain CT does not show a large stroke or bleed. If a significant amount of time has passed since initial presentation, an MRI can be utilized to assess infarct burden. However, the prognosis of an acute basilar artery occlusion is very poor if not revascularized as soon as possible. Due to presence of contralateral vertebral artery and vertebral artery luminal size, a balloon catheter for proximal occlusion is typically not used. Otherwise the technique can be similar to thrombectomy for the anterior circulation. When symptoms are mild, thrombotic occlusion secondary to a plaque rupture of intracranial atherosclerotic disease (ICAD) is the most likely etiology. In this scenario close attention should be given to the CT angiography looking for proximal cervical occlusion or multiple segmental ICAD. On the other hand, young patients with a history of trauma or cervical manipulation suggest dissection. No matter the etiology, adequate access to the BA needs to be achieved. In most cases, since BA occlusion has less tortuosity, pure aspiration by accessing the proximal clot can be achieved without crossing the clot. A trial with primary aspiration thrombectomy using the Direct Aspiration First-Pass Technique (ADAPT) should always be considered first. A retrospective review of 436 acute ischemic stroke patients who underwent mechanical thrombectomy using ADAPT included 57 (13%) patients with vertebrobasilar occlusions, and the posterior circulation group had a similar likelihood of good outcome compared with the anterior group (42.9% vs. 43.2%, respectively). A stent retriever can also be utilized for thrombectomy. Oftentimes, it may be necessary to access the proximal PCA in order to deploy the stent or to be able to get a more distal position for the aspiration catheter. A retrospective review of 161 patients with large vessel occlusion who underwent thrombectomy with stent retriever included a total of 24 BAOs. In this study, mortality was higher in the group with a BA occlusion, but successful recanalization was associated with a more favorable mRS at 90 days [36]. If the aspiration catheter is unable to access the face of the clot without crossing the lesion with microcatheter and microwire, a stent retriever deployment can be achieved after delivery of the microcatheter distal to the assumed location of the clot. Challenging cases such as those presenting with chronic bilateral vertebral artery occlusions have limited anterograde access. In this case, a retrograde access though a trans-PCom may be considered a feasible alternative. Another challenging case may be seen when an embolic basilar occlusion is secondary to a thrombotic occlusion of the vertebral ostium. A contralateral approach should be used to open the BA. However, a revascularization of the larger vertebral ostium is often required with upfront stenting allowing a large-bore aspiration catheter through the stenotic segment to continue to the intracranial occlusion.

Anticoagulation and Antiplatelet Therapy After Endovascular Treatment of Acute Basilar Artery Occlusion

Dual antiplatelet therapy (DAT) was found to reduce the incidence of early neurological deterioration and early recurrent ischemic strokes by 15% in patients with posterior circulation or basilar artery stenosis.

After thrombectomy in patients with an acute BAO, some hospitals elect to start adjunctive anticoagulation therapy in the hyperacute setting. A study conducted at the University of Helsinki examined 211 patients with angiography-proven basilar artery occlusion who were subsequently treated with IV thrombolysis and either unfractionated heparin (UFH) or LMWH. The study concluded that in patients with BAO, the rate of symptomatic intracranial hemorrhage (sICH) was 0% vs. 14.9% in LMWH and UFH, respectively, in patients with an mRS score of 0–2. On the other hand, patients with an mRS score of 5–6 showed a significant difference in the risk of ending up bedridden or deceased with 34.5% vs. 63% in favor of LMWH [37]. In another study at the Semmelweis University Heart and Vascular Center in Budapest, it was concluded that the immediate treatment of occlusion underlying stenosis, particularly BAO, with stents and DAT correlated to an overall improved survival and better functional outcomes [38]. Thus the role of DAT and anticoagulation therapy is quite promising in the overall prognosis of patients with basilar artery occlusion.

References

1. Nouh A, Remke J, Ruland S. Ischemic posterior circulation stroke: a review of anatomy, clinical presentations, diagnosis, and current management. Front Neurol. 2014;5:30.
2. Schonewille W, Algra A, Serena J, Molina C, Kappelle L. Outcome in patients with basilar artery occlusion treated conventionally. J Neurol Neurosurg Psychiatry. 2005;76:1238–41.
3. Mattle HP, Arnold M, Lindsberg PJ, Schonewille WJ, Schroth G. Basilar artery occlusion. Lancet Neurol. 10:1002–14.
4. Goyal M, Menon BK, van Zwam WH, Dippel DWJ, Mitchell PJ, Demchuk AM, et al. Endovascular thrombectomy after large-vessel ischaemic stroke: a meta-analysis of individual patient data from five randomised trials. Lancet. 2016;387:1723–31.
5. Berkhemer OA, Fransen PSS, Beumer D, van den Berg LA, Lingsma HF, Yoo AJ, et al. A randomized trial of intraarterial treatment for acute ischemic stroke. N Engl J Med. 0:null.
6. Goyal M, Demchuk AM, Menon BK, Eesa M, Rempel JL, Thornton J, et al. Randomized assessment of rapid endovascular treatment of ischemic stroke. N Engl J Med. 2015;372:1019–30.
7. Saver JL, Goyal M, Bonafe A, Diener H-C, Levy EI, Pereira VM, et al. Stent-retriever thrombectomy after intravenous t-pa vs. T-pa alone in stroke. N Engl J Med. 2015;372:2285–95.
8. Jovin TG, Chamorro A, Cobo E, de Miquel MA, Molina CA, Rovira A, et al. Thrombectomy within 8 hours after symptom onset in ischemic stroke. N Engl J Med. 2015;372:2296–306.
9. Campbell BCV, Mitchell PJ, Kleinig TJ, Dewey HM, Churilov L, Yassi N, et al. Endovascular therapy for ischemic stroke with perfusion-imaging selection. N Engl J Med. 2015;372:1009–18.
10. Powers WJ, Derdeyn CP, Biller J, Coffey CS, Hoh BL, Jauch EC, et al. 2015 aha/asa focused update of the 2013 guidelines for the early management of patients with acute ischemic stroke regarding endovascular treatment: a guideline for healthcare professionals from the American Heart Association/American Stroke Association. Stroke. 2015;46:3020.
11. Mokin M, Sonig A, Sivakanthan S, Ren Z, Elijovich L, Arthur A, et al. Clinical and procedural predictors of outcomes from the endovascular treatment of posterior circulation strokes. Stroke. 2016;47:782–8.
12. Liu X, Xu G, Liu Y, Zhu W, Ma M, Xiong Y, et al. Acute basilar artery occlusion: endovascular interventions versus standard medical treatment (best) trial-design and protocol for a randomized, controlled, multicenter study. Int J Stroke. 2017;12:779–85.
13. Hong JM, Chung C-S, Bang OY, Yong SW, Joo IS, Huh K. Vertebral artery dominance contributes to basilar artery curvature and peri-vertebrobasilar junctional infarcts. J Neurol Neurosurg Psychiatry. 2009;80:1087–92.
14. Wake-Buck AK, Gatenby JC, Gore JC. Hemodynamic characteristics of the vertebrobasilar system analyzed using mri-based models. PLoS One. 2012;7:e51346.
15. Lasjunias P, Beresntein A. Clinical vascular anatomy and variations. Berlin Heidelberg: Springer-Verlag; 2001.
16. Stephens R, Stilwell D. Arteries and veins of the human brain. Springfield, IL: Thomas; 1969.
17. Perren F, Poglia D, Landis T, Sztajzel R. Vertebral artery hypoplasia. A predisposing factor for posterior circulation stroke? Neurology. 2007;68:65–7.
18. van Raamt AF, Mali WP, van Laar PJ, van der Graaf Y. The fetal variant of the circle of Willis and its influence on the cerebral collateral circulation. Cerebrovasc Dis. 2006;22:217–24.
19. Gao LY, Guo X, Zhou JJ, Zhang Q, Fu J, Chen WJ, et al. Basilar artery fenestration detected with ct angiography. Eur Radiol. 2013;23:2861–7.

20. Griessenauer CJ, Loukas M, Tubbs RS, Cohen-Gadol AA. The artery of percheron: an anatomic study with potential neurosurgical and neuroendovascular importance. Br J Neurosurg. 2014;28:81–5.
21. Shaban A, Albright KC, Boehme AK, Martin-Schild S. Circle of Willis variants: fetal pca. Stroke Res Treat. 2013;2013:6.
22. Goldmakher GV, Camargo EC, Furie KL, Singhal AB, Roccatagliata L, Halpern EF, et al. Hyperdense basilar artery sign on unenhanced ct predicts thrombus and outcome in acute posterior circulation stroke. Stroke. 2009;40:134–9.
23. Da Ros V, Meschini A, Gandini R, Del Giudice C, Garaci F, Stanzione P, et al. Proposal for a vascular computed tomography-based grading system in posterior circulation stroke: a single-center experience. J Stroke Cerebrovasc Dis. 2016;25:368–77.
24. Maus V, Kalkan A, Kabbasch C, Abdullayev N, Stetefeld H, Barnikol UB, et al. Mechanical thrombectomy in basilar artery occlusion : presence of bilateral posterior communicating arteries is a predictor of favorable clinical outcome. Clin Neuroradiol. 2019;29:153–60.
25. Pallesen LP, Gerber J, Dzialowski I, van der Hoeven EJ, Michel P, Pfefferkorn T, et al. Diagnostic and prognostic impact of pc-aspects applied to perfusion ct in the basilar artery international cooperation study. J Neuroimaging. 2015;25:384–9.
26. Strbian D, Sairanen T, Silvennoinen H, Salonen O, Kaste M, Lindsberg PJ. Thrombolysis of basilar artery occlusion: impact of baseline ischemia and time. Ann Neurol. 2013;73:688–94.
27. Puetz V, Khomenko A, Hill MD, Dzialowski I, Michel P, Weimar C, et al. Extent of hypoattenuation on ct angiography source images in basilar artery occlusion: prognostic value in the basilar artery international cooperation study. Stroke. 2011;42:3454–9.
28. Alemseged F, Shah DG, Diomedi M, Sallustio F, Bivard A, Sharma G, et al. The basilar artery on computed tomography angiography prognostic score for basilar artery occlusion. Stroke. 2017;48:631–7.
29. Saver JL, Goyal M, van der Lugt A, et al. Time to treatment with endovascular thrombectomy and outcomes from ischemic stroke: a meta-analysis. JAMA. 2016;316:1279–89.
30. Albers GW. Late window paradox. Stroke. 2018;49:768.
31. Schonewille WJ, Wijman CA, Michel P, Rueckert CM, Weimar C, Mattle HP, et al. Treatment and outcomes of acute basilar artery occlusion in the basilar artery international cooperation study (basics): a prospective registry study. Lancet Neurol. 2009;8:724–30.
32. Singer OC, Berkefeld J, Nolte CH, Bohner G, Haring HP, Trenkler J, et al. Mechanical recanalization in basilar artery occlusion: the endostroke study. Ann Neurol. 2015;77:415–24.
33. Bracard S, Ducrocq X, Mas JL, Soudant M, Oppenheim C, Moulin T, et al. Mechanical thrombectomy after intravenous alteplase versus alteplase alone after stroke (thrace): a randomised controlled trial. Lancet Neurol. 2016;15:1138–47.
34. Gory B, Mazighi M, Blanc R, Labreuche J, Piotin M, Turjman F, et al. Mechanical thrombectomy in basilar artery occlusion: influence of reperfusion on clinical outcome and impact of the first-line strategy (ADAPT vs stent retriever). J Neurosurg. 2018;129:1482–91.
35. van Houwelingen RC, Luijckx GJ, Mazuri A, Bokkers RP, Eshghi OS, Uyttenboogaart M. Safety and outcome of intra-arterial treatment for basilar artery occlusion. JAMA Neurol. 2016;73:1225–30.
36. Hu SY, Yi HJ, Lee DH, Hong JT, Sung JH, Lee SW. Effectiveness and safety of mechanical thrombectomy with stent retrievers in basilar artery occlusion: comparison with anterior circulation occlusions. J Korean Neurosurg Soc. 2017;60:635–43.
37. Ritvonen J, Strbian D, Silvennoinen H, Virtanen P, Salonen O, Lindsberg PJ, et al. Thrombolysis and adjunct anticoagulation in patients with acute basilar artery occlusion. Eur J Neurol. 2019;26:128–35.
38. Nardai S, Kis B, Gubucz I, Berentei Z, Vajda Z, Orosz P, et al. Coronary stent implantation in acute basilar artery occlusion with underlying stenosis: potential for increased effectiveness in endovascular stroke therapy. Euro Interv: journal of EuroPCR in collaboration with the Working Group on Interventional Cardiology of the European Society of Cardiology. 2019.

Chapter 14
Carotid Terminus Occlusion

Sami Al Kasab, Eyad Almallouhi, and Alejandro M. Spiotta

Characteristics and Classification

Acute carotid terminus occlusion (CTO) causes about 5% of ischemic strokes secondary to emergent large vessel occlusion (ELVO) and about 20% of internal carotid artery (ICA) occlusions [1–4]. The term"CTO" has also been used to describe ICA occlusions in the supra-clinoid segment or ICA bifurcation [3, 5]. Previous studies have reported that approximately 80% of CTOs are caused by cardioembolic etiology [3]. Patients with CTO present with higher stroke severity and infarction volume compared to patients who present with proximal middle cerebral artery (MCA) or more proximal ICA occlusions [1–3, 6–9], likely as an end result of disruption of direct circle of Willis collaterals across the anterior communicating artery (Acom). However, collateral cerebral circulation plays an important role in determining outcomes of CTO, and multiple classifications have been proposed depending on the clot morphology and the collaeral circulation at the circle of Willis [9, 10]. One classification categorized CTOs on conventional cerebral angioram into (1) ICA-I clot, occlusion of the ICA terminus with reconstitution of the proximal portions of the MCA and anterior cerebral artery (ACA); (2) ICA-L clot, occlusion of the ICA terminus and proximal portion of the MCA with a partial or complete patency of the ipsilateral proximal ACA; and (3) ICA-T clot, occlusion of ICA terminus with the proximal portions of MCA and ACA [10]. A study by Liebenskind et al. included 72 patients with CTO and found that ICA-I occlusions required a smaller average number of attempts to recanalize with the MERCI device [10]. Also, the authors

S. Al Kasab · E. Almallouhi
Medical University of South Carolina, Department of Neurology, and Neurosurgery, Charleston, SC, USA

A. M. Spiotta (✉)
Department of Neurosurgery, Medical University of South Carolina, Charleston, SC, USA
e-mail: spiotta@musc.edu

F. K. Hui et al. (eds.), *12 Strokes*, https://doi.org/10.1007/978-3-030-56857-3_14

found that collateral flow through the Acom was a strong predictor of recanalization success and long-term independence.

Another classification suggested by Lee et al. categorized CTO into (1) simple CTO, with patent A2 segment of ACA (via Acom) and posterior cerebral artery (PCA) (via posterior communicating artery (Pcom) of P1 segment of PCA), or (2) complex CTO, if they do not meet any of the previous criteria [9]. The authors found that infarction volume for simple CTO was about one-fifth and favorable outcome was about five times higher compared to complex CTO [9].

Imaging

Although CTOs are commonly seen in daily practice, diagnosis remains a challenge without invasive cerebral vascular imaging [11–15]. Originally described by Kniemeyer et al., multiple studies evaluated the cervical carotid "pseudo-occlusion" phenomenon, which describes non-opacification of contrast on single-phase computed tomography angiography (CTA) in the cervical portion of ICA, resulting from a downstream occlusion in distal portions of the intracranial ICA [14, 16]. The resultant stagnant column of blood in the cervical ICA without an outlet creates an apparent filling defect on CTA by lack of contrast penetration, giving the appearance that the cervical carotid is occluded just beyond the bifurcation. As a result, CTA may overestimate the extent of occlusion compared with conventional cerebral angiogram [16]. One suggested solution to determine a real cervical occlusion vs. pseudo-occlusion is to use delayed contrast-enhanced computed tomography (CT) [16]. However, Wareham et al. showed that delayed imaging was able to show contrast beyond the cervical segment in only 2 out of 11 acute stroke patients with cervical pseudo-occlusion [12]. On the other hand, Munich et al. were able to identify CTO in three out of three patients who had cervical pseudo-occlusion on traditional CTA using time-resolved whole-head CTA (4D CTA). Finally, color Doppler-assisted duplex imaging (CDDI) or magnetic resonance angiography (MRA) can be used to identify cervical pseudo-occlusion, but their use may not be feasible in the setting of acute stroke in most centers [17, 18]. In addition, Furst et al. found that the specificity and sensitivity for traditional CDDI, 2D MRA, and 3D MRA in identifying cervical pseudo-occlusion vs. complete occlusion were 0.92 and 0.70, 1.0 and 0.65, and 0.89 and 0.47, respectively.

A study by Diouf et al. included 37 stroke patients with CTA showing lack of attenuation in the cervical portion of ICA, and 12 (32.4%) of them had pseudo-occlusion [11]. Another study in the United Kingdom evaluated the imaging characteristics of 26 patients with CTO, 13 of which had cervical pseudo-occlusion, and found that predictors of having this phenomenon are thrombus extension to the ophthalmic segment of ICA and patency of the posterior communicating artery and ophthalmic artery [12]. Importantly, Grossberg et al. found that while patients with cervical pseudo-occlusion had significantly lower chances of achieving complete reperfusion with mechanical thrombectomy, there was no difference in the long-term mortality and functional independence [13].

Prognosis and Response to Treatment

Acute ischemic strokes secondary to CTO are associated with worse prognosis compared to other ELVOs in general [1, 2, 6–8]. In a study by Lee et al., three out of ten patients with acute CTO achieved complete recanalization with mechanical thrombectomy (using a combination of the stent retriever and Penumbra system), and none of the patients who received intravenous thrombolysis without mechanical thrombectomy achieved complete recanalization [6].

Another study evaluated the recanalization rate with intravenous thrombolysis according to the occlusion site [1]. Authors found that the odds of achieving complete recanalization for a proximal MCA was seven times higher than CTO [1]. In addition, none of the 14 patients with CTO who were included achieved early recovery (National Institutes of Health Stroke Scale ≤ 2 at 24 hours), and only 2 of them had favorable functional outcome (modified Rankin scale ≤ 1) at 90 days [1]. In addition, von Kummer et al. demonstrated that the recanalization rate for patients with CTO is about half compared to patients with proximal MCA occlusion with a combination of intraarterial and intravenous thrombolysis [19]. The authors hypothesized that CTO clots are more likely to be organized or calcified which can explain the poor response rate to thrombolysis [19].

In our experience, we have found that successful recanalization of CTO can be achieved with a similar approach to M1 occlusions utilizing a direct aspiration first-pass technique (ADAPT). With ADAPT, the most common protocol we use is an 8 French sheath, commonly a Neuron 088 Max (Penumbra, Oakland, California, USA) or 088 Infinity (Stryker Neurovascular, Fremont, California, USA). This is advanced to the distal cervical internal carotid artery over an insert and guidewire. The insert and guidewire are then removed, and a large-bore aspiration catheter is advanced over a microcatheter and microwire to the level of clot. We commonly use a 3MAX microcatheter (Penumbra) and 0.016 inch Fathom wire (Boston Scientific Corp., Natick, Massachusetts, USA). Most commonly used aspiration catheters in our practice are a JET 7 0.072 (Penumbra) and AXS Vecta 0.071 (Stryker). First the microcatheter and microwire are advanced past the clot to the distal M1 segment in cases of CTO. Then, as the large-bore aspiration catheter is approaching the clot, the microcatheter and microwire are withdrawn while advancing the aspiration catheter "railroad technique." The simultaneous pushing forward of the aspiration catheter while removing the 3MAX and wire helps deliver the catheter smoothly and navigate tortuosity including the carotid siphon. As the aspiration catheter is advanced to the level of the occlusion and beyond, the 3MAX and microwire should be withdrawn into the aspiration catheter so the clot is ingested with an "open mouth" catheter tip. As the 3MAX and microwire are withdrawn entirely from the catheter system, gentle forward pressure on the aspiration catheter will allow it to travel another 0.5–1 cm into the M1 segment. At this point, the aspiration catheter has entirely ingested the thrombus, and connecting the proximal end of the catheter to aspiration tubing and applying negative pressure via the pump will purge the catheter of the thrombus. In our experience, this technique helps in better engagement of the clot with the aspiration catheter and prevents distal embolization. It is critical to size the aspiration catheter closely to the target vessel and select the largest catheter that the vessel can safely accommodate.

Case Presentation

Case 1

A middle-aged man presented with acute-onset left-sided weakness. Patient had a past medical history of hypertension, hyperlipidemia, diabetes mellitus, atrial fibrillation, congestive heart failure, and end-stage renal disease. He was last seen well 40 minutes prior to arrival to the emergency department. His National Institutes of Health Stroke Scale (NIHSS) was 21. Computed tomography of the head showed hypoattenuation of the gray-white matter junction in the right frontal area. Computed tomography angiography (CTA) of the head and neck showed tapered occlusion of the cervical right internal carotid artery (Fig. 14.1a). Patient received intravenous alteplase and was taken for mechanical thrombectomy. Angiography of the common carotid artery showed sluggish antegrade flow of the cervical internal carotid artery with complete occlusion at the carotid terminus (Fig. 14.1b, c). Aspiration thrombectomy was performed with resultant TICI 3 flow (Fig. 14.1d).

Case 2

A middle-aged woman presented with right-sided weakness and inability to speak. Patient had a history of hypertension, coronary artery disease, and end-stage renal disease. She was last seen well 11 hours prior to presenting to the hospital. Her National Institutes of Health Stroke Scale (NIHSS) was 22. Computed tomography of the head showed subtle loss of the gray-white matter differentiation in the left insular region. Computed tomography angiography of the head and neck showed occlusion at the left carotid terminus and M1 segment (Fig. 14.2a). Patient was taken for mechanical thrombectomy with resultant TICI 3 revascularization following 1-pass aspiration (Figs. 14.2b, c).

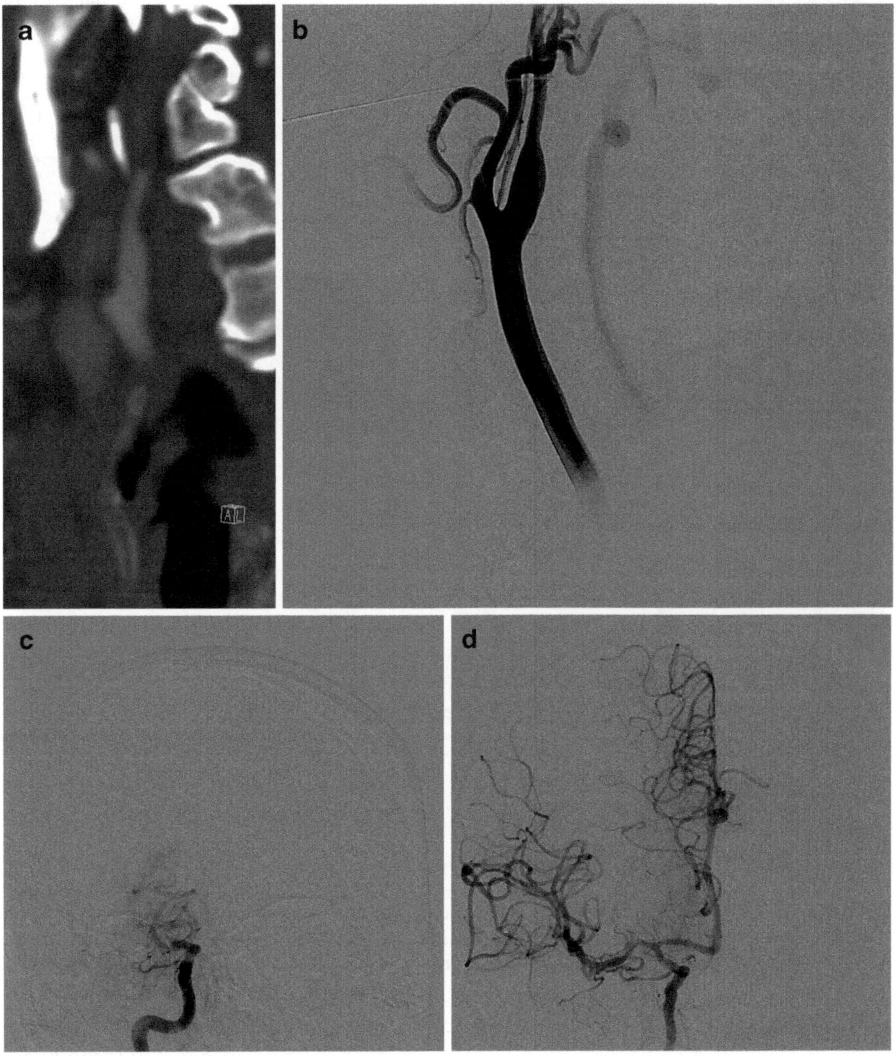

Fig. 14.1 (**a**) CTA of the neck shows tapered occlusion of the internal carotid artery just distal to the bifurcation. (**b**) DSA shows patent cervical internal carotid artery. (**c**) DSA shows complete occlusion at the carotid terminus. (**d**) DSA shows complete revascularization of the carotid terminus following mechanical thrombectomy

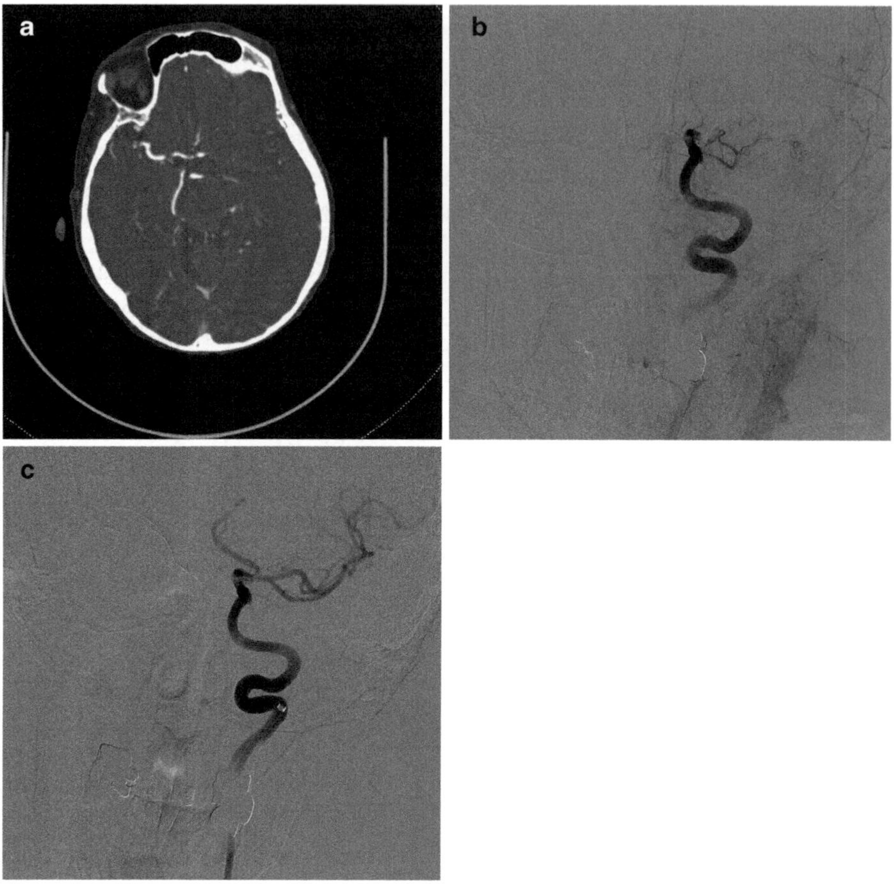

Fig. 14.2 (**a**) CTA of the head showing complete occlusion of the left carotid terminus. (**b**) DSA shows complete occlusion of the left carotid terminus. (**c**) Complete revascularization of the carotid terminus following mechanical thrombectomy

References

1. Saqqur M, Uchino K, Demchuk AM, et al. Site of arterial occlusion identified by transcranial Doppler predicts the response to intravenous thrombolysis for stroke. Stroke. 2007;38:948–54.
2. Zaidat OO, Suarez JI, Santillan C, et al. Response to intra-arterial and combined intravenous and intra-arterial thrombolytic therapy in patients with distal internal carotid artery occlusion. Stroke. 2002;33:1821–6.
3. Hong JM, Lee SE, Lee SJ, Lee JS, Demchuk AM. Distinctive patterns on CT angiography characterize acute internal carotid artery occlusion subtypes. Medicine (Baltimore). 2017;96:e5722.
4. Bhatia R, Hill MD, Shobha N, et al. Low rates of acute recanalization with intravenous recombinant tissue plasminogen activator in ischemic stroke. Stroke. 2010;41:2254–8.
5. Gibo H, Lenkey C, Rhoton AL Jr. Microsurgical anatomy of the supraclinoid portion of the internal carotid artery. J Neurosurg. 1981;55:560–74.

6. Lee JS, Hong JM, Lee SJ, Joo IS, Lim YC, Kim SY. The combined use of mechanical thrombectomy devices is feasible for treating acute carotid terminus occlusion. Acta Neurochir. 2013;155:635–41.
7. Jansen O, von Kummer R, Forsting M, Hacke W, Sartor K. Thrombolytic therapy in acute occlusion of the intracranial internal carotid artery bifurcation. AJNR Am J Neuroradiol. 1995;16:1977–86.
8. Christou I, Felberg RA, Demchuk AM, et al. Intravenous tissue plasminogen activator and flow improvement in acute ischemic stroke patients with internal carotid artery occlusion. J Neuroimaging. 2002;12:119–23.
9. Lee SU, Hong JM, Kim SY, Bang OY, Demchuk AM, Lee JS. Differentiating carotid terminus occlusions into two distinct populations based on Willisian collateral status. J Stroke. 2016;18:179–86.
10. Liebeskind DS, Flint AC, Budzik RF, et al. Carotid I's, L's and T's: collaterals shape the outcome of intracranial carotid occlusion in acute ischemic stroke. J Neurointerv Surg. 2015;7:402–7.
11. Diouf A, Fahed R, Gaha M, et al. Cervical internal carotid occlusion versus pseudo-occlusion at CT angiography in the context of acute stroke: an accuracy, Interobserver, and Intraobserver Agreement Study. Radiology. 2018;286:1008–15.
12. Wareham J, Crossley R, Barr S, Mortimer A. Cervical ICA pseudo-occlusion on single phase CTA in patients with acute terminal ICA occlusion: what is the mechanism and can delayed CTA aid diagnosis? J Neurointerv Surg. 2018;10:983–7.
13. Grossberg JA, Haussen DC, Cardoso FB, et al. Cervical carotid pseudo-occlusions and false dissections: intracranial occlusions masquerading as extracranial occlusions. Stroke. 2017;48:774–7.
14. Kniemeyer HW, Aulich A, Schlachetzki F, Steinmetz H, Sandmann W. Pseudo- and segmental occlusion of the internal carotid artery: a new classification, surgical treatment and results. Eur J Vasc Endovasc Surg. 1996;12:310–20.
15. Marquering HA, Nederkoorn PJ, Beenen LF, et al. Carotid pseudo-occlusion on CTA in patients with acute ischemic stroke: a concerning observation. Clin Neurol Neurosurg. 2013;115:1591–4.
16. Kim JJ, Dillon WP, Glastonbury CM, Provenzale JM, Wintermark M. Sixty-four-section multidetector CT angiography of carotid arteries: a systematic analysis of image quality and artifacts. AJNR Am J Neuroradiol. 2010;31:91–9.
17. Regina G, Testini M, Fullone M, et al. Pseudo-occlusion of the internal carotid artery: report of 15 cases and review of the literature. Int Angiol. 1997;16:147–50.
18. Fürst G, Saleh A, Wenserski F, et al. Reliability and validity of noninvasive imaging of internal carotid artery pseudo-occlusion. Stroke. 1999;30:1444–9.
19. Kummer RV, Holle R, Rosin L, Forsting M, Hacke W. Does arterial recanalization improve outcome in carotid territory stroke? Stroke. 1995;26:581–7.

Chapter 15
Thrombectomy for Acute Occlusion in Intermediate-Sized Distal Arteries

Angelique Sao Mai S. Do, Robin M. Babadjouni, and Michael J. Alexander

Introduction

The evolution of endovascular treatment for acute stroke due to large vessel occlusion (LVO) has rapidly progressed since the publication of the major mechanical thrombectomy trials in 2015 and subsequent studies [1–5]. This has provided class 1, level A evidence that mechanical thrombectomy should be performed in patients with acute large vessel occlusion within 6 hours if there is not already a large completed infarction and in patients within 24 hours of onset of stroke symptoms if their brain perfusion profile is favorable and they have met other clinical criteria [6, 7]. Most mechanical thrombectomy studies have focused on LVO within the intracranial internal carotid artery and M1 segment of the middle cerebral artery (MCA) (Table 15.1). Several trials have also included M2 MCA occlusions [8–15] and vertebral artery or basilar artery occlusions. There has been less emphasis on acute stroke due to intermediate-sized arterial occlusions, such as anterior cerebral artery (ACA), M3 or M4 MCA, or posterior cerebral artery (PCA) occlusions [16, 17].

Occlusions in the more distal intermediate-sized arteries are less likely to have very high National Institutes of Health Stroke Scale (NIHSS) scores, but can have very functionally incapacitating strokes. ACA occlusions can result in hemiparesis or hemiplegia, abulia, supplementary motor region strokes, and other symptoms. M3–M4 occlusions may result in aphasia or hemiplegia, particularly if the occlusions are in frontal opercular or rolandic branches, respectively. PCA occlusions may lead to severe thalamic strokes, cortical neglect syndromes, pronounced visual

A. S. M. S. Do · R. M. Babadjouni
Department of Neurosurgery, Cedars-Sinai Medical Center, Los Angeles, CA, USA

M. J. Alexander (✉)
Department of Neurosurgery, Neurovascular Center, Cedars-Sinai Medical Center, Los Angeles, CA, USA
e-mail: michael.alexander@cshs.org

F. K. Hui et al. (eds.), *12 Strokes*, https://doi.org/10.1007/978-3-030-56857-3_15

Table 15.1 Early mechanical thrombectomy trials for LVO (large vessel occlusion) and the incidence of distal artery thrombectomies in these trials

	Intervention	Location (number and percentage)
MR CLEAN [1]	SOC vs SOC + IA treatment Intra-arterial thrombolytic (alteplase or urokinase) +/− thrombectomy	Intracranial ICA = 1/233 (0.4) ICA with M1 = 59/233 (25.3) M1 = 154/233 (66.1) **M2 = 18/233 (7.7)** **A1 or A2 = 1/233 (0.4)** Extracranial ICA = 75/233 (32.2)
ESCAPE [2]	SOC vs. SOC + thrombectomy	ICA with M1 = 45/163 (27.6) M1 or all M2 = 111/163 (68.1) **Single M2 = 6/163 (3.7)**
REVASCAT [3]	SOC vs. SOC + thrombectomy with solitaire stent retriever	ICA with M1 = 26/102 (25.5) M1 = 66/102 (64.7) **M2 = 10/102 (9.8)** Ipsilateral cervical carotid = 19/102 (18.6)
SWIFT PRIME [4]	IV tPA vs. IV tPA + thrombectomy with stent retriever	ICA = 17/93 (18) M1 = 62/93 (67) **M2 = 13/93 (14)**
EXTEND IA [5]	IV tPA vs. IV tPA + thrombectomy with solitaire stent retriever	ICA = 11/35 (31) M1 = 20/35 (57) **M2 = 4/35 (11)**
DEFUSE [6]	SOC vs. SOC + thrombectomy	ICA = 32/92 (35) M1 = 60/92 (65)
DAWN [7]	SOC vs. SOC + thrombectomy	ICA = 22/107 (21) M1 = 83/107 (78) **M2 = 2/107 (2)**

Note the very low enrollment of patients with distal artery occlusions (in bold)
SOC standard of care, *IA* intra-arterial, *ICA* internal carotid artery, *tPA* tissue plasminogen activator

field deficits, and others. Distal artery occlusions may present primarily, or may occur as a sequela of an LVO thrombectomy. The latter may be distal embolus from the primary occlusion, e.g., M4 occlusion following an M1 thrombectomy, or an incipient embolus from thrombectomy of an adjacent vessel, e.g., de novo A1 occlusion following an M1 thrombectomy.

Intravenous lytic therapy for intermediate-sized arteries is more effective than for treatment of large vessel occlusions, since the clot burden is considerably less [18]. However, intravenous lytics may still be an ineffective therapy for revascularization, or patients may be out of the time window for such treatment. This leaves endovascular thrombectomy as the only interventional treatment for these patients.

While several studies included a sparse number of these intermediate artery occlusions within the larger studies, the AHA/ASA (American Heart Association/American Stroke Association) guidelines only gave recommendation for thrombectomy in LVO (large vessel occlusion) strokes. For more distal, intermediate-sized arteries, the AHA/ASA does not state that thrombectomy is recommended but does state that it may be reasonable [19].

Grossberg et al. [16] retrospectively analyzed a single-institution series of 69 patients with distal occlusions. This included 45 patients with the distal occlusion as the primary treatment location, 23 patients with a distal occlusion following an LVO thrombectomy, and 1 patient who had both primary and rescue treatment. The vessels treated included 32 M3 segments, 25 ACA segments, and 7 PCA segments, with the remainder being a combination of arterial locations. In this series, they obtained a TICI (thrombolysis in cerebral infarction) revascularization grade of TICI 2b or TICI 3 in 83% of the patients and a rate of intraparenchymal hematoma in the region of the treated artery of 4%. The primary thrombectomy method in these distal occlusions included 56% stent retrievers and 45% aspiration.

The recently reported multi-center STAR (Stroke Thrombectomy and Aneurysm Registry) data [20] analyzed the treatment of patients with distal arterial occlusions who underwent mechanical thrombectomy. Although it was a retrospective analysis of registry data, it did provide interesting insight into some of the key differences between large vessel and distal vessel thrombectomy. In their series of 2819 patients undergoing mechanical thrombectomy for acute stroke, 130 patients (4.6%) were distal occlusions. They defined a distal artery as M3 or M4 segments of the MCA, any segment of the ACA, and any segment of the PCA. The breakdown of the locations is as follows: M3, 41 cases; A1/A2, 23 cases; P1, 37 cases; and P2, 20 cases. The study found that patients presented with generally lower NIHSS scores than the LVO cohort, as would be expected. The mean NIHSS was 16 in the LVO group and 11 in the distal artery group, which was statistically significant ($p < 0.001$). In their series, they were more likely to use the ADAPT (A Direct Aspiration First-Pass Technique) [21] for revascularization in the distal group (57%) compared to ADAPT cases in the LVO group (44%), versus use of a stent retriever.

Interestingly, the procedural complication rate of 5% was the same in both the LVO and distal artery thrombectomy cases. Post-procedure successful revascularization rates of TICI 2b or TICI 3 were similar between the LVO thrombectomy group (84%) and the distal artery thrombectomy group (82%). Regarding clinical outcomes, the rate of mRS (modified Rankin Scale) score 0–2 was better in the distal group compared to the LVO group (51% vs. 40%), but since the distal groups started with a better functional baseline, the p value in the adjusted analysis did not show a statistical difference in good outcomes.

We will review several of the more common distal artery segments in this chapter. While each has its unique clinical presentation and angiographic anatomy, there are certain principles that are universal in the thrombectomy procedures of the distal vessels. (1) Thoughtful consideration should be given regarding whether thrombectomy is prudent. Just because we can technically perform the procedure does not necessarily mean we should do it. The benefit must clearly outweigh the risk and the patient or family should be thoroughly consented that there is a relative paucity of data on distal vessel thrombectomy. (2) Either a short-length stent retriever or aspiration catheter alone may be used. In our practice, this is fairly dependent on regional arterial anatomy and the interventionalist's preference. (3) Microwire access to the distal circulation should be seamless, and if the microwire cannot be advanced easily through and past the clot, it should not be advanced.

Arterial perforation in these smaller distal vessels has the potential for making patient's worse clinically. (4) We universally inject a vasolytic agent, such as nitroglycerin, into the artery before advancing the microcatheter and wire. Even a small amount of mechanically induced vasospasm can increase the difficulty in these small vessels exponentially.

M2 Segment Occlusion

Several of the mechanical thrombectomy studies focused specifically on M2 segment vessels (Table 15.2). While the percentage of cases treated with aspiration alone and stent retriever is variable in these studies, the revascularization rates and complication rates are very similar to, if not better than, M1 revascularizations. Because an M2 segment vessel may supply 50% or more of the entire MCA territory, an occlusion of this branch can lead to a significant neurologic deficit. Often, if the occlusion is in the dominant M2 branch, it may even be the same diameter as the M1 segment (Fig. 15.1a). As the M2 segment is vertical and the M1 segment is horizontal, however, the added hurdle of overcoming the angulation of the stent retriever or aspiration catheter with respect to the intermediate catheter is involved in the M2 vessel. Situating the aspiration intermediate catheter either in the distal M1 or very proximal M2 helps obviate this problem. Most interventionalists, from a technical standpoint, treat M1 and M2 occlusions similarly, although some prefer to use large-bore catheters directly on the M1 clots and somewhat smaller, more flexible, intermediate catheters for M2 to negotiate the 90-degree angulation and engage the M2 clot with the intermediate catheter. Either technique can result in

Table 15.2 Mechanical thrombectomy studies focused on the treatment of M2 occlusions

Study	Number of patients	Thrombectomy mode	TICI 2b or TICI 3
Flores, 2015 [8]	65	86% stent retriever, 4.6% IA tPA, 9% none (angiogram only)	78%
Dorn, 2015 [9]	15	Stent retriever	93%
Park, 2016 [10]	32	Aspiration 4MAX	84%
Countinho, 2016 [11]	50	Stent retriever	85%
Kim, 2017 [12]	41	25 aspiration, 16 stent retriever	64% aspiration, 81% stent retriever
Sarraj, JAMA Neurol, 2017 [13]	288	Stent retriever or aspiration	78%
Saber, 2017 [14]	337	200 stent retriever, 156 aspiration	87% stent retriever, 80% aspiration
Salahuddin, 2018 [15]	59	Stent retriever or aspiration	85%

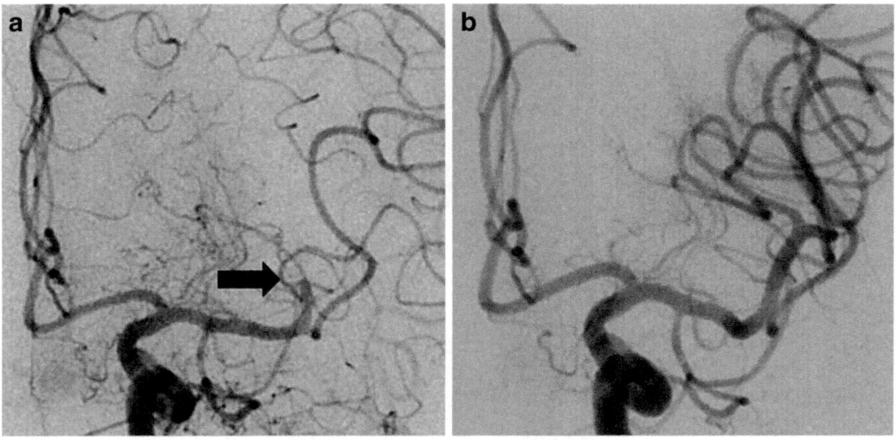

Fig. 15.1 Case example 1 – M2 segment occlusion. This nonagenarian patient presented with a left M2 occlusion (**a**); however, this branch supplied over 75% of the entire MCA territory as the dominant M2 branch. There is a 90% angulation between M1 and M2, but successful revascularization was achieved (**b**) with the intermediate aspiration catheter advanced to the end of the M1 segment and stent retriever past the M2 thrombus

TICI 3 revascularization (Fig. 15.1b). Kim et al. [12] reported a lower success rate of aspiration thrombectomy if the M2 occlusion was distal to the angulation of M2, presumably due to less effective engagement with the face of the clot.

M3–M4 Occlusions

The decision to perform a thrombectomy in patients with M3–M4 occlusions must be engaged with a greater reliance on the perceived risk-benefit ratio. There is currently no good randomized data on these distal occlusions. In our practice, if the deficit is pronounced, such as aphasia or monoplegia, then we believe thrombectomy is merited, particularly if tPA is not an option. However, more subtle deficits, such as a pronator drift, would not merit intervention.

Technical Considerations

We will often use a smaller intermediate catheter (1.65 mm outer diameter) that can access the distal M2 branch, which makes it technically easier to perform a stent retriever thrombectomy in the distal M3 or M4 vessel. In very tortuous anatomy, a "grappling hook" technique [22] can be used to anchor the stent retriever in the distal artery, pull some backward force on the stent retriever, and push forward force on the intermediate catheter to advance it closer to the face of the clot.

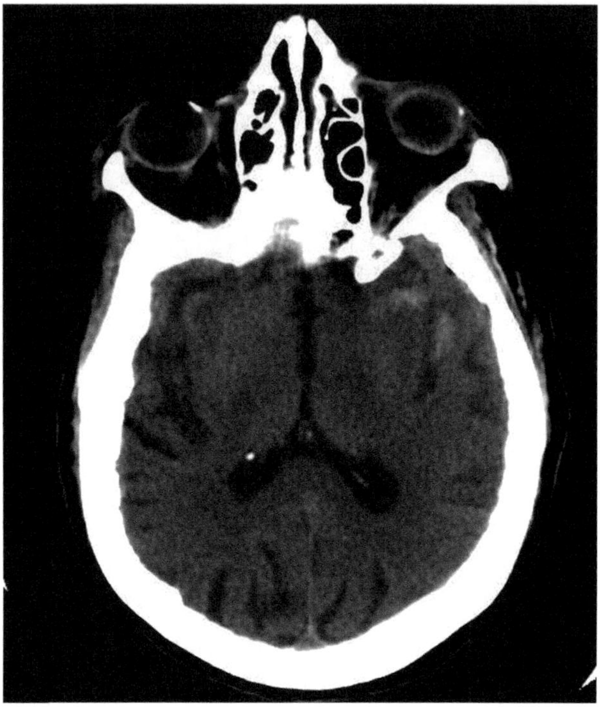

Fig. 15.2 Subarachnoid hemorrhage seen post-thrombectomy within the left Sylvian fissure following a left M3 segment mechanical thrombectomy. No contrast extravasation was seen during the procedure, and the bleed did not extend on follow-up scanning

Particularly in older patients with rigid, atherosclerotic vessels, the use of a stent retriever may transiently straighten or stretch a vessel that is not particularly mobile. In these more distal vessels, altering the shape of these arteries when retrieving the stent retriever may tear a small perforator vessel in the area, leading to subarachnoid hemorrhage. These may not be seen on the post-thrombectomy angiogram, but easily diagnosed on the post-intervention head CT (Fig. 15.2). Fortunately, these are typically self-limited bleeds, usually not requiring any additional intervention.

Likewise, ADAPT can be used in an M3–M4 branch using a smaller-sized aspiration catheter. A 4.7 French catheter will fit into vessels in the 1.2-mm range. These clots are typically small, so if one can get the catheter up to or slightly beyond the proximal face of the clot, then aspiration alone is highly successful with a single pass (Fig. 15.3).

Anterior Cerebral Artery Occlusions

A proximal A1 segment occlusion may potentially be of no clinical significance if there is an ample anterior communicating artery that supplies the distal ACA territory. One key exception would be if the artery of Heubner originated from the

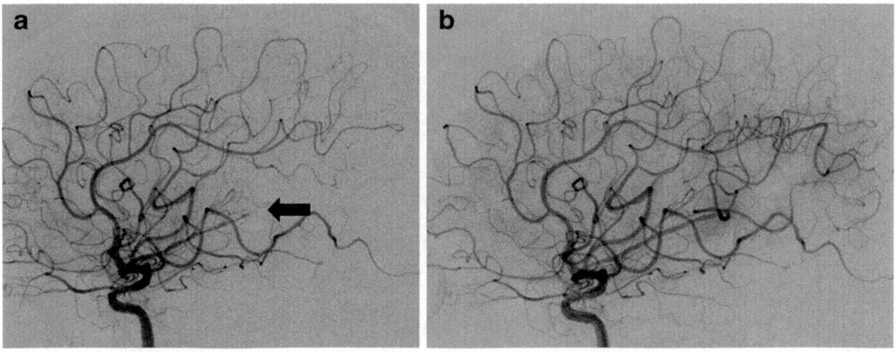

Fig. 15.3 Case example 2 – M4 segment occlusion. The patient presented with aphasia from this left M4 angular artery branch occlusion (**a**, arrow). The occluded artery appears very straight; however, the post-ADAPT thrombectomy angiogram demonstrates that the artery branches are very angulated past the initial occlusion, but full revascularization was possible with aspiration only (**b**)

occluded A1 segment. If the clot extends to the A1–A2 junction, however, then the opportunity for collateral flow from the anterior communicating artery is obviated. Typically, collateral blood flow from the pial MCA vessels or the PCA collaterals via the pericallosal artery is insufficient with acute ACA occlusion.

It may be more challenging to advance an intermediate aspiration catheter into the ACA as often this vessel originates at an acute angle from the ICA, whereas the MCA originates at an obtuse angle (Fig. 15.4). Smaller intermediate catheters have a better chance of accessing the A1 segment, especially if the "grappling hook" technique, which was described above, is employed. If A1 access with the intermediate catheter cannot be achieved, then it is best to leave the aspiration catheter in the distal ICA in an effort to engage at least the origin of the ACA as the stent retriever is being pulled back, to avoid inadvertent secondary embolization of the clot into the MCA branches.

Once the microcatheter is navigated into the A2 segment, the distal ACA is typically not tortuous, so it can be navigated fairly distal into the pericallosal artery, if needed. Typically, we will infuse 100 μg of intra-arterial nitroglycerin into the ACA prior to advancing the microcatheter to avoid mechanically induced vasospasm. Although it is still oversized, we prefer using a short, 3-mm-diameter stent retriever in the ACA to avoid arterial injury to the intima.

In more distal ACA occlusions in the A2 or distal pericallosal arteries, it is important to place the long sheath (with 0.088-inch inner lumen or larger) as distal as possible in the internal carotid artery and the intermediate catheter (in the 1.65-mm-outer-diameter range) in at least the A1 segment. This will not only give more support for the retrieval system but also will make it technically easier to track the stent retriever or small aspiration catheter to the distal clot. Particularly in cases of distal ACA occlusions or in the distal pericallosal artery, extra support and length is necessary to access distal vasculature (Fig. 15.5).

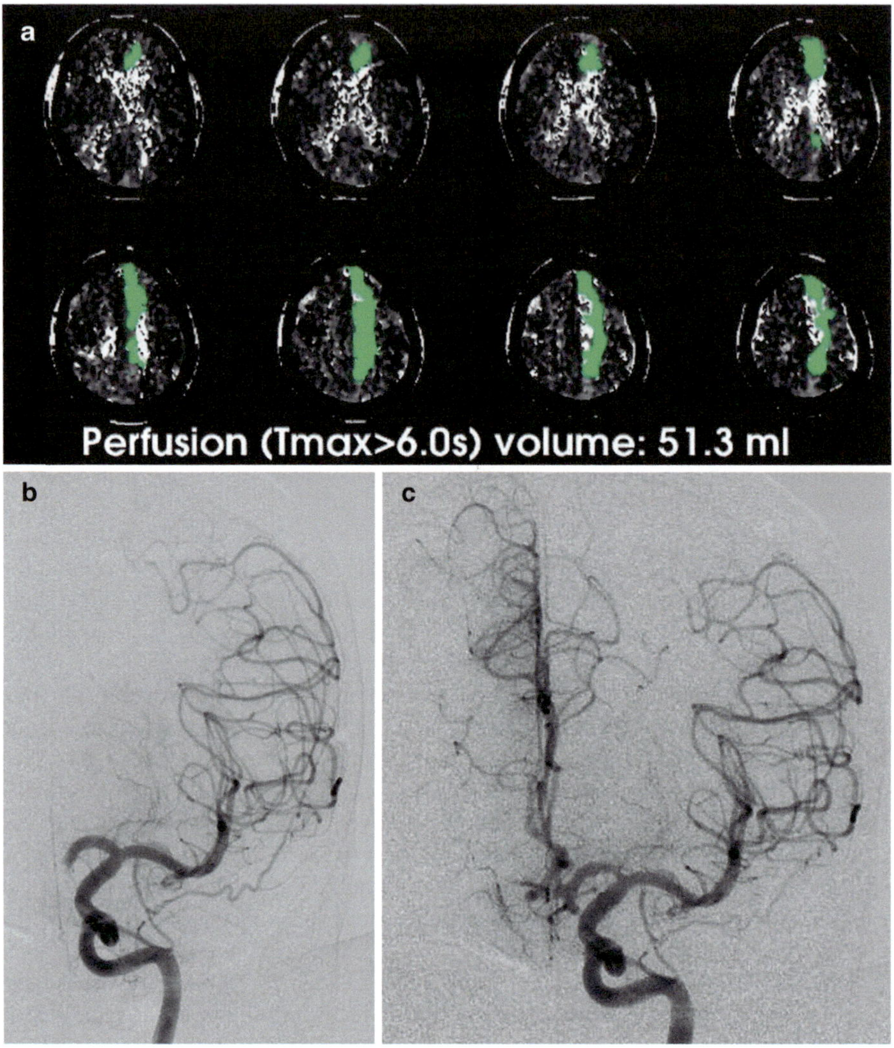

Fig. 15.4 Case example 3 – A1 segment ACA occlusion – The patient presented with abulia, did not speak or follow commands, and demonstrated right arm and leg weakness. CT perfusion demonstrated penumbra tissue along the entire ACA distribution (**a**). The initial angiogram demonstrated a distal A1 segment occlusion of a large ACA (**b**). Following a single-pass stent retriever and aspiration thrombectomy, there was revascularization of the ACA territory (**c**) with resolution of the patient's symptoms

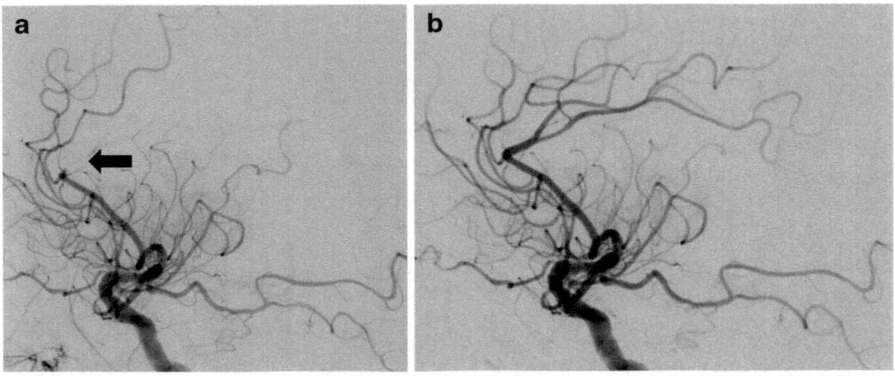

Fig. 15.5 Case example 4 – distal ACA segment occlusion – The patient presented with right-sided weakness and was found to have a distal ACA occlusion at the genu (**a**, arrow). Following the use of a 1.65-mm-outer-diameter intermediate catheter to the proximal A2 segment and 3-mm stent retriever, we obtained full revascularization of the ACA territory (**b**)

Posterior Cerebral Artery Occlusions

Occlusion of the PCA may initially present as a top of the basilar syndrome, and as the clot advances, it occludes the PCA (Fig. 15.6). Therefore, the patient may appear to improve significantly, but still have persistent unilateral deficits. The P1 segment occlusions are often the most devastating occlusions, particularly if they obstruct the thalamoperforators, which can result in a significant unilateral thalamic stroke, or in the rare occasions in which patients have an artery of Percheron, a bilateral thalamic stroke. If the clot is small, then the posterior communicating artery may supply blood to the distal PCA, but often the clot will transverse the P1–P2 junction or the posterior communicating artery is small or absent, so the entire PCA territory is at risk. The P1 segments, however, are often in the 2-mm-diameter range, so performing a thrombectomy is very similar to that of an M1 thrombectomy, with the exception that access through the vertebral arteries is smaller and more tortuous than that of ICA access. Also, similar to an M1 thrombectomy, in which a perfect TICI 3 revascularization can still have lenticulostriate perforator strokes in the basal ganglia, a technically perfect P1 thrombectomy could still have a thalamus stroke, due to the thalamoperforator vessel occlusion (Fig. 15.6d).

More distal PCA occlusions have no thalamic stroke symptoms but may have hemianopsia or hemi-sensory deficit or neglect which is significant for the patient. Thrombectomy in the more distal PCA branches technically is somewhat dependent on the distal tortuosity and size of the vessels (Fig. 15.7). With minimal deficits intervention is likely not indicated; however, reversal of visual and sensory deficits is achievable if the artery is of significant size.

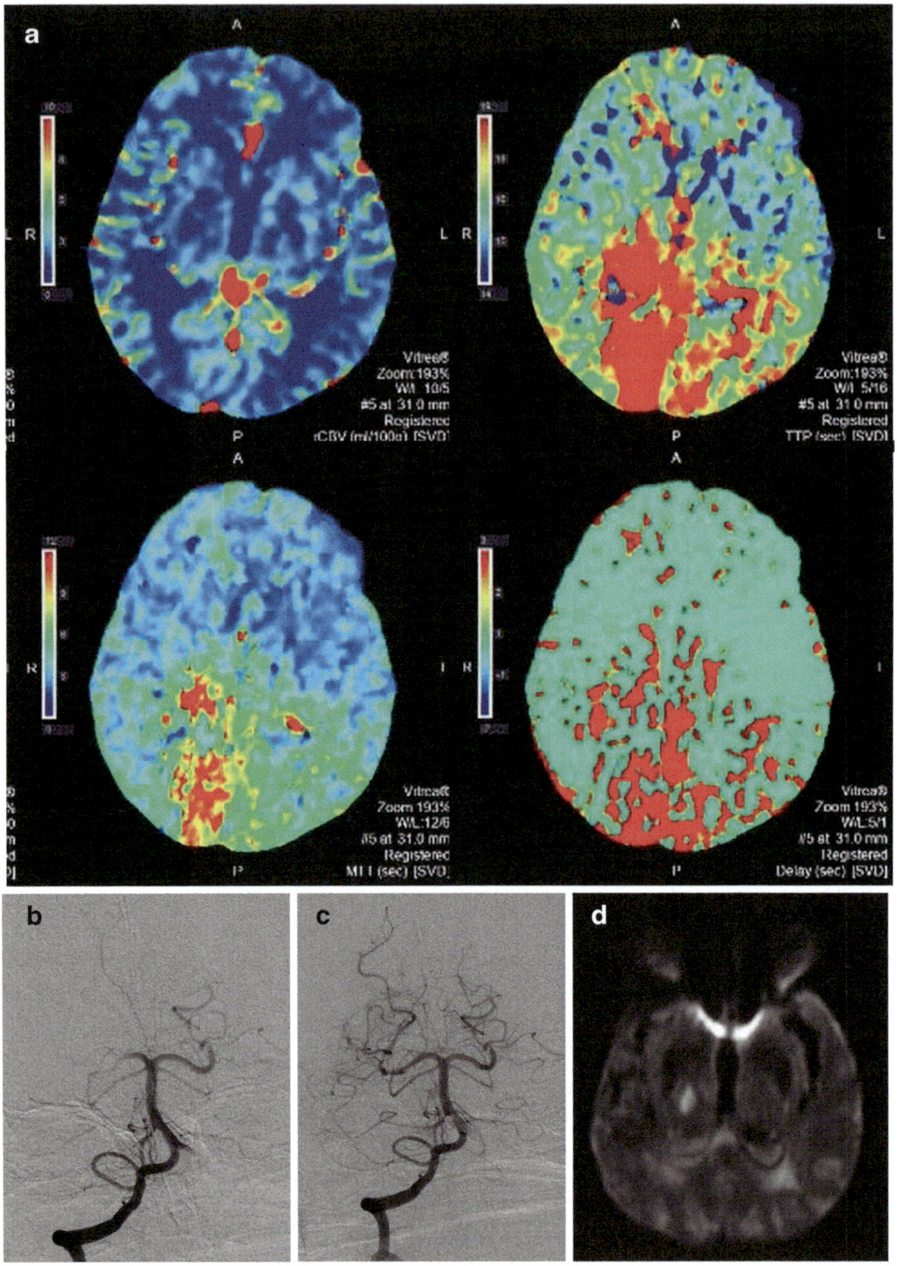

Fig. 15.6 Case example 5 – P1 segment PCA occlusion – The patient presented with confusion, left-sided neglect, hemi-sensory loss, visual field deficit, and left-sided weakness. The CTP demonstrated a right PCA perfusion deficit, including the thalamus (**a**). The initial angiogram showed a right P1 PCA occlusion (**b**). Following a single pass with a stent retriever and large-bore (0.072-inch inner diameter) aspiration catheter in the P1 segment, there was full revascularization of the PCA territory (**c**). Post-thrombectomy MRI at 24 hours shows no distal PCA infarct; however, there is a right thalamic infarct seen (**d**)

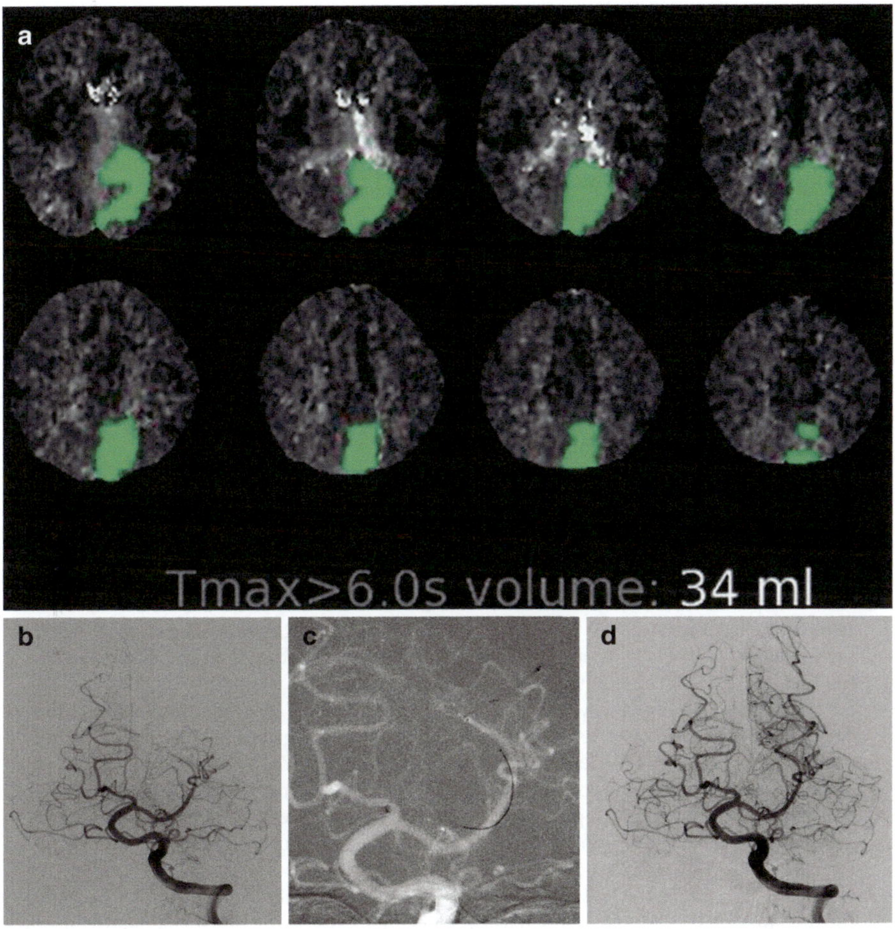

Fig. 15.7 Case example 6 – distal PCA segment occlusion. The patient presented with an acute right hemianopsia as well as right-sided neglect. CTP showed a large penumbra area in the left PCA territory (**a**). The angiogram showed a left P3–P4 occlusion (**b**); however, the P1 and P2 segments are large and not tortuous, making access of the M3–M4 branch occlusion possible with the stent retriever (**c**). The post-thrombectomy angiogram demonstrated full extensive revascularization of the entire PCA territory (**d**), and the patient's symptoms immediately resolved

Conclusions

While the use of mechanical thrombectomy of the M2 segment in the initial thrombectomy trials was less focused upon, compared to other LVO occlusions, the subsequent literature places thrombectomy of the vessel more likely in the LVO occlusion category, than distal or intermediate-sized artery. Thrombectomy in the more distal vessels, such as M3 and M4, the ACA branches, and the PCA branches is far less common in most series and clinical experiences. This may partially be due to the fact that IV tPA is more effective at lysing these smaller clots quickly, compared to LVO. Therefore, we generally encounter persistent distal vessel occlusions less frequently. However, in situations in which either IV tPA is not possible or has not lysed the distal clot, mechanical thrombectomy of distal arteries appears to be as safe and as effective as thrombectomy in LVO, based on the STAR registry data.

Either a stent retriever with aspiration or ADAPT with a smaller intermediate aspiration catheter than the ones used in LVO appears to be a viable treatment option in these distal vessels. As our experience with intermediate-sized, distal vessel occlusions grows, we will likely be able to help more patients with distal artery occlusions in which management options are limited.

References

1. Berkhemer OA, Fransen PS, Beumer D, van den Berg LA, Lingsma HF, Yoo AJ, The MR CLEAN Investigators, et al. A randomized trial of intraarterial treatment for acute ischemic stroke. N Engl J Med. 2015;372:11–20.
2. Goyal M, Demchuk AM, Menon BK, Eesa M, Rempel JL, Thornton J, et al. Randomized assessment of rapid endovascular treatment of ischemic stroke. N Engl J Med. 2015;372:1019–30.
3. Jovin TG, Chamorro A, Cobo E, de Miquel MA, Molina CA, Rovira A, The REVASCAT Trial Investigators, et al. Thrombectomy within 8 hours after symptom onset in ischemic stroke. N Engl J Med. 2015;372(24):2296–306.
4. Saver JL, Goyal M, Bonafe A, Diener HC, Levy EI, Pereira VM, et al. Stent-retriever thrombectomy after intravenous t-PA vs. t-PA alone in stroke. N Engl J Med. 2015;372:2285–95.
5. Campbell BC, Mitchell PI, Kleinig TI, Dewey HM, Churilov I, Yassi N, et al. Endovascular therapy for ischemic stroke with perfusion imaging selection. N Engl J Med. 2015;372:1009–18.
6. Albers GW, Marks MP, Kemp S, Christensen S, Tsai JP, Ortega-Gutierrez S, The DEFUSE 3 Investigators, et al. Thrombectomy for stroke at 6 to 16 hours with selection by perfusion imaging. N Engl J Med. 2018;378(8):708–18.
7. Nogueira RG, Jadhav AP, Haussen DC, Bonafe A, Budzik RF, Bhuva P, The DAWN Investigators, et al. Thrombectomy 6 to 24 hours after stroke with a mismatch between deficit and infarct. N Engl J Med. 2018;378:11–21.
8. Flores A, Tomasello A, Cardona P, Angeles de Miquel M, Gomis M, Garcia Bermejo P, Catalan Stroke Code and Reperfusion Consortium (Cat-SCR), et al. Endovascular treatment for M2 occlusions in the era of stentrievers: a descriptive multicenter experience. J Neurointerv Surg. 2015;7:234–7.
9. Dorn F, Lockau H, Stetefeld H, Kabbasch C, Kraus B, Dohmen C, et al. Mechanical thrombectomy of M2-occlusion. J Stroke Cerebrovasc Dis. 2015;24:1465–70.
10. Park JS, Kwak HS. Manual aspiration thrombectomy using penumbra catheter in patients with acute M2 occlusion: a single-center analysis. J Korean Neurosurg Soc. 2016;59:352–6.
11. Countinho JM, Liebeskind DS, Slater LA, Nogueira RG, Baxter BW, Levy EI, et al. Mechanical thrombectomy for isolated M2 occlusions: a post hoc analysis of the STAR, SWIFT, and SWIFT PRIME studies. AJNR Am J Neuroradiol. 2016;37:667–72.
12. Kim YW, Son S, Kang DH, Hwang YH, Kim YS. Endovascular thrombectomy for M2 occlusions: comparison between forced arterial suction thrombectomy and stent retriever thrombectomy. J Neurointerv Surg. 2017;9:626–30.
13. Sarraj A, Sangha N, Hussain MS, Wisco D, Vora N, Elijovich L, et al. Endovascular therapy for acute ischemic stroke with occlusion of the middle cerebral artery M2 segment. JAMA Neurol. 2017;74:488–9.

14. Saber H, Narayanan S, Palla M, Saver JL, Nogueira RG, Yoo AJ, et al. Mechanical thrombectomy for acute ischemic stroke with occlusion of the M2 segment of the middle cerebral artery: a meta-analysis. J Neurointerv Surg. 2018;10:620–4.
15. Salahuddin H, Ramaiah G, Slawski DE, Shawver J, Buehler M, Zaidi SF, et al. Mechanical thrombectomy of M1 and M2 middle cerebral artery occlusions. J Neurointerv Surg. 2018;10:330–4.
16. Grossberg JA, Rebello LC, Haussen DC, Bouslama M, Bowen M, Barreira CM, et al. Beyond large vessel occlusion strokes: distal occlusion thrombectomy. Stroke. 2018;49:1662–8.
17. Vargas J, Spiotta AM, Fargen K, Turner RD, Chaudry I, Turk A. Experience with a direct aspiration first pass technique (ADAPT) for thrombectomy in distal cerebral artery occlusions causing acute ischemic stroke. World Neurosurg. 2017;99:31–6.
18. Meyne JK, Zimmermann PR, Rohr A, Riedel C, Hansen HC, Pulkowski U, et al. Thrombectomy vs. systemic thrombolysis in acute embolic stroke with high clot burden: a retrospective analysis. Rofo. 2015;187:555–60.
19. Powers WJ, Rabinstein AA, Ackerson T, Adeoye OM, Bambakidis NC, Becker K, et al. Guidelines for the early management of patients with acute ischemic stroke: 2019 update to the 2018 guidelines for the early management of acute ischemic stroke: a guideline for healthcare professionals from the American Heart Association/American Stroke Association. Stroke. 2019;50:e344–418.
20. Anadani M, Alawieh A, Arthur AS, Kim JT, De Leacy R, Maier I, The STAR Collaborators, et al. Mechanical thrombectomy for distal occlusions: efficacy, functional and safety outcomes: insight from the STAR collaboration. Presented at the International Stroke Conference, Los Angeles, CA, February 2020.
21. Turk AS, Spiotta A, Frei D, Mocco J, Baxter B, Fiorella D, et al. Initial clinical experience with the ADAPT technique: a direct aspiration first pass technique for stroke thrombectomy. J Neurointerv Surg. 2014;6:231–7.
22. Hui FK, Hussain MS, Spiotta A, Bhalla T, Toth G, Moskowitz SI, et al. Merci retrievers as access adjuncts for reperfusion catheters: the grappling hook technique. Neurosurgery. 2012;70:456–60.

Chapter 16
The Tandem Occlusion

Charlotte Y. Chung, Liwei Jiang, Ferdinand K. Hui, and Blaise William Baxter

The treatment approaches for large vessel anterior circulation acute ischemic strokes with concomitant extracranial internal carotid artery tandem occlusions remain controversial. Our first area of debate surrounds the "what to tackle first" dilemma and deciding on the treatment order of approach. This order of approach dilemma encompasses all possible technique combinations and permutations for addressing the intracranial and extracranial target lesions. The order is not the only debated issue, however. How best to treat the extracranial carotid occlusion is also debated – whether to use the Dotter technique, angioplasty alone, or angioplasty plus carotid stenting. Our second area of debate is similar to Hamlet's Shakespearean dilemma, but in this setting to stent or not to stent, that is the question. The main concern surrounding the "to stent or not to stent" controversy is unrelated to technical difficulty of stent placement in this clinical setting. The hesitancy to definitively treat the carotid occlusive stenosis by stenting lies in committing the patient to dual antiplatelet therapy (DAPT). The antiplatelet regime and the symptomatic hemorrhagic transformation rate in this acute stroke patient population are debated and have not

C. Y. Chung (✉)
Department of Radiology and Imaging Sciences, Emory University School of Medicine, Atlanta, GA, USA
e-mail: charlotte.yuk-yan.chung@emory.edu

L. Jiang
Department of Radiology, Brigham and Women's Hospital, Boston, MA, USA

F. K. Hui
Department of Radiology, Division of Interventional Neuroradiology, The Johns Hopkins Hospital, Baltimore, MD, USA

B. W. Baxter
Department of Radiology, Lehigh Valley Health Network, Allentown, PA, USA

F. K. Hui et al. (eds.), *12 Strokes*, https://doi.org/10.1007/978-3-030-56857-3_16

been the specific focus of endovascular stroke trials. Here we present cases from our practices to highlight several of the technique options for approaching the typical as well as the more complex tandem occlusions.

Case 1

First, we describe the commonly used proximal-to-distal (extracranial-first) strategy for treating tandem occlusions.

Presentation

A 42-year-old woman presented 5 hours after onset of aphasia, right-sided weakness, and right facial droop, with a National Institutes of Health Stroke Scale (NIHSS) score of 12. Pertinent history included hypertension and smoking. Initial non-contrast CT of the head revealed a hyperdense MCA sign on the left, with no appreciable parenchymal hypodensities (ASPECTS 10) (Fig. 16.1a). CT angiography of the head and neck showed tandem occlusions of the left cervical internal carotid artery (ICA) (Fig. 16.1b) and carotid terminus (Fig. 16.1c).

The patient was brought to the angiography suite 7 hours after symptom onset. Initial angiogram showed occlusion of the left ICA at its origin (Fig. 16.2a). Intracranially, the left MCA and ACA were non-opacified, consistent with concomitant carotid T occlusion (Fig. 16.2b).

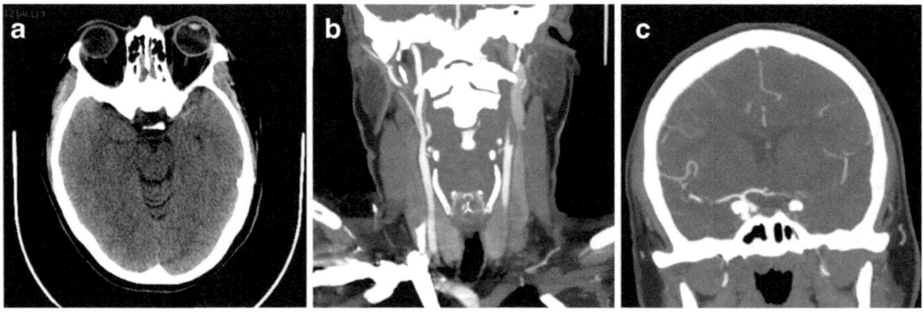

Fig. 16.1 Tandem occlusions of the left cervical ICA and ICA terminus in a woman with left MCA syndrome. (**a**) Axial non-contrast CT of the head shows a dense left MCA. (**b**) Coronal CT angiogram of the neck demonstrates tapering occlusion of the proximal left cervical ICA. (**c**) Concomitant non-opacification of the left ICA cavernous segment and terminus with minimal opacification of the left A1 and M1 segments is seen on coronal CT angiogram of the head. Reconstitution of the distal territories from the contralateral circulation is noted

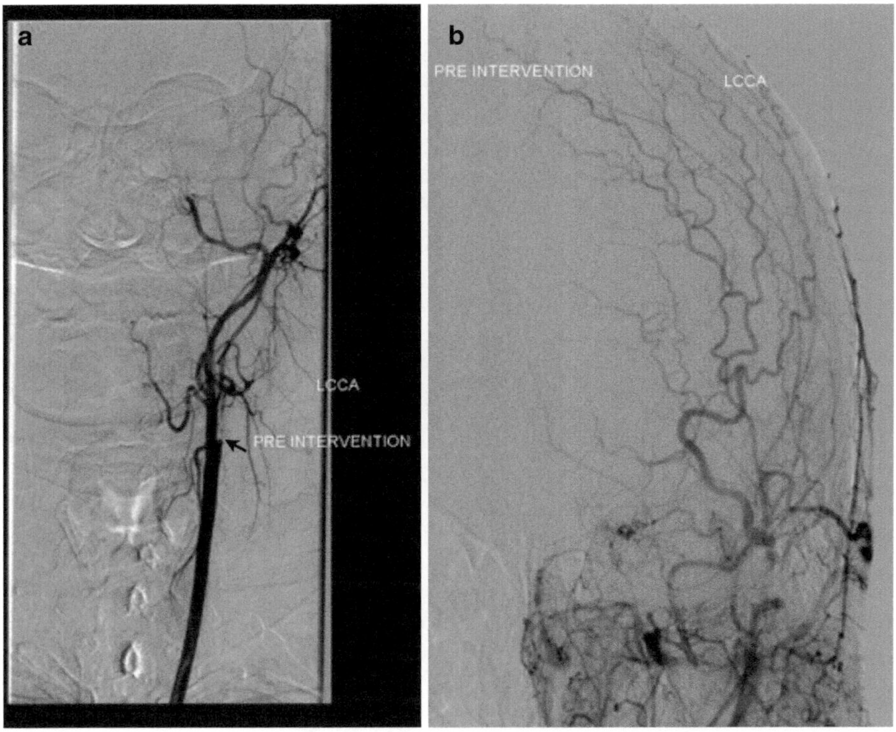

Fig. 16.2 Pre-intervention angiogram with AP views at the neck and head. (**a**) Cervical view of left CCA injection shows abrupt cutoff at the left ICA origin (arrow). The left ECA and distal branches are opacified. (**b**) Cranial view demonstrates no filling of the intracranial left ICA, MCA, ACA, or their distal branches, with absent retrograde flow to distal ICA vasculature. Distal branches of the left ECA are opacified

Technique

Treatment of the tandem occlusion was approached in a proximal-to-distal manner. An 8F (10 cm length) Terumo Pinnacle (Terumo Corporation, Tokyo, Japan) femoral access sheath was placed. 6F (80 cm length) straight-tip Penumbra Neuron MAX 088 sheath (Penumbra Inc., Alameda, California, USA) was then advanced coaxially over a 6F (125 cm length) Penumbra Berenstein Select catheter and angled-tip 035 (180 cm length) standard Terumo glidewire. With the Neuron MAX tip in the distal left common carotid artery (CCA), an arteriogram was performed to identify the site of the occlusion at the origin of the left internal carotid artery (ICA) (Fig. 16.3a). A 4F (120 cm length) angled Terumo Glidecath tip was pointed at the ICA stump and the 035 Terumo glidewire advanced across the occlusive stenosis. With the Glidewire beyond the occlusive stenosis, the 4F Glidecath was then advanced over the wire until the catheter tip was in the distal cervical segment of the left ICA. The glidewire was then exchanged for a 014 J-tip (300 cm length) Boston

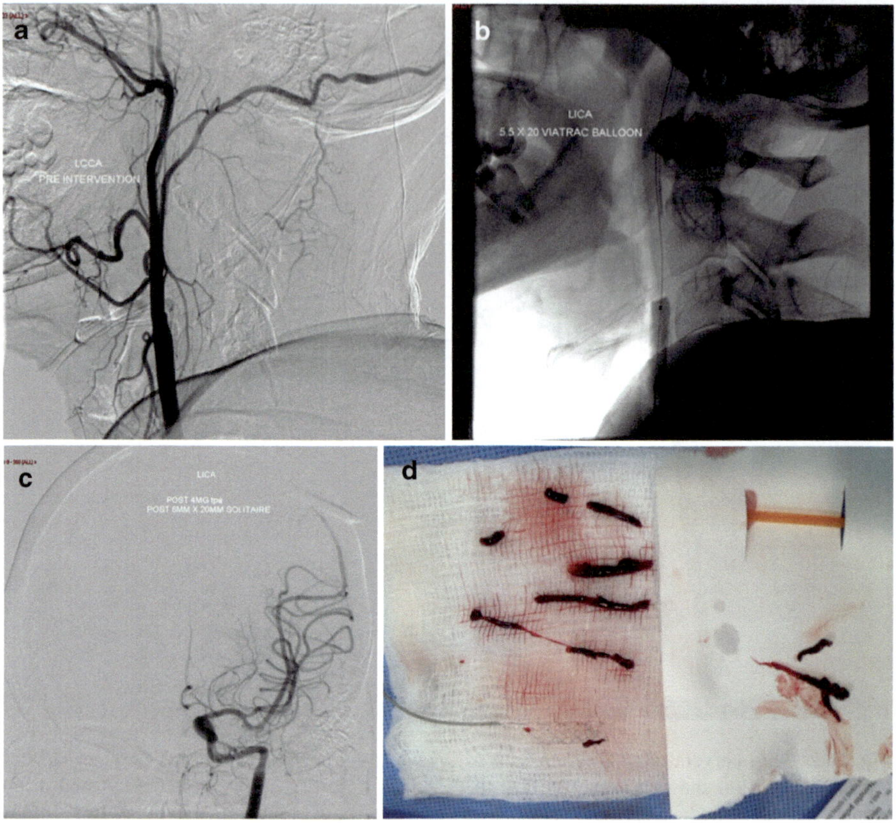

Fig. 16.3 Angioplasty of the proximal cervical left ICA occlusion followed by intracranial thrombectomy. (**a**) Complete occlusion at the ICA origin is seen on pre-interventional lateral cervical view of the left CCA injection. (**b**) Non-subtracted lateral cervical view demonstrates the inflated Viatrac 5.5 × 20 mm balloon across the expected location of the left ICA origin, when compared to the pre-intervention subtracted view (**a**). (**c**) AP cranial view of left ICA injection after 4 mg intra-arterial tPA and one pass of the 6 × 20 mm Solitaire FR stent retriever shows improved flow at the left carotid terminus, ACA, MCA, and distal vasculature. (**d**) Multiple passes with the stent retriever were performed with removal of significant clot burden

Scientific PT Graphix intermediate guidewire (Boston Scientific, Marlborough, Massachusetts, USA). The occlusive stenosis at the left ICA origin was then angioplastied using a 5.5 × 20 mm Abbott RX Viatrac 14 plus peripheral dilatation balloon (Abbott Laboratories, Abbott Park, Illinois, USA) (Fig. 16.3b). During balloon deflation the Neuron MAX tip was advanced across the stenosis. A Medtronic 027 Marksman microcatheter (ev3/Medtronic Plc, Dublin, Ireland) was advanced over a 014 (205 cm length) Transcend soft-tip guidewire (Stryker, Kalamazoo, Michigan, USA). When the microcatheter tip reached the clot, the guidewire was removed and 4 mg of tissue plasminogen activator (tPA) were administered intra-arterially within the clot. Two thrombectomy passes were then performed using a Medtronic 6 × 20 mm Solitaire FR stent retriever and a large clot burden was removed (Fig. 16.3d).

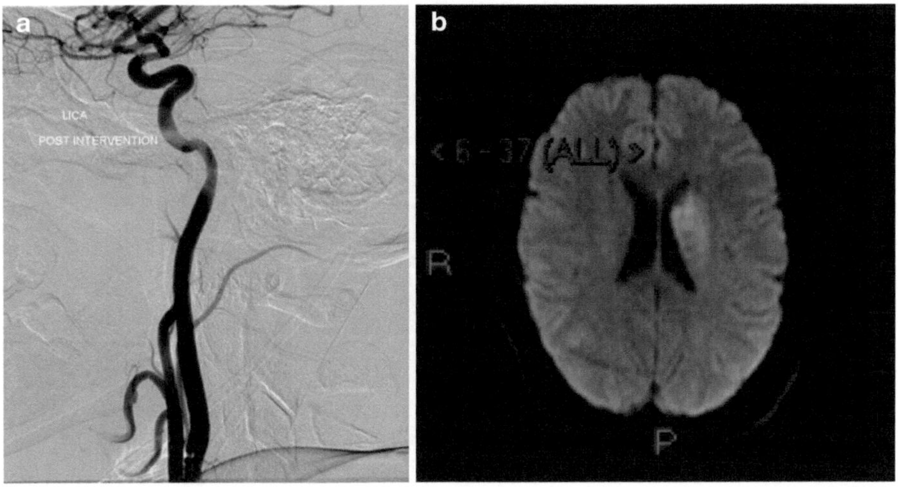

Fig. 16.4 Post-intervention outcome. (**a**) Lateral cervical view of left ICA injection demonstrates widely patent left ICA at the site of prior occlusion and angioplasty. (**b**) Axial diffusion-weighted MRI of the brain obtained 24 hours after intervention demonstrated residual restricted diffusion at the left basal ganglia, consistent with acute infarction

Post-two passes, TICI 2B cerebral revascularization was achieved (Fig. 16.3c). The sheath tip was then withdrawn into the distal left CCA. Arteriogram was performed to assess patency of the angioplastied occlusive stenosis at the origin of the left ICA (Fig. 16.4a). With there being patency at the stenosis and robust flow within the ICA, stent placement was deemed unnecessary and the procedure was terminated. Total procedural time was 50 minutes. The patient recovered uneventfully and was discharged on post-procedural day 4, with NIHSS score of 1 and residual infarct involving only the left basal ganglia (Fig. 16.4b). On follow-up, 30- and 90-day mRS were 0.

Comments from Authors: Extracranial-First Approach

The proximal-to-distal (or extracranial-first) approach was employed in this case by first addressing the proximal lesion with balloon angioplasty. Since the proximal lesion can be recanalized easily and quickly in the majority of cases with angioplasty alone, this is a straightforward approach to gain rapid access to the intracranial occlusion. Following treatment of the intracranial occlusion, re-examining the recanalized proximal occlusion allows one to determine the need for further angioplasty and/or stenting. Instead of aiming for complete vessel patency, the objective at this juncture is to eliminate significant flow limitation, which would predispose to re-thrombosis and possible recurrent distal embolization. Angioplasty alone is our preferred recanalization technique for the emergent

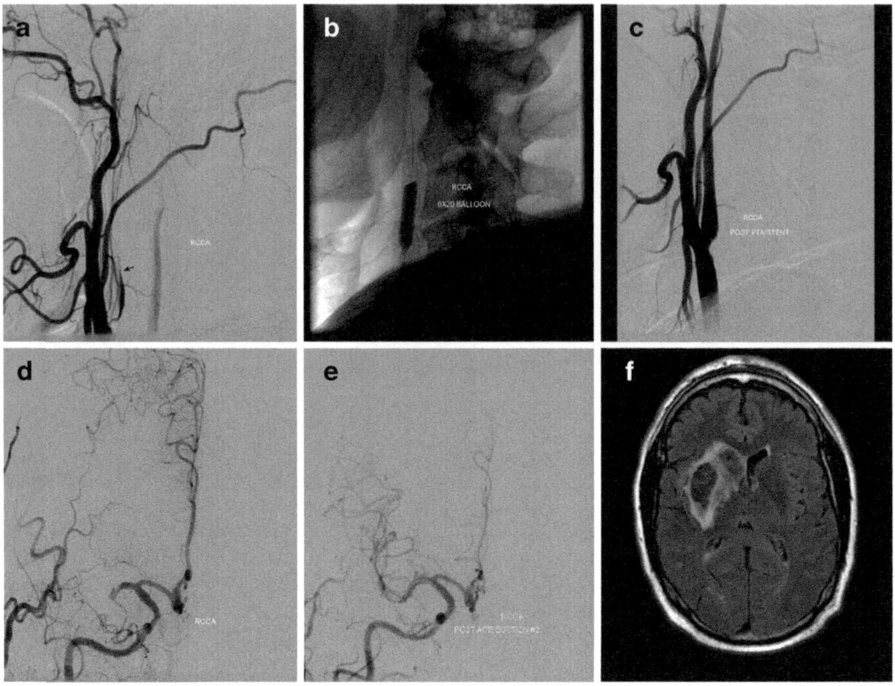

Fig. 16.5 A 55-year-old man presents with right MCA syndrome and an NIHSS score of 14. Initial lateral cervical angiogram (**a**) shows complete occlusion of the cervical right ICA (arrow). Treatment with balloon angioplasty, stenting, and post-stenting balloon dilation (**b**) resulted in resolution of the occlusion (**c**). Subsequent AP cranial angiogram (**d**) demonstrates tandem occlusion of the right MCA M1 segment, which was successfully revascularized with two-pass direct aspiration with a Penumbra ACE reperfusion catheter (**e**). (**f**) MRI axial FLAIR image of the brain obtained post-intervention demonstrates an infarct limited to the right basal ganglia

procedure. (The need for an antiplatelet regimen, which potentially increases the risks of hemorrhagic conversion and intracranial bleeding, makes stenting a less attractive option in the acute peri-stroke period.) Vessels with residual stenosis can subsequently be interrogated with noninvasive imaging (CT or MR angiogram) and definitive treatment with stenting (if necessary) deferred until the risks of initiating DAPT are deemed reasonable. However, if maintaining patency of the ICA is of concern at the time of the thrombectomy procedure, then antiplatelet therapy can be initiated and stent placement performed (Fig. 16.5a–f). The rationale for each procedural step described above and the materials/devices selected will now be addressed. In gaining femoral access, the choice to place a short femoral sheath rather than use the Neuron MAX as the stand-alone sheath is twofold. Firstly, it allows the long sheath to be placed in a one-step fashion coaxially over the Select diagnostic catheter, and this one-step approach is often a time-saving procedural maneuver. If there is challenging arch anatomy, then the short sheath allows the operator to address the challenging access with their favorite "tough arch" catheter and exchange over a "stiffer" exchange-length guidewire for placement of the long carotid access sheath. Secondly, the occluded ICA may have a significant clot burden to address. The long sheath can be used to aspirate and remove this ICA clot. If the long sheath becomes occluded, then it is easily removed to clear the lumen with the short sheath maintaining femoral access. When attempting to cross the occlusive stenosis, the support of a 035 guidewire vs. a 014 guidewire is often required. The angled 035 Glidewire already opened for the long carotid sheath placement often works well. The angled tip in some cases may catch on the underlying plaque and may make crossing the narrowed lumen at the stenosis site difficult. In these cases, pointing the tip of the 4F angled catheter at the apex of the ICA stump and using a straight-tip 035 Glidewire to explore the stenosis can often be successful to gain access across the occlusion. Once across the occlusive stenosis, the 014 J-tip (300 cm length) Boston Scientific PT Graphix intermediate guidewire was employed as the exchange-length 014 guidewire for angioplasty. The PT Graphix guidewire was selected as it provides good support during angioplasty and subsequent sheath advancement across the stenosis. Sheath advancement across the stenosis is also facilitated by using a "balloon anchoring" technique. When the balloon is inflated to angioplasty the stenosis, the operator can begin advancing the Neuron MAX tip. When the Neuron MAX tip gets to the proximal end of the balloon, deflation is initiated and simultaneously the Neuron MAX tip is advanced over the partially deflated balloon. This "balloon anchoring" technique helps protect the stenotic site and reduces the shoulder that is present if the Neuron MAX is advanced over the bare wire. With access to treat the intracranial occlusion gained, a small dose of intra-arterial tissue plasminogen activator (tPA) was delivered into the intracranial occlusive clot. Presently, the shorter procedural times and improved TICI 2B/3 revascularization scores with thrombectomy devices alone have largely eliminated this practice of adjunctive administration of intra-arterial tPA. During performance of the thrombectomy passes, a balloon guide catheter was felt to be unnecessary as the sheath advanced across the proximal ICA stenosis was occlusive providing arrest of antegrade flow within the ICA. During withdrawal of the stent retriever into the sheath tip, sheath aspiration was applied in order to help deliver the clot into the sheath lumen and avoid stripping the clot from the thrombectomy device. Once successful intracranial revascularization was achieved, the sheath tip was withdrawn into the distal left CCA and an arteriogram performed in order to ensure patency of the left ICA (Fig. 16.4a). With there being patency of the stenosis and robust flow within the ICA, stent placement was deemed unnecessary.

Case 2

Alternatively, tandem occlusions can be approached in a distal-to-proximal (intracranial-first) fashion, first targeting the distal occlusion. In this case we describe the modified Dotter technique for proximal recanalization.

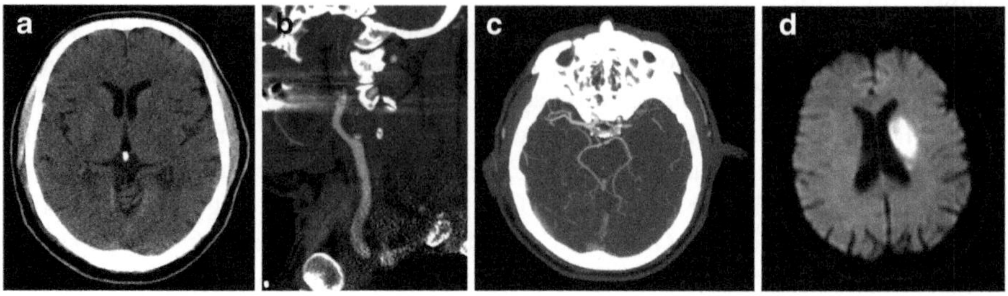

Fig. 16.6 Left basal ganglia infarct in a patient with left ICA origin and M1 segment tandem occlusions. (**a**) Axial non-contrast CT image of the head demonstrates loss of gray-white differentiation and hypoatttenuation of the left putamen and globus pallidus. (**b**) Sagittal CT angiogram image of the neck shows non-opacification of the left ICA at the carotid bifurcation, with atherosclerotic calcifications of the proximal ICA, suggestive of atherosclerotic disease as the underlying cause of the proximal occlusion. (**c**) Axial CT angiogram of the head shows arterial cutoff of the left MCA proximal M1 segment, with reconstitution of the distal M3 territory (likely from ACA-MCA leptomeningeal collaterals). (**d**) Axial diffusion-weighted MRI image of the brain obtained 1.5 hours after arrival demonstrates restricted diffusion limited to the left basal ganglia, consistent with infarction

Presentation

A 73-year-old man was found down in the early morning with symptoms consistent with left MCA syndrome and an NIHSS score of 24. On arrival, non-contrast CT of the head showed a subtle hypodensity at the left basal ganglia and no intracranial hemorrhage (Fig. 16.6a). He was deemed not to be a candidate for IV-tPA due to uncertain symptom onset time. Arterial cutoffs at the left ICA origin and the M1 segment of the left MCA were seen on CT angiogram, consistent with a tandem occlusion (Fig. 16.6b, c). A relatively small area of restricted diffusion isolated to the left basal ganglia on MRI (Fig. 16.6d) was a mismatch to the severity of his clinical deficits, prompting the decision for endovascular intervention. Initial diagnostic angiograms showed occlusions of the left ICA origin (Fig. 16.7a) extending to the petrous portion and the proximal M1 segment of the left MCA (Fig. 16.7b).

Technique

The modified Dotter technique [1] was employed. A coaxial system of a Penumbra Neuron MAX, a Penumbra 054 reperfusion catheter, a Marksman microcatheter (ev3/Medtronic Plc, Dublin, Ireland), and a 016 Fathom guidewire (Boston Scientific, Marlborough, Massachusetts, USA) was used to select the left common carotid artery proximal to the occlusion. The proximal left ICA occlusion was tunneled through sequentially with the guidewire and then the microcatheter. The Penumbra 054 reperfusion catheter was then advanced through the occlusion. Control angiogram with the catheter tip distal to the proximal occlusion demonstrated the proximal left M1 occlusion (Fig. 16.8a). Mechanical thrombectomy of

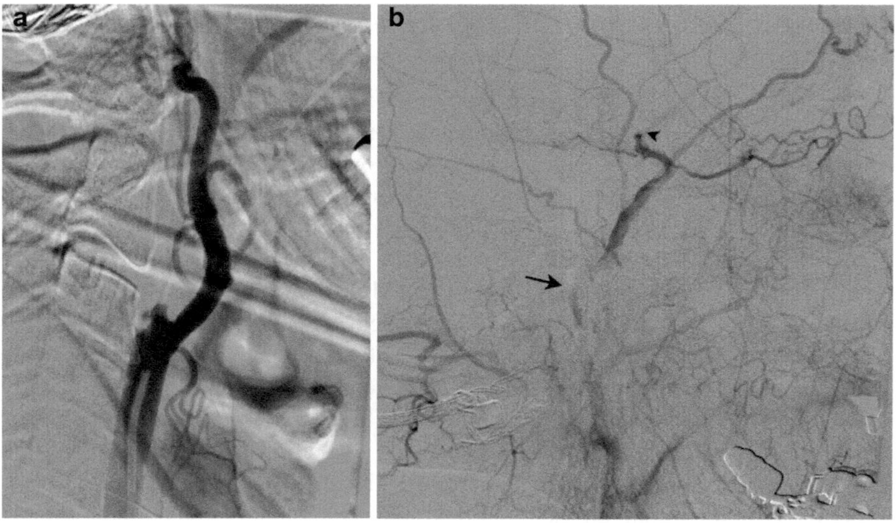

Fig. 16.7 Pre-intervention angiogram with lateral views at the neck and head. (**a**) Cervical view of left CCA injection shows abrupt occlusion of the left ICA origin. (**b**) Cranial view demonstrates distal reconstitution from the ophthalmic artery, with occlusive thrombus at the left ICA petrous segment (arrow) and proximal left M1 segment (arrowhead)

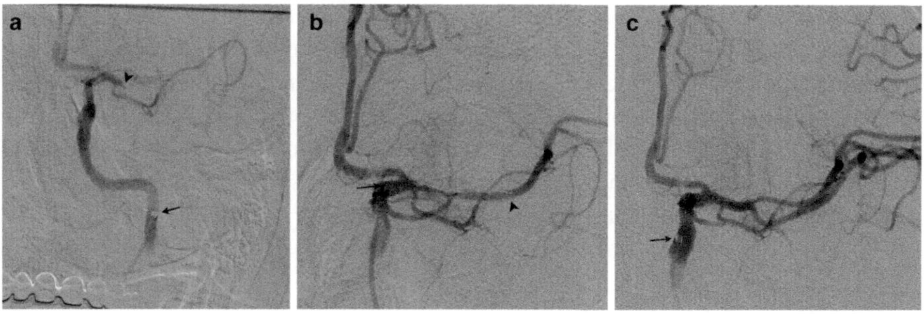

Fig. 16.8 Injections and thrombectomy after advancement of the 0.054″ aspiration catheter beyond the proximal left ICA occlusion. (**a**) AP cranial view shows the tip of the 0.054″ catheter at the left ICA petrous segment (arrow). Tapering occlusion of the proximal left M1 segment is seen just distal to an early anterior temporal branch (arrowhead). (**b**) The 0.054″ catheter was further advanced until the tip was at the supraclinoid segment (arrow). The Solitaire FR stent retriever was deployed under aspiration across the proximal M1 occlusion (arrowhead). (**c**) Repeat angiogram with 0.054″ catheter (arrow) pulled back to the clinoidal segment demonstrates resolution of the proximal M1 occlusion

the M1 occlusion was performed with a Medtronic Solitaire FR stent retriever under aspiration (Fig. 16.8b), with successful TICI 3 recanalization (Fig. 16.8c). No further intervention was needed for the proximal ICA occlusion. Aspiration time was 2 minutes, with total case time of 1.25 hours. Post-procedure, the patient's symptoms completely resolved and he was discharged to home with an NIHSS score of 0.

Comments from Authors: Modified Dotter Technique

In this case, the tandem occlusion was approached in a distal-to-proximal (intracranial-first) manner. Using the modified Dotter technique allowed recanalization of the proximal occlusion without balloon angioplasty or stenting. Traditionally, the intracranial-first strategy involves first treating the distal occlusion and then addressing the proximal occlusion with balloon angioplasty and/or stenting. Those in favor of the intracranial-first strategy cite a shorter time from groin puncture to end-organ reperfusion [2]. In treating tandem occlusions, MCA flow improvement post-thrombolysis was strongly associated with clinical benefit, even in the setting of failed ICA recanalization [3], supporting the importance of addressing the distal lesion. One should be aware that treating the extracranial occlusion after restoring flow distally risks distal embolization of dislodged thrombi. Lockau et al. state that continuous clot aspiration may reduce this risk [2], while Hui et al. advocate deploying an embolic protection device distal to the carotid occlusion [4]. Woodward et al. describe a modified Dotter technique that achieves proximal patency without stenting and thus obviates the need for antiplatelet therapy, akin to the manner in which Dotter and Judkins in the 1960s crossed an occlusion with a guidewire and recanalized the vessel with progressively larger stiff catheters [5]. The modified Dotter technique employs a hydrophilic guidewire (or a microwire, if desired) to cross the occluded segment, followed by sequential forceful advancement of a diagnostic catheter and then a sheath over the guidewire through the occlusion while under vigorous aspiration; once proximal patency is achieved, the intracranial clot is treated with catheter aspiration. Limitations of the modified Dotter technique include unknown long-term proximal patency, the possibility of extending an occlusion due to dissection, and the risk of iatrogenic clot embolization. Woodward et al. contend that the risk of distal embolization is low, given the combination of vigorous aspiration and a state of flow arrest created by the long carotid sheath filling the lumen at the stenotic site [1].

Case 3

Tandem occlusions secondary to cervical carotid dissection with intracranial emboli often require definitive emergent treatment with stenting, necessitating initiation of DAPT in the acute peri-stroke period.

Presentation

A 37-year-old woman with several days of headache suddenly collapsed with symptoms of lethargy, right hemiparesis, aphasia, and left gaze preference. NIHSS score was 24.

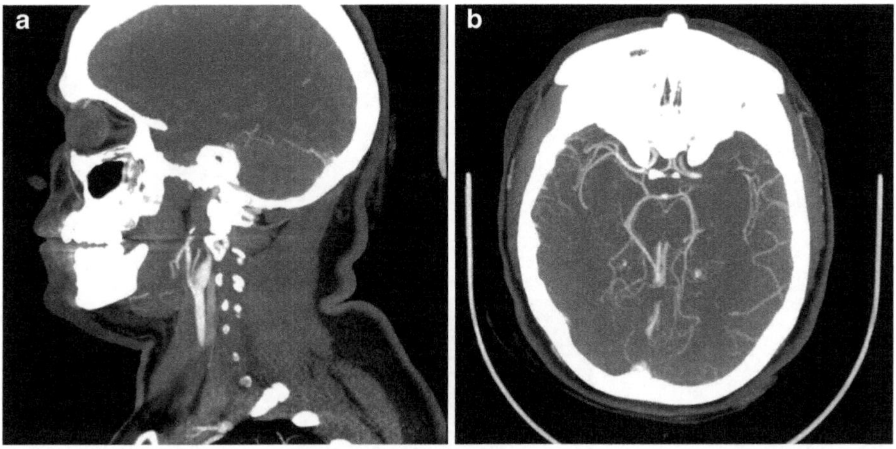

Fig. 16.9 Tandem occlusion with proximal left ICA carotid dissection in a 37-year-old woman presenting with altered mental status and left MCA syndrome. (**a**) Lateral CT angiogram of the neck demonstrates eccentric tapering of the proximal left ICA. (**b**) Axial CT angiogram of the head shows an arterial cutoff at the left MCA proximal M1 segment

On arrival, non-contrast CT of the head showed a hyperdense left MCA with basal ganglia parenchymal hypodensity consistent with ASPECTS of 7. CT angiogram of the head and neck revealed eccentric tapering stenosis of the proximal cervical left ICA (Fig. 16.9a) and cutoff of the left M1 (Fig. 16.9b). The patient's age, clinical presentation, and imaging findings were consistent with a tandem occlusion caused by cervical carotid dissection. Initial diagnostic angiogram demonstrated tapered occlusion of the proximal cervical left ICA characteristic of dissection (Fig. 16.10a). A gentle repeat injection was performed within the occluded ICA (Fig. 16.10b). This arteriogram was used to better define the dissection site at the cervico-petrous junction of the ICA and help guide coaxially a Penumbra ACE64 reperfusion catheter over a Penumbra Velocity microcatheter and a 014 Transcend soft-tip guidewire. With the ACE64 positioned as a distal access catheter to address the intracranial occlusion, an arteriogram was performed defining the left M1 origin cutoff (Fig. 16.10c).

Technique

Given the ability to navigate across the segment of stenotic/occluded left ICA dissection, an intracranial-first approach was used to first revascularize the left M1 occlusion. The base catheter was a Neuron MAX catheter. A Solitaire FR stent retriever and ACE64 catheter system was advanced into the left MCA (Fig. 16.10d, e), and one-pass thrombectomy under aspiration was performed with restoration of TICI 3 flow (Fig. 16.10f). The Solitaire was removed through the ACE64 leaving

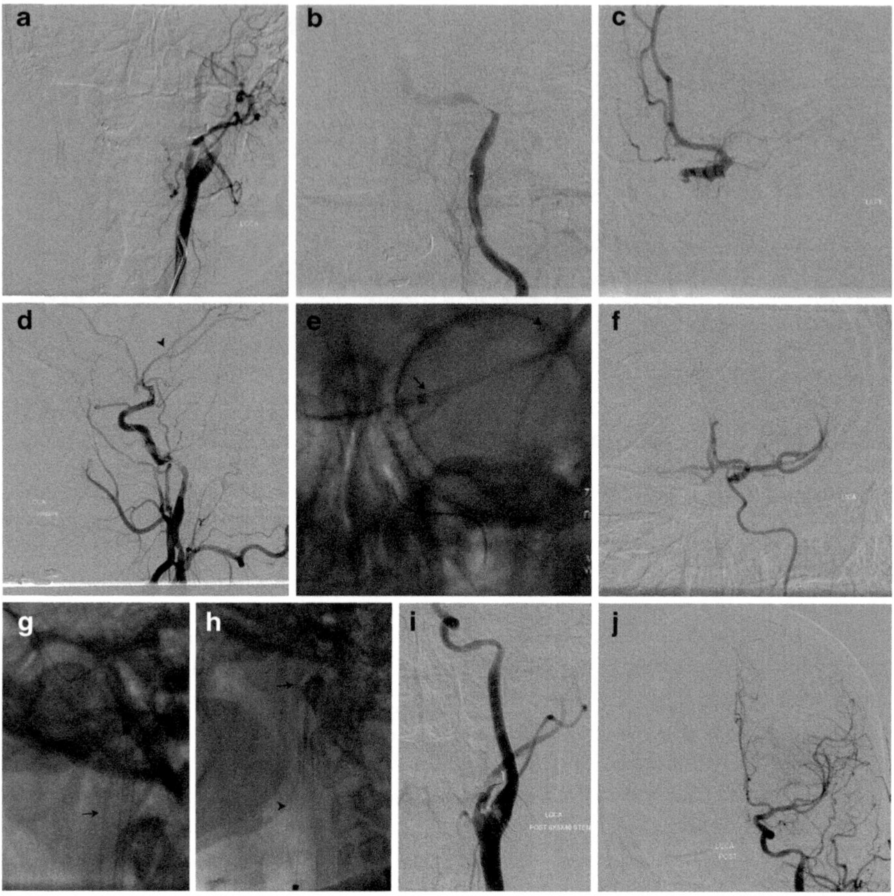

Fig. 16.10 Intracranial-first approach requiring stenting of the proximal carotid dissection. (**a**) AP cervical view of left CCA injection demonstrating eccentric luminal narrowing of the proximal cervical left ICA, similar in appearance to that seen on CT angiogram. (**b**) AP cervical view of repeat angiogram through the microcatheter now advanced into the petrous segment of the left ICA shows long left ICA cervical and petrous segment irregular narrowing with a focal area of severe stenosis in the distal petrous segment. (**c**) AP cranial view of left CCA injection shows retrograde flow opacifying the left ICA terminus and ACA. Occlusions at the left ICA supraclinoid segment and left MCA origin are seen. (**d**) On lateral view, a Solitaire FR stent retriever was successfully navigated into the left MCA with distal markers (arrowhead) at the M2 bifurcation. (**e**) Non-subtracted AP cranial view showed advancement of a large-bore aspiration catheter (arrow) into the proximal M1 segment. Distal markers of the Solitaire FR stent retriever are noted (arrowhead). (**f**) Following one-pass thrombectomy under aspiration, there is successful revascularization of the left M1 and M2 branches as seen on AP cervical angiogram through the 0.054″ catheter at the distal cervical left ICA. (**g**, **h**) Non-subtracted cervical views demonstrate sequential placement of an Enterprise 4.0 × 30 mm stent (arrow) and a 6 × 8 × 40 mm taper stent (arrowhead) along the petrous and cervical segments of the left ICA. (**i**) Repeat left CCA injection after stenting shows a widely patent proximal left ICA on AP cervical view. (**j**) Post-intervention, AP cranial view of a left CCA injection demonstrates successful TICI 3 revascularization

the aspiration catheter tip distal to the dissected ICA segment in order to maintain distal access. The proximal carotid dissection was then addressed. A 014 J-tip (300 cm length) Boston Scientific PT Graphix intermediate guidewire was advanced through the ACE64 and the ACE64 exchanged for a Medtronic 027 Marksman microcatheter. An Enterprise 4.0 × 30 mm stent was deployed across the leading edge of the dissection at the cervico-petrous junction. Abbott Acculink 6 × 40 mm and 6 × 8 × 40 mm carotid stents were then deployed over the microwire in series covering the entire length of the cervical segment of the ICA to create a full metal jacket (Fig. 16.10g, h). Post-stenting, the left ICA was widely patent (Fig. 16.10i) and there remained TICI 3 intracranial revascularization (Fig. 16.10j). Post-procedure MRI revealed infarction predominantly within the left basal ganglia, with minimal involvement of the left insula region.

Comments from Authors: Approach to Antiplatelet Therapy

In this case employing the intracranial-first approach, a large-bore aspiration catheter was advanced across the carotid dissection and then maintained distal to that segment, doubling as a guide catheter for Solumbra technique thrombectomy. For reconstruction of the proximal carotid dissection, we recommend deploying a flexible stent that would conform to the curvature of the vessel, for example, an Enterprise intracranial stent, across the cervical-petrous junction. Overlapping straight carotid stents in the more proximal cervical segment can be used to tack down the dissection flap and obliterate the false lumen.

Definitive treatment of the proximal carotid dissection at the time of emergent intervention prevents persistent minimal flow (with the potential of recurrent distal emboli) or complete occlusion (which may compromise intracranial circulation). One may entertain the idea of delaying treatment of an occluded carotid dissection if contralateral or collateral flow is sufficient to maintain perfusion in the immediate period; however, success of this strategy is uncertain with scarring of the dissection flap over time. Medical treatment with anti-coagulation is contraindicated in the acute peri-stroke period; thus, most would employ endovascular angioplasty followed by stenting.

Regardless of the choice between extracranial-first and intracranial-first strategies, carotid stenting requires the initiation of an antiplatelet regimen, which increases the risk of hemorrhagic conversion. The meta-analysis by Wilson et al. demonstrated a slightly higher rate of symptomatic intracranial hemorrhage after endovascular treatment of tandem occlusions compared to the general mechanical thrombectomy population in the HERMES collaboration (8% versus 4.4%), attributing the difference to the need for more aggressive antiplatelet therapy after stenting, which was performed for the majority of the patients included in the analysis [6]. Antiplatelet regimens usually involve aspirin and/or clopidogrel and have been highly variable across published studies.

Angioplasty alone would theoretically reduce the risk of bleeding. When both stenting and angioplasty alone are viable strategies, the decision for one over the other is controversial. Wilson et al. found no significant difference in outcome, complication rate, technical success rate, or procedural time between the two extracranial treatment approaches, although the sample size in the angioplasty-only group is small [6]. The angioplasty alone strategy is preferred in our practices, primarily driven by the desire to minimize risk of intracranial hemorrhage associated with antiplatelet therapy.

Case 4

In certain situations, both the extracranial-first approach and modified Dotter technique may not be feasible due to rigidity or size of the proximal clot. In these complex cases, innovative approaches may be required, as presented in the following case.

Presentation

A 65-year-old woman presented with left-sided hemiplegia and an NIHSS score of 25. MRI on arrival demonstrated sparse diffusion restriction in the left basal ganglia, and the patient was brought directly to the angiography suite.

Technique

Initial diagnostic angiograms showed a large occlusive thrombus at the distal left CCA extending into the proximal left ICA, with non-opacification of the ECA (Fig. 16.11a). A microwire followed by a 0.054″ Penumbra reperfusion catheter was advanced through the proximal occlusive thrombus. Angiogram performed with the catheter distal to the left distal CCA/ICA origin thrombus revealed extensive sub-occlusive thrombus throughout the petrous and cavernous segment, occlusive thrombus of the clinoid segment, and complete non-opacification of the left ICA terminus, left MCA, ACA, and distal branches (Fig. 16.11b, c). Given the large thrombus burden within the left ICA, decision was made to proceed with mechanical thrombectomy of the extracranial left ICA at this point. Several passes were made with ensemble suction and withdrawal of an aspiration catheter and Solitaire stent retriever together (6 mm diameter) while applying suction also in the 7F guide catheter, and recanalization of the left MCA was eventually achieved (Fig. 16.11d). Repeat angiogram demonstrated resolution of the intracranial left ICA thrombus with TICI 3 revascularization (Fig. 16.11e). The 0.054″ catheter was pulled back into the proximal left CCA for a repeat angiogram, which showed no appreciable residual distal left CCA/proximal left ICA thrombus (Fig. 16.11f). The left ECA remained occluded at its origin; however, given the low risk of ischemic

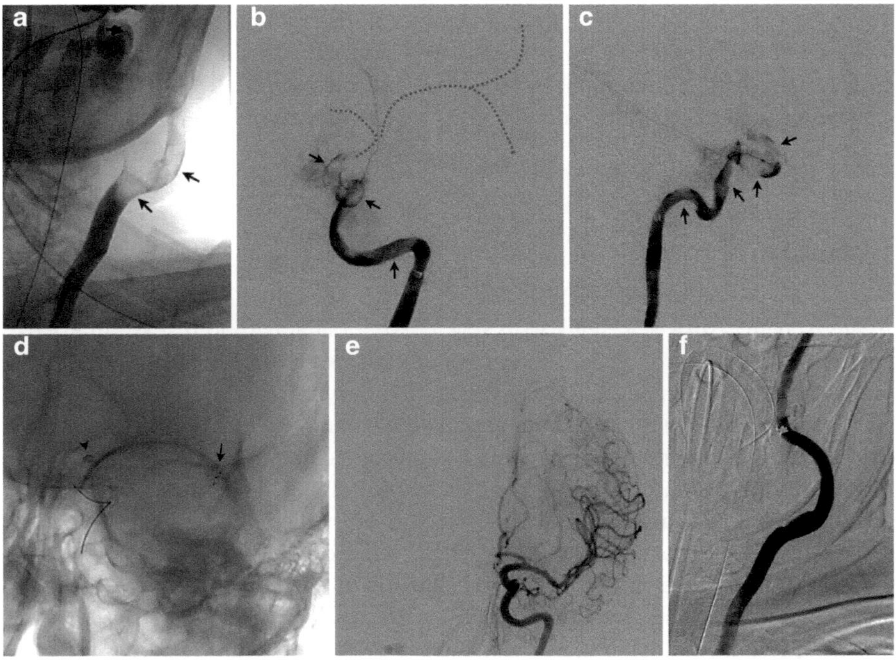

Fig. 16.11 Massive left CCA to MCA occlusion requiring multiple thrombectomy attempts. (**a**) Non-subtracted AP cervical view of left CCA injection demonstrates occlusive thrombus at the distal left CCA extending into the proximal left ICA (arrows). The left ECA is also non-opacified. A 0.054″ aspiration catheter was advanced through the proximal occlusion until its distal tip was at the petrous segment. Repeat angiogram in the AP (**b**) and lateral (**c**) views shows sub-occlusive and occlusive thrombus throughout the petrous, cavernous, and clinoid segments of the ICA. The ICA terminus and distal MCA and ACA are not opacified (gray dotted line in **b**). Multiple passes with the Solitaire FR stent retriever (arrow) under aspiration from the 0.054″ catheter (arrowhead) within the left ICA were performed, with eventual advancement of the reperfusion system into the left MCA, as shown in (**d**). Post-intervention, repeat injection with AP cranial view of the head (**e**) demonstrates resolution of the large clot burden with the intracranial left IC, with TICI 3 cerebral blood flow. (**f**) AP view of the neck on left CCA injection shows widely patent distal left CCA and cervical ICA. The left ECA remains completely occluded at its origin

complications due to robust collaterals and the possibility of re-embolization when mobilizing the ECA clot, further interventions were not pursued to avoid distal emboli into previously normal territories. Post-intervention, the patient's symptoms completely resolved. She was discharged in stable condition with NIHSS score of 0.

Comments from Authors: Management of Extensive Occlusions

Endovascular management of acute ischemic stroke remains a young procedure. Encountering unusual anatomy, mechanisms of occlusion, and frankly surprisingly large clot burdens remain definite possibilities. Remembering the goal of therapy – efficient, safe restoration of flow – will help the operator decide the best among uncertain options. In this case, recognizing that the clot burden likely required the largest-bore catheter possible, and that direct suction through both catheters would be useful in reducing clot re-embolization, resulted in the favorable outcome.

Discussion

Acute ischemic stroke presents with severe extracranial carotid disease in 20% of patients and acute carotid occlusion in 2% of patients [7, 8]. Atherosclerotic disease or dissection occluding the extracranial carotid artery can concurrently cause occlusive emboli in the distal intracranial vasculature, resulting in acute stroke symptoms [8, 9]. In contrast to intracranial occlusion alone, tandem occlusions respond poorly to IV-tPA therapy, and its presence predicts poor clinical outcome [3, 10, 11]. As open embolectomy can only be directed toward the extracranial occlusion, the intracranial lesion in a tandem occlusion would require treatment with endovascular thrombectomy. However, the proximal occlusion blocks access to the distal occlusion, complicating the approach to such lesions. Indeed, increased severity of the proximal lesion (occlusion versus stenosis) is associated with lower rates of complete reperfusion [12].

In 2015, five randomized stroke intervention trials – MR CLEAN [13], ESCAPE [14], SWIFT PRIME [15], EXTEND-IA [16], and REVASCAT [17] – showed superiority of endovascular thrombectomy (primarily utilizing stent retrievers) over standard medical care. Patients with tandem occlusions were notably included in all five trials, although SWIFT PRIME excluded tandem occlusions on a case-by-case basis if the operator felt that the proximal occlusion would require stenting. The HERMES collaboration, which pooled data from the five trials, found overall treatment benefit in not only the 1132 patients with single intracranial occlusions but also in the 122 patients with tandem occlusions, concluding that the tandem occlusions should be treated [18].

Despite technical challenges to the interventionalist, tandem occlusions are amenable to endovascular mechanical thrombectomy [19–21]. Effective and, importantly, safe restoration of flow is the ultimate goal. There is controversy in whether the extracranial or the intracranial occlusion should be treated first. A 2018 meta-analysis of greater than 1000 patients found no significant difference in outcome, complication rate, technical success rate, or procedural time between extracranial-first and intracranial-first strategies [6]. The recent TITAN (Thrombectomy in TANdem Lesions) registry showed similar conclusions [22].

Additionally, it remains unclear how exactly the extracranial lesion should be treated, although growing evidence suggests acute stenting of the proximal lesion as an effective and safe strategy [23–26]. Currently, avoidance of the antiplatelet therapy required with stenting drives our preference toward angioplasty alone or the modified Dotter strategies. Further prospective and randomized trials to define an optimal antiplatelet regimen that minimizes reperfusion injury and hemorrhagic risks while adequately preventing thrombotic complications would greatly expand the feasibility of strategies involving metal implants/devices such as stenting. There is continued room for high-quality evidence and innovation that not only looks to break new ground but also pays homage to the masters of the past.

Quick Reference

Extracranial-First Approach:

1. Cross proximal occlusion with wire (0.016″ or even 0.035″).
2. Treat proximal occlusion: Angioplasty with balloon catheter and stent if needed.
3. Obtain stable guide catheter access across treated proximal occlusion.
4. Stent retriever/aspiration thrombectomy of distal occlusion.
5. Verify patency of proximal occlusion.

Modified Dotter Approach:

1. Select the occluded common carotid artery with a coaxial system of an outer sheath/catheter (e.g., Penumbra Neuron MAX/0.054″ reperfusion catheter), inner catheter/microcatheter (e.g., Marksman microcatheter), and a guidewire/microwire (e.g., 0.016″ Fathom).
2. Tunnel through the occlusion with the guidewire.
3. Tunnel through the occlusion with the inner catheter.
4. Tunnel through the occlusion with the outer catheter and obtain stable access across proximal occlusion.
5. Stent retriever/aspiration thrombectomy of distal occlusion.
6. Verify patency of proximal occlusion.

References

1. Woodward K, Wegryn S, Staruk C, Nyberg EM. The Dotter method revisited: early experience with a novel method of rapid internal carotid artery revascularization in the setting of acute ischemic stroke. J Neurointerv Surg. 2016;8:360–6.
2. Lockau H, Liebig T, Henning T, Neuschmelting V, Stetefeld H, Kabbasch C, et al. Mechanical thrombectomy in tandem occlusion: procedural considerations and clinical results. Neuroradiology. 2015;57:589–98.
3. Christou I, Felberg RA, Demchuk AM, Burgin WS, Malkoff M, Grotta JC, et al. Intravenous tissue plasminogen activator and flow improvement in acute ischemic stroke patients with internal carotid artery occlusion. J Neuroimaging. 2002;12:119–23.
4. Hui FK, Hussain MS, Elgabaly MH, Sivapatham T, Katzan IL, Spiotta AM. Embolic protection devices and the Penumbra 054 catheter: utility in tandem occlusions in acute ischemic stroke. J Neurointerv Surg. 2011;3:50–3.
5. Dotter CT, Judkins MP. Percutaneous transluminal treatment of arteriosclerotic obstruction. Radiology. 1965;84:631–43.

6. Wilson MP, Murad MH, Krings T, Pereira VM, O'Kelly C, Rempel J, et al. Management of tandem occlusions in acute ischemic stroke – intracranial versus extracranial first and extracranial stenting versus angioplasty alone: a systematic review and meta-analysis. J Neurointerv Surg. 2018;10:721–8.
7. Tallarita T, Lanzino G, Rabinstein AA. Carotid intervention in acute stroke. Perspect Vasc Surg Endovasc Ther. 2010;22:49–57.
8. Rahme R, Abruzzo TA, Ringer AJ. Acute ischemic stroke in the setting of cervical carotid occlusion: a proposed management strategy. World Neurosurg. 2011;76:S60–5.
9. Spiotta AM, Lena J, Vargas J, Hawk H, Turner RD, Chaudry MI, et al. Proximal to distal approach in the treatment of tandem occlusions causing an acute stroke. J Neurointerv Surg. 2015;7:164–9.
10. Rubiera M, Ribo M, Delgado-Mederos R, Santamarina E, Delgado P, Montaner J, et al. Tandem internal carotid artery/middle cerebral artery occlusion: an independent predictor of poor outcome after systemic thrombolysis. Stroke. 2006;37:2301–5.
11. Kim YS, Garami Z, Mikulik R, Molina CA, Alexandrov AV. Early recanalization rates and clinical outcomes in patients with tandem internal carotid artery/middle cerebral artery occlusion and isolated middle cerebral artery occlusion. Stroke. 2005;36:869–71.
12. Anadani M, Spiotta A, Alawieh A, Turjman F, Piotin M, Steglich-Arnholm H, et al. Effect of extracranial lesion severity on outcome of endovascular thrombectomy in patients with anterior circulation tandem occlusion: analysis of the TITAN registry. J Neurointerv Surg. 2019;11:970–4.
13. Berkhemer OA, Fransen PSS, Beumer D, van den Berg LA, Lingsma HF, Yoo AJ, et al. A randomized trial of intraarterial treatment for acute ischemic stroke. N Engl J Med. 2015;372:11–20.
14. Goyal M, Demchuk AM, Menon BK, Eesa M, Rempel JL, Thornton J, et al. Randomized assessment of rapid endovascular treatment of ischemic stroke. N Engl J Med. 2015;372:1019–30.
15. Saver JL, Goyal M, Bonafe A, Diener H-C, Levy EI, Pereira VM, et al. Stent-retriever thrombectomy after intravenous t-PA vs. t-PA alone in stroke. N Engl J Med. 2015;372:2285–95.
16. Campbell BCV, Mitchell PJ, Kleinig TJ, Dewey HM, Churilov L, Yassi N, et al. Endovascular therapy for ischemic stroke with perfusion-imaging selection. N Engl J Med. 2015;372:1009–18.
17. Jovin TG, Chamorro A, Cobo E, de Miquel MA, Molina CA, Rovira A, et al. Thrombectomy within 8 hours after symptom onset in ischemic stroke. N Engl J Med. 2015;372:2296–306.
18. Goyal M, Menon BK, van Zwam WH, Dippel DWJ, Mitchell PJ, Demchuk AM, et al. Endovascular thrombectomy after large-vessel ischaemic stroke: a meta-analysis of individual patient data from five randomised trials. Lancet. 2016;387:1723–31.
19. Behme D, Mpotsaris A, Zeyen P, Psychogios MN, Kowoll A, Maurer CJ, et al. Emergency stenting of the extracranial internal carotid artery in combination with anterior circulation thrombectomy in acute ischemic stroke: a retrospective multicenter study. Am J Neuroradiol. 2015;36:2340–5.
20. Malik AM, Vora NA, Lin R, Zaidi SF, Aleu A, Jankowitz BT, et al. Endovascular treatment of tandem extracranial/intracranial anterior circulation occlusions: preliminary single-center experience. Stroke. 2011;42:1653–7.
21. Gory B, Haussen DC, Piotin M, Steglich-Arnholm H, Holtmannspötter M, Labreuche J, et al. Impact of intravenous thrombolysis and emergent carotid stenting on reperfusion and clinical outcomes in patients with acute stroke with tandem lesion treated with thrombectomy: a collaborative pooled analysis. Eur J Neurol. 2018;25:1115–20.
22. Haussen DC, Turjman F, Piotin M, Labreuche J, Steglich-Arnholm H, Holtmannspötter M, et al. Head or neck first? Speed and rates of reperfusion in thrombectomy for tandem large vessel occlusion strokes. Interv Neurol. 2019;8:92–100.
23. Papanagiotou P, Haussen DC, Turjman F, Labreuche J, Piotin M, Kastrup A, et al. Carotid stenting with antithrombotic agents and intracranial thrombectomy leads to the highest recanalization rate in patients with acute stroke with tandem lesions. J Am Coll Cardiol Intv. 2018;11:1290–9.

24. Jadhav AP, Zaidat OO, Liebeskind DS, Yavagal DR, Haussen DC, Hellinger FR, et al. Emergent management of tandem lesions in acute ischemic stroke: analysis of the STRATIS registry. Stroke. 2019;50:428–33.
25. Zhu F, Bracard S, Anxionnat R, Derelle A-L, Tonnelet R, Liao L, et al. Impact of emergent cervical carotid stenting in tandem occlusion strokes treated by thrombectomy: a review of the TITAN collaboration. Front Neurol. 2019;10:206. Available from: https://www.ncbi.nlm.nih.gov/pmc/articles/PMC6421313/.
26. Anadani M, Spiotta AM, Alawieh A, Turjman F, Piotin M, Haussen DC, et al. Emergent carotid stenting plus thrombectomy after thrombolysis in tandem strokes. Stroke. 2019;50:2250–2.

Chapter 17
Acute Stroke Thrombectomy and Emergent Management of Tandem Cervical Dissections

Madhav Sukumaran, Ramez N. Abdalla, Donald R. Cantrell, Matthew B. Potts, and Sameer A. Ansari

Introduction

Cervical dissections are a rare etiology of acute ischemic stroke accounting for approximately 2% of all cases. However, cervical dissections remain the most common cause of ischemic stroke among younger patients (16–45 years of age), contributing to 10–25% of thromboembolic mechanisms [1]. Various spontaneous, traumatic, and iatrogenic etiologies of cervical dissections may be related to underlying genetic and inherited connective tissue disorders such as fibromuscular dysplasia, osteogenesis imperfecta type 1, Ehler-Danlos type 4, Marfan, and Loyes-Dietz syndromes. In general, the prognosis of isolated cervical dissections is favorable, and medical management with anticoagulation or antiplatelet therapy is the standard of care with spontaneous healing or stable imaging findings in the vast majority of patients. Delayed endovascular treatment of isolated cervical internal carotid artery (ICA) dissections is reserved for patients presenting with (1) recurrent ischemic symptoms and/or thromboembolic strokes refractory to medical management, (2) progression of dissection-related stenoses at risk for occlusion, or (3) symptomatic/enlarging dissecting aneurysms or pseudoaneurysms.

M. Sukumaran · D. R. Cantrell · M. B. Potts
Departments of Radiology and Neurological Surgery, Northwestern University, Feinberg School of Medicine, Chicago, IL, USA

R. N. Abdalla
Departments of Radiology and Neurological Surgery, Northwestern University, Feinberg School of Medicine, Chicago, IL, USA

Department of Radiology, Ain Shams University, Cairo, Egypt

S. A. Ansari (✉)
Departments of Radiology, Neurology, and Neurological Surgery, Northwestern University, Feinberg School of Medicine, Chicago, IL, USA
e-mail: s-ansari@northwestern.edu

F. K. Hui et al. (eds.), *12 Strokes*, https://doi.org/10.1007/978-3-030-56857-3_17

Emergent endovascular treatment may be required for cervical ICA dissections presenting with concomitant large vessel occlusion (LVO), flow-limiting and long-segment lesions with impending occlusion, and/or hypoperfusion-related ischemia at risk for infarction. Since superimposed extracranial carotid/intracranial atherosclerotic disease or dissections are often an etiology of emergent LVO, it may be necessary to combine cervical angioplasty and/or stenting techniques with intracranial thrombectomy. Endovascular angioplasty/stenting techniques are valuable adjunctive treatments to mechanical thrombectomy in tandem carotid-intracranial occlusions secondary to acutely ruptured carotid atherosclerotic plaques or cervical dissection related intimal tears with in situ thrombosis/occlusions or severe flow-limiting stenoses resulting in distal intracranial emboli. Furthermore, extracranial carotid angioplasty/stent placement may be necessary in emergent settings to provide distal access for intracranial thrombectomy, vessel salvage, and/or revascularization in hypoperfusion ischemic syndromes without sufficient intracranial collaterals [2–5].

Due to the importance of cervical revascularization in these settings, several groups have demonstrated the feasibility of emergency ICA angioplasty and/or stenting combined with intracranial thrombectomy for tandem ICA-middle cerebral artery (MCA) occlusions with acceptable rates of successful recanalization, complications, and clinical outcomes. In the recent randomized controlled trials that demonstrated a benefit of endovascular thrombectomy for acute ischemic stroke, carotid artery stent placement was performed in 8.6–12.9% of patients [6]. These studies suggest that emergent endovascular treatment of extracranial ICA pathology with concomitant intracranial thrombectomy may be safe and effective. However, there is no consensus or standardization regarding the indications or techniques for emergent endovascular treatment of cervical dissections. Few studies have focused on the management of cervical dissections with or without tandem intracranial ELVOs in the acute ischemic stroke setting, often limited to small sample sizes and non-standardized treatment techniques. For example, there are no clear thresholds or definitions of flow-limiting cervical dissections that would warrant emergent endovascular stenting over medical management, with various approaches reported in the literature including symptomatic or clinical ischemia assessment, perfusion imaging-based selection, long segment pathology, and/or inadequate intracranial collaterals. In addition, the basic procedural methodology whether to first revascularize the intracranial occlusion (distal-to-proximal) or cervical stenosis/occlusion (proximal-to-distal) remains controversial.

We describe our protocol and techniques for the emergent stenting of cervical dissections presenting with tandem intracranial occlusions in the setting of acute ischemic stroke. We present three cases that presented to our institution and the treatment strategies employed. Each case highlights important considerations for the endovascular management of cervical dissections. We hope the following applications will be of general interest and utility to neurointerventionalists in their practice/.

Patient Selection/General Procedural Considerations

As for all interventional procedures, the impact of appropriate patient selection for endovascular therapy cannot be overstated. While there have been multiple randomized controlled trials demonstrating the benefit of mechanical thrombectomy for acute ELVO in both early [6] and delayed presentations (DAWN and DEFUSE-3), [7, 8] patients presenting with tandem lesions were limited or excluded from these trials. In our practice, we evaluate tandem pathology patients with analogous clinical and imaging inclusion/exclusion criteria to the mechanical stroke thrombectomy trials for isolated ELVO.

Following femoral or alternative arterial access, we advance a 6 French guide sheath (0.088 inch inner diameter) coaxially over a guidewire into the affected common carotid/vertebral artery, proximal to the cervical dissection. Alternatively, an 8F balloon guide catheter may be utilized for protective flow arrest techniques during both intracranial thrombectomy and cervical stent reconstruction. We then perform digital subtraction angiography (DSA) with craniocervical projections to assess the cervical and intracranial vasculature. Depending on the severity of the cervical dissection, the distal cervical pathology and intracranial vasculature may or may not be visualized. Through the guide sheath/catheter, we carefully probe and advance a guidewire/microwire (0.014–0.035 inch) and coaxial catheter complex (including an outer large bore distal access aspiration catheter and stent retriever microcatheter for intracranial thrombectomy) across the narrowed true lumen of the dissection under biplane fluoroscopic guidance. It is imperative to advance cautiously across the cervical dissection, remaining within the true vessel lumen to avoid progression of subintimal pathology. If intramural thrombus with intraluminal extension is suspected, the thrombectomy aspiration catheter can be advanced under aspiration to reduce the thrombus burden. Intermittent proximal guide and/or microcatheter check angiograms with gentle contrast hand injections are used to confirm access and progress through the true lumen, opacifying the normal distal cavernous carotid and intracranial vasculature. Additionally, the entire length of the dissection flap, presence of flow-limitation, mural thrombus, and/or associated dissecting aneurysms may be better appreciated on DSA after coaxial catheter recanalization, which may not have been clearly opacified on initial CTA findings.

Following successful access across the cervical dissection flap, we are typically able to perform mechanical thrombectomy effectively. We prefer to target the intracranial occlusion first and reestablish cerebral blood flow for time-sensitive tissue salvage using traditional aspiration and/or stent retriever thrombectomy techniques. Since we typically utilize 6 French flexible distal guide sheaths (DGSs) with > 0.088 inch inner diameters for proximal carotid or vertebral access, we attempt to safely advance these trackable guide sheaths across the entire carotid dissection flap, even across the skull base into the ICA petrocavernous segments, coaxially over both the large bore distal access aspiration catheter and stent retriever microcatheter system for efficient intracranial thrombectomy (GUARD technique) [9]. In the setting of a tandem dissection, this technique further augments coaxial catheter recanalization across a severe dissection, expanding the true lumen, promoting realignment of the intimal flap, improving antegrade flow, and potentially avoiding stent reconstruction in the emergent setting.

After intracranial thrombectomy, cervical and intracranial angiograms are repeated to plan further intervention of the cervical dissection, if needed, as flow limitation across the dissection can be best evaluated after reestablishing intracranial outflow. Cervical dissection pathology must be carefully evaluated as a large bore coaxial microcatheters or distal guide sheath is retracted across the intimal flap over an exchange length safety guide/microwire to maintain access and under aspiration if any residual intraluminal thrombus associated with the dissection is suspected. Consideration of treatment options include stent reconstruction, angioplasty alone, or conservative medical management with anticoagulation/antiplatelet therapy if sufficient coaxial catheter recanalization and antegrade flow has been restored. Various clinical and imaging criteria have been described in the literature to assess if stent reconstruction of a carotid dissection will be required or whether conservative medical management can be initiated: (1) persisting severe neurological symptoms and/or cerebral ischemia (as per CT/MR perfusion imaging) despite intracranial thrombectomy or no large vessel occlusion; (2) long segment >3.5 cm and severe flow-limiting dissections at risk for impending occlusion; (3) angiographic observation for 30–60 minutes with interval vessel occlusion despite intraprocedural heparin anticoagulation or antiplatelets (IV cangrelor/eptifibatide or pre-existing ASA/thienopyridine therapy); (4) flow-limiting dissections with inadequate circle of Willis collaterals resulting in an angiographic venous delay >2 seconds in the downstream cerebral hemisphere [4, 5].

Stent Reconstruction of Cervical Dissections

If stent reconstruction is deemed necessary, we precisely calculate the degree of dissection related stenosis, normal arterial diameter measurements proximal and distal to the dissection pathology, length of the injured vessel segment and stent construct (single vs. tandem/partially overlapping stents) required to cover the proximal inflow zone and the distal intimal flap, using both CTA and intraoperative DSA measurements. 3D DSA techniques may be helpful in visualization and measurement of complex dissection pathology such as spiral intimal flaps, dissecting aneurysms, and tortuous vascular anatomy.

Self-expanding carotid stents have been designed for atraumatic deployment with decreased, yet adequate, radial force to treat atherosclerotic lesions. Successful treatment of internal carotid artery dissections with these stents has been extensively described with single or partially overlapping tandem stent constructs. We perform stent reconstruction of proximal and mid cervical carotid dissections predominantly with self-expanding, open cell carotid stents (e.g., Precise stent, Cordis, Miami Lakes, FL or Acculink, Abbott Vascular, Galway, Ireland), which are flexible, atraumatic, and relatively trackable into mildly tortuous cervical vasculature. Stent deployment expands the true lumen, tacking the intimal flap to the outer vessel wall, and immediately improves vessel diameter and antegrade flow. Alternatively, if anatomy permits, the higher metal-mesh ratio of stiffer, closed cell self-expanding carotid stents may further decrease the porosity across the inflow zone to allow intimal healing, promote pseudoaneurysm thrombosis, and secure pre-existing thrombus along the dissected vessel wall preventing intracranial migration. Self-expanding carotid stents have also been designed with both enhanced radial force and/or greater metal matrix with closed cell (e.g., Wallstent, Boston Scientific,

Marlborough, MA, X-Act, Abbott Vascular, Galway, Ireland) or hybrid (NexStent, Boston Scientific, Marlborough, MA, Protégé, Medtronic, Plymouth, MN) nitinol construction, providing equally effective and safer alternatives to balloon-expanding stents in proximal to mid cervical dissections and dissecting aneurysms.

Although lower-profile peripheral stent delivery systems are promising developments, the high profile and rigid construction of self-expanding (open or closed cell) carotid stents or balloon-expanding peripheral stents prevents their utilization in distal cervical or skull base lesions (petrocavernous ICA or V2-V3 segment vertebral arteries), which are often involved in long segment, flow-limiting dissections requiring emergent revascularization. The limited flexibility and trackability of these stents prohibits deployment in the tortuous anatomy and redundant vascular loops of high cervical/skull base segments. In these situations, the off-label utilization of self-expanding intracranial stents for aneurysm or atherosclerotic diseases have been shown to be effective in the treatment of distal cervical and intracranial dissections due to their inherent lower-profile, flexible nitinol construction, and trackable delivery systems. Furthermore, intracranial stents provide sufficient radial force and atraumatic luminal expansion for the treatment of distal cervical, skull base, and intracranial dissection pathology [10]. Newer flow diverter intracranial stent technology may also be employed for the salvage of distal cervical and skull base dissections, albeit with relatively decreased radial force and more challenging deployment than traditional intracranial stents. However, these braided flow-diverting intracranial stents provide markedly improved metal coverage for flow remodeling to induce dissecting aneurysm thrombosis, flexibility for deployment in tortuous anatomy/vascular loops without kinking, and availability of stent diameters approaching 5.5–6 mm for large caliber vasculature.

Lower profile balloon-expanding coronary and peripheral stents have been described in the treatment of cervical dissections, but they are relatively inflexible and less trackable in tortuous or redundant vasculature in comparison to self-expanding intracranial stents. Since balloon-expanding coronary stents are more rigid than intracranial stents, they may be predisposed to kinking and deformation, especially in tortuous and mobile distal cervical segments with neck flexion, rotation, or extension. Although they possess enhanced radial force with balloon expansion delivery systems with advantages in severe dissections with intramural hemorrhage in the osseous petrous canal, excessive radial force during deployment in dissected, fragile distal cervical or intracranial vasculature can lead to complications of propagating dissection or vessel rupture. Furthermore, balloon-expanding stents do not possess metal memory like nitinol-based self-expanding stents, and therefore, problems in stent sizing of segments with non-uniform diameters could result in poor apposition proximally or overinflation/vessel injury distally. Finally, the greater metal matrix and radial force of coronary stents may predispose to increased foreign body reaction and platelet aggregation resulting in thromboembolic complications or myointimal proliferation, especially in the setting of pre-existing endothelial injury. If drug-eluting coronary stents are utilized to minimize effects of intimal hyperplasia, extended dual antiplatelet therapy >1 year is required due to delayed stent endothelialization.

Covered stent grafts have shown utility in the simultaneous treatment of dissections and dissecting aneurysms and are convenient devices in excluding giant pseudoaneurysms [1]. Adverse properties include large-profile delivery systems, limited trackability in tortuous vasculature, occlusion risk to perforating arteries, and lack of long-term patency data. For these reasons, covered stent grafts are not typically employed in the emergency setting of tandem dissections/dissecting aneurysms and stroke thrombectomy.

During stent deployment, we avoid distal filter protection devices in the treatment of cervical dissections, unlike carotid atherosclerotic lesions, which have a greater potential for thromboemboli during carotid angioplasty/stenting. If utilized in the treatment of dissections, filter protection devices may risk further intimal injury or dissection progression during advancement of relatively rigid delivery systems over less supportive rapid exchange/monorail systems. Furthermore, a safe landing zone for a filter protection device within a normal vessel segment may not be possible in symptomatic cervical dissections requiring stent reconstruction, that often involve long segments extending to the skull base and tortuous vasculature. Proximal flow arrest techniques using large profile balloon guide catheters with concomitant aspiration during carotid stent deployment may be feasible and offer advantages over filter protection devices in the treatment of cervical dissection. Pre- and post-stent balloon angioplasty has been reported in the endovascular treatment of carotid artery dissections. However, the indications for angioplasty alone in the treatment of dissections are limited, usually reserved to obtain access across a severe stenosis, or for salvage of an incompletely expanded stent.

Final cervical and intracranial angiograms assess interval changes status post stent reconstruction of a cervical dissection: adequacy of luminal expansion, stent coverage across the inflow zone and entire intimal flap, uniform stent apposition to the vessel wall with overlapping coverage of tandem stents, improvement in flow dynamics and intracranial flow, and complications of in-stent thrombus, in-stent kinking/stenosis, or distal intracranial thromboembolic complications. Stent placement expands the true lumen of a dissected vessel to immediately re-establish blood flow, realign the intimal flap, and trap the subintimal hematoma. Over the next several weeks to months, hematoma resorption, intimal healing, and stent endothelialization reconstructs the parent artery.

Post-procedure Antiplatelets and Follow-Up Imaging

Acute/subacute thromboembolic stroke, in-stent thrombosis, and parent vessel occlusion are well-documented complications following metallic stent placement in the cervical and intracranial vasculature. Preventing thromboembolic complications entails the routine use of systemic heparin (activated clotting time 2.0–2.5 times baseline) during endovascular procedures. Patients undergoing elective stenting procedures are invariably placed on pre-procedural dual antiplatelet therapy for prophylaxis, but emergent presentation of an acute ischemic stroke with tandem cervical dissection and large vessel occlusion is a high risk setting for both thromboembolic complications post-stent reconstruction and intracranial hemorrhage complications post-thrombectomy. Our emergent antiplatelet loading protocol has evolved from an oral/rectal administration of clopidogrel 600 mg and aspirin 300–600 mg to safer shorter-acting agents with intravenous (IV) cangrelor (~15 μg/kg loading dose and 2 μg/kg maintenance, titrated with P2Y12 assays) or glycoprotein IIb/IIIa inhibitors (eptifibatide 180 μg/kg loading dose). We reserve the transition from IV antiplatelet therapy to aspirin/clopidogrel loading until post-procedure or serial CT head studies exclude reperfusion or infarct transformation hemorrhagic complications. Subsequently, dual antiplatelet therapy (clopidogrel 75 mg and aspirin 81–325 mg daily) is continued for at least 12 weeks after stenting depending on the metallic stent construct burden and follow-up imaging results. Due to a non-negligible population that may be resistant to clopidogrel, P2Y12 testing is recommended to assess antiplatelet efficacy and increased dosing or alternative potent thienopyridines (ticagrelor 180 mg loading dose and 90mg BID) may be required.

If a tandem cervical dissection after stroke thrombectomy is managed medically, we will attempt loading immediately with at least aspirin 325 mg and consider delayed loading with a dual antiplatelet (clopidogrel) or transition to oral anticoagulation after stable serial CT head imaging findings.

We perform early (<1 month) post-procedure MRA/CTA and carotid Doppler ultrasound imaging for either baseline assessment or to identify unstable progression of severe pathology (especially for cervical dissections that are managed conservatively with medical management). Serial follow-up MRA/CTA imaging at 1 month, 3–6 months, and every 1–2 years can be performed until resolution, but allows interval assessment of vessel wall healing, normalization of vessel caliber, residual dissection related stenosis/subintimal hematoma, in-stent thrombus, delayed intimal hyperplasia/in-stent stenosis, and stability or thrombosis of associated dissecting aneurysms. MRA may be a suboptimal technique in the evaluation of cervical dissections status post stent reconstruction secondary to metallic susceptibility artifact, but if utilized to minimize CT radiation exposure, contrast enhanced techniques are recommended. For proximal cervical lesions status post stent reconstruction, routine carotid Doppler ultrasound studies may be sufficient follow-up at 3-month intervals for 1 year and then biannually similar to post-carotid stenting algorithm for atherosclerotic lesions.

Case 1: Stent Reconstruction of Severe Flow Limiting and Long Segment Cervical Dissection Restores Cerebral Perfusion

A 37-year-old male presented to our institution after acute onset of severe neurological deficits, left middle cerebral artery (MCA) syndrome with an NIH Stroke Scale of 19, and transient improvement of symptoms after intravenous r-tPA (recombinant tissue plasminogen activator) thrombolysis. CTA head/neck studies demonstrated a severe left ICA cervical dissection without an intracranial LVO, but poor circle of Willis collaterals. Subsequent MR DWI/PWI studies identified small foci of acute infarcts in the left frontal and parietal-temporal lobes (watershed and/or embolic), but a large peripheral region of elevated mean transit time and decreased cerebral blood flow consistent with an ischemic penumbra and salvageable tissue

(Fig. 17.1a). Due to the patient's relatively young age and persisting, fluctuating symptoms not responsive to hemodynamic augmentation, emergent endovascular recanalization and stent reconstruction of the acute cervical dissection was initiated to prevent left MCA infarct progression.

In this case, general anesthesia was induced with a goal systolic blood pressure of 160–180 mm Hg to augment pial collaterals and cerebral perfusion during attempted revascularization. Intravenous heparin anticoagulation was administered throughout the procedure.

A 6 French standard guide sheath (0.088 inch inner diameter, 90 cm) was advanced into the distal left common carotid artery over a 5 French vertebral diagnostic catheter; initial angiograms redemonstrated the acute left ICA cervical dissection with the characteristic tapered "flame sign" and "string sign" extending to the C1–C2 level resulting in complete occlusion and no antegrade intracranial flow (Fig. 17.1b). Retrograde reconstitution of the cavernous and supraclinoid segments was noted through external carotid collaterals via the middle meningeal-ophthalmic arteries and internal maxillary artery (foramen rotundum)-inferolateral trunk consistent in a setting of poor circle of Willis collaterals.

The 5 French vertebral diagnostic catheter was removed and microcatheter/0.014 inch microwire complex were carefully advanced through the 6F guide sheath across the true lumen of the left ICA cervical dissection to the C1–C2 level. Intermittent biplane check angiograms demonstrated recanalization and improved visualization of the severely narrowed and irregular proximal to mid cervical segments of the left ICA terminating in a large dissecting pseudoaneurysm in the distal cervical segment, just proximal to the skull base. We carefully advanced the microwire through the true lumen to achieve recanalization of the long segment LICA dissection extending past the skull base into the petrocavernous segments, again using intermittent check angiograms, until the microcatheter was advanced safely into the intracranial M2 segment of the left MCA (Fig. 17.1b). For adequate access and purchase across the nearly occlusive and flow-limiting left ICA dissection, the microcatheter was removed over a 300 cm 0.014 inch exchange microwire with a safe distal J loop for planned stent reconstruction and revascularization of the cervical LICA dissection.

Following loading bolus of intravenous eptifibatide (0.18 mg/kg), a Neuroform 4 × 20 mm intracranial stent (Stryker Neurovascular, Fremont, CA) was deployed across the posterior genu segment of the cavernous left ICA to trap the distal extension of the intimal flap. Next, a Wingspan 4.5 × 20 mm intracranial stent (Stryker Neurovascular, Fremont, CA) was advanced and deployed with partial overlap from the precavernous segment distally and across the horizontal petrous segment proximally. Finally, a Neuroform 4.5 × 20 mm intracranial stent was deployed with

grams demonstrate successful and complete stent reconstruction of the cervical and petrocavernous left ICA dissection with robust antegrade flow into the intracranial circulation consistent with TICI 3 reperfusion. Note decreased inflow into the distal cervical pseudoaneurysm after stent remodeling, but a 50% residual dissection-related stenosis related to the intramural hematoma. (**e**) Follow-up biplane cervical angiograms at 6 months demonstrate vessel wall healing of the long segment ICA dissection status post stent reconstruction with near-complete restoration of vessel caliber, interval involution of the distal cervical pseudoaneurysm with no residual stenosis, and robust antegrade flow into the intracranial circulation

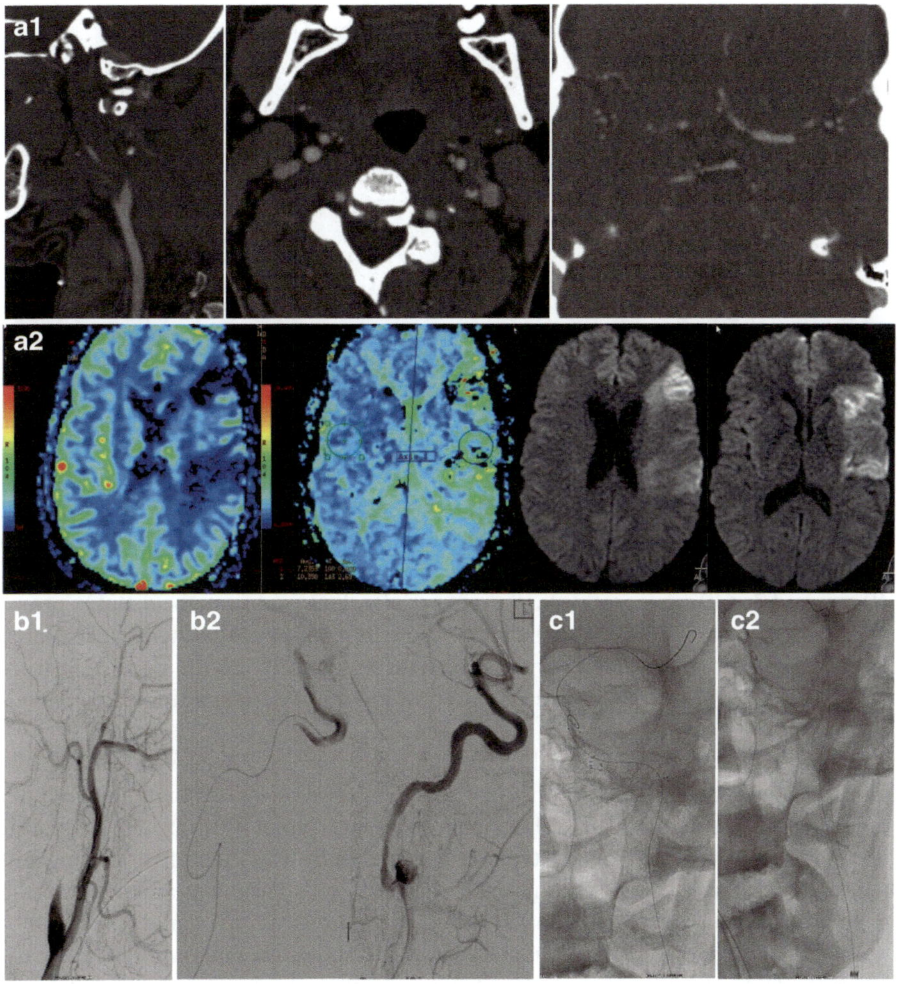

Fig. 17.1 Stent reconstruction of severe flow limiting and long segment cervical dissection restores cerebral perfusion. (**a1**) CTA head/neck studies with coronal MIP and axial images demonstrate long segment, severe internal carotid artery dissection/occlusion without intracranial LVO, but poor circle of Willis collaterals due to hypoplastic anterior communicating and posterior communicating arteries. (**a2**) MR DWI/PWI axial images identify acute embolic frontal-temporal infarcts with large region of elevated mean transit time (MTT) and decreased cerebral blood flow (CBF) in the left MCA distribution consistent with an ischemic penumbra. (**b1**) Lateral DSA image of left common carotid artery injection demonstrates a severe flow-limiting/occlusive dissection, just past the proximal cervical segment of the left ICA with a characteristic flame sign. (**b2**) During microcatheter recanalization of the long segment cervical dissection extending into the petrocavernous segments, lateral DSA images identify re-establishment of slow antegrade flow with prominent subintimal contrast extravasation and dissecting pseudoaneurysm in the distal cervical segment. (**c1**) Oblique radiographs demonstrate partially overlapping intracranial stent reconstruction of the distal intimal flap in the petrocavernous segments with deployed Neuroform 4 × 20 mm and Wingspan 4.5 × 20 mm stents over an exchange length microwire in the MCA. (**c2**) Further stent reconstruction of the vertical petrous segment with a Neuroform 4.5 × 20 mm intracranial stent at the skull base as well as distal to proximal cervical intimal flap reconstruction with self-expanding Precise 6 × 40 mm and 7 × 40 mm carotid stents. (**d**) Final biplane cervical angio-

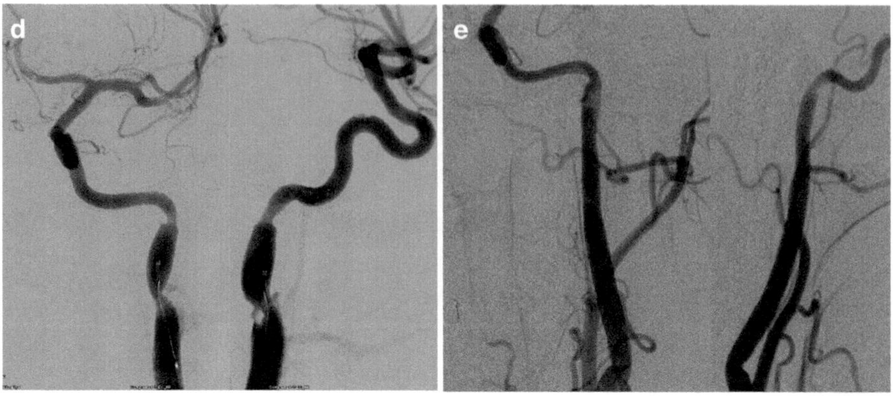

Fig. 17.1 (continued)

partial overlap within the Wingspan stent and across the vertical petrous segment, extending just below the skull base, enabling proximal vessel reconstruction with traditional self-expanding carotid stents. Two partially overlapping Precise 6 × 40 mm and 7 × 40 mm carotid stents were serially deployed from the distal to proximal cervical segments covering the most severe dissection related stenosis and large pseudoaneurysm in the distal cervical segment resulting in intimal flap reconstruction of the cervical left ICA and impaired inflow into the dissecting pseudoaneurysm (Fig. 17.1c).

Final cervical and intracranial angiograms demonstrated successful recanalization and stent reconstruction of the long segment left ICA dissection with markedly improved vessel diameter and robust antegrade intracranial flow through the multiple, tandem carotid/intracranial stents, consistent with TICI 3 reperfusion. A prominent 50% residual stenosis remains in the distal cervical segment at the site of the prior pseudoaneurysm and severe dissection-related stenosis with mild residual subintimal opacification, probably due to a large intramural hematoma. Improved caliber in the vertical petrous segment is also noted with mild residual 20–30% stenosis at the skull base transition of the carotid and intracranial stents (Fig. 17.1d).

Case 2: Mechanical Thrombectomy with Coaxial Catheter Revascularization of Tortuous Tandem Cervical Dissection

A 65-year-old male was transferred to our institution approximately 10 hours after his last known well with severe neurological deficits of global aphasia, right facial droop, hemiplegia, and left gaze preference consistent with an NIH Stroke Scale of 17. CTA head/neck and CT brain perfusion studies demonstrated a small core infarct limited to the lentiform nucleus (ASPECTS 9), secondary to suspected tandem cervical and intracranial left ICA occlusions extending into the left M1 MCA, but with a large ischemic penumbra suggestive of salvageable tissue. Since the patient was eligible for intervention as per the DAWN and DEFUSE-3 trial criteria, emergent mechanical stroke thrombectomy was initiated.

As the patient's airway was secure and he appeared cooperative, monitored anesthesia care was provided with arterial line monitoring and systolic blood pressures of 160–180 mm Hg to augment pial collaterals until revascularization could be achieved. Intravenous heparin anticoagulation was provided throughout the procedure.

A 6 French flexible DGS (0.088 inch inner diameter, 100 cm) was advanced into the left common carotid artery over a 5 French vertebral diagnostic catheter. Initial angiograms revealed abrupt tapering of the proximal cervical left internal carotid artery, resulting in complete occlusion secondary to severe, flow-limiting left ICA dissection involving the mid and distal cervical segments (Fig. 17.2a).

After multiple attempts, a shapeable 0.038 inch glidewire was able to achieve access across the compressed true lumen and prominent intimal flap involving a 360 degree loop of the distal cervical ICA dissection, eventually migrating into the normal petrous segment of the left ICA. Next, a 0.068 inch reperfusion/aspiration thrombectomy catheter was advanced across the cervical ICA segments over the glidewire to maintain recanalization of the severe dissection-related stenosis/occlusion. Furthermore, coaxial advancement of the 6 French DGS was performed across the cervical dissection to augment dilatation of the true lumen, maintain intimal flap realignment, and provide support for planned stroke thrombectomy (Fig. 17.2b).

With 6 French DGS access across the cervical dissection, intracranial thrombectomy was initiated using a 0.068 inch reperfusion catheter, 0.027 inch microcatheter, and a 0.016 inch microwire. The triaxial catheter system was advanced past the normal petrocavernous segments, traversing the supraclinoid ICA and M1 MCA occlusions into the M2 inferior division segment, confirmed on intermittent check angiograms. A 6 × 40 mm stent retriever was deployed across the large thromboembolic burden for several minutes to optimize clot integration. Mechanical thrombectomy was performed with 2 serial stent retriever passes under vacuum aspiration via the 0.068 inch reperfusion catheter abutting the proximal aspect of the clot as well as manual aspiration via the triaxial 6 French DGS, which was further advanced into the distal petrous segment consistent with the GUARD technique [9], resulting in TICI 2c reperfusion (Figs. 17.2c).

The DGS was retracted under vacuum aspiration to retrieve any extraneous thrombus along the left ICA into the proximal cervical segment, but a safety exchange length 0.035 inch glidewire was maintained across the dissection pathology. Delayed cervical and intracranial angiograms were performed over 15–30 minutes to confirm successful intracranial thrombectomy and stability of cervical revascularization, especially across the severe distal cervical dissection and tortuous vascular loop segment. Although a prominent residual dissection flap with subintimal opacification remained in the mid and distal cervical ICA (possibly with early dissecting aneurysm formation), there was stable vessel caliber with no residual flow-limitation or intraluminal thrombus (Fig. 17.2d). Therefore, we deferred stent reconstruction of the cervical dissection, that would have also been difficult or impossible with existing stent technology at the time, due to distal cervical tortuosity and large vessel diameter. The patient was medically treated with

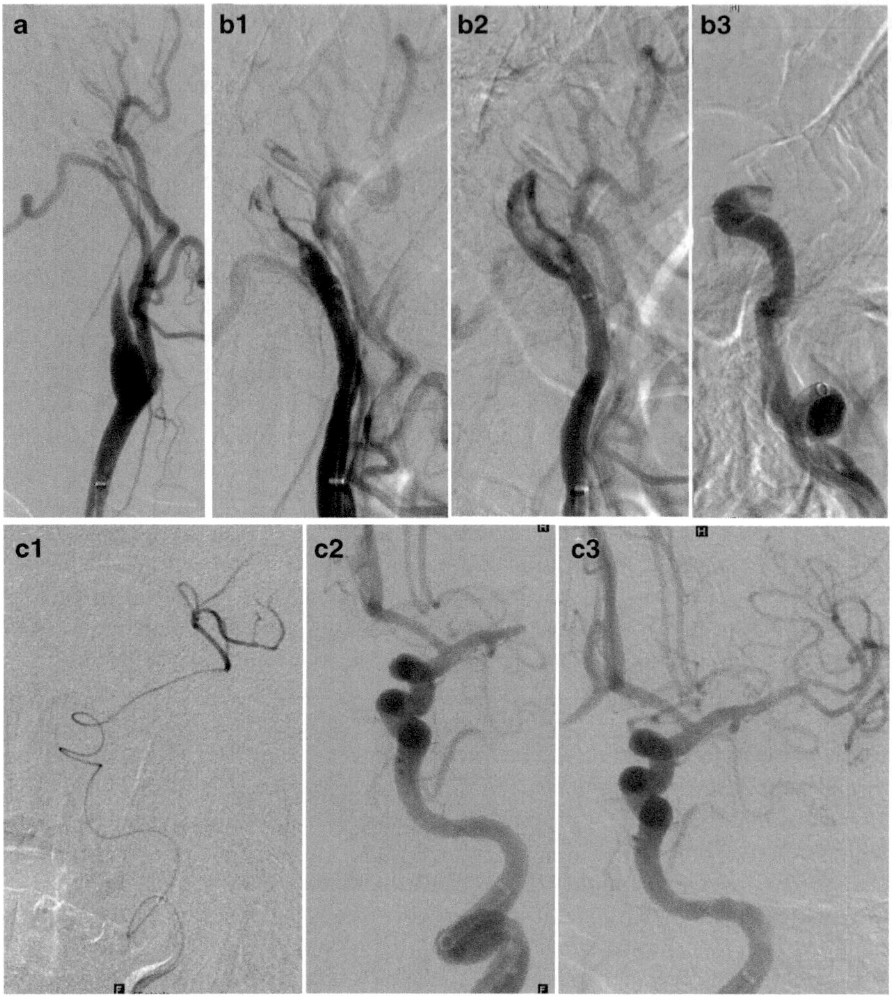

Fig. 17.2 Mechanical thrombectomy with coaxial catheter revascularization of tortuous tandem cervical dissection. (**a**) Lateral DSA image of left common carotid artery injection demonstrates a severe flow-limiting/occlusive, mid to distal cervical left ICA dissection with the characteristic flame sign on initial angiography. (**b1**–**b3**) Serial oblique DSA images after coaxial catheter and flexible DGS recanalization of distal cervical ICA dissection with a prominent intimal flap, and progressive advancement across the involved 360 degree cervical loop, but persisting distal intracranial thromboembolic occlusion of the supraclinoid ICA and M1 left MCA. (**c1**–**c3**) AP DSA images demonstrate intracranial microcatheter access into the left MCA and two serial post-thrombectomy passes with stent retrieval under proximal aspiration, resulting in successful TICI 2c reperfusion. (**d1**–**d4**) Final serial AP/lateral DSA images status post revascularization of cervical dissection and intracranial thrombectomy confirm a stable intimal flap without flow limitation or reocclusion over 30 minutes, obviating the need for stent reconstruction

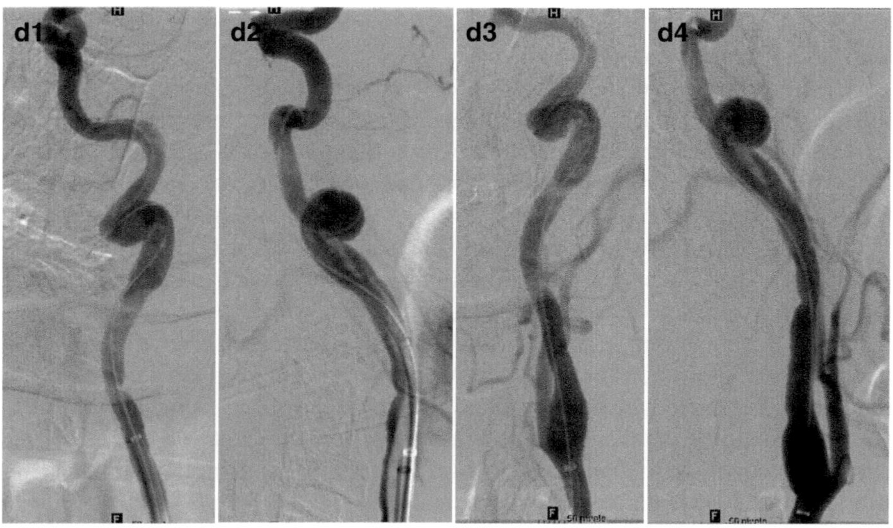

Fig. 17.2 (continued)

anticoagulation for 3 months and subsequent transition to aspirin antiplatelets with stable CTA and carotid Doppler ultrasound imaging findings on serial follow-up studies.

Case 3: Mechanical Thrombectomy with Stent Reconstruction of Unstable Tandem Cervical Dissection

A 54-year-old male with a history of hyperlipidemia presented 23 hours after last known well with severe neurological deficits consisting of left facial droop, hemiparesis, hemineglect, dysarthria, and right sided gaze deviation, consistent with an NIH Stroke Scale of 13. Noncontrast CT and CTA head/neck studies demonstrated early ischemic changes (ASPECTS 6), suspected tandem LVO of the mid cervical right ICA, and large thromboembolic burden in the cavernous/supraclinoid intracranial ICA extending into the M1–M2 segments of the right MCA. Additionally, CT brain perfusion studies confirmed a small core infarct volume (~20 mL) and large ischemic penumbra as per quantitative post-processing analysis software. Due to the salvageable tissue profile as per the DAWN trial criteria, emergent mechanical thrombectomy was initiated.

Since the patient was able to follow simple commands and remain stationary for the procedure, monitored anesthesia care was provided with arterial line monitoring and goal systolic blood pressures of 160–180 mm Hg to augment pial collaterals until revascularization could be achieved.

A 6 French, flexible DGS was coaxially advanced into the proximal cervical right ICA over a 5 French vertebral catheter. Initial angiography demonstrated contrast reflux into the carotid bifurcation with normal antegrade opacification of the right external carotid artery, but with tapering of the mid cervical right ICA segment that terminated in a complete distal cervical ICA occlusion (Fig. 17.3a).

An 0.035 inch glidewire was carefully navigated across the occluded true lumen of the mid and distal cervical ICA dissection for vessel recanalization and placed in the distal horizontal petrous segment for purchase and support. A 0.072 inch reperfusion/aspiration thrombectomy catheter was then advanced over the glidewire under vacuum aspiration for local thrombectomy, yielding a significant burden of intraluminal clot. Subsequently, coaxial advancement of the 6 French DGS was performed into the petrous segment of the right internal carotid artery across the entire dissection flap to maintain vessel recanalization, potential intimal flap stabilization via its large diameter, and guide sheath support for planned intracranial thrombectomy. Intermittent angiography demonstrated complete recanalization of the mid and distal cervical ICA segments with reflux opacification of a large 10 × 15 mm fusiform carotid pseudoaneurysm associated with the tortuous distal cervical segment and significant proximal vessel irregularity in the mid cervical segment, consistent with dissection-related stenoses. Additionally, a small dissection flap was observed extending into the junction of the vertical-horizontal petrous segments, but antegrade flow remains obstructed distally due to an extensive intracranial thrombus burden in the cavernous/supraclinoid ICA extending into the MCA (Fig. 17.3b).

Intracranial thrombectomy was initiated with coaxial advancement of the 0.072 inch reperfusion catheter and 0.027 inch microcatheter over a 0.016 inch microwire across the cavernous/supraclinoid ICA and M1–M2 MCA occlusions. A 6 × 40 mm stent retriever was deployed across the thromboembolus for several minutes to optimize clot integration. Mechanical thrombectomy was performed with 3 serial stent retrieval passes under vacuum aspiration via 0.072 inch reperfusion catheter abutting the proximal aspect of the clot. Additionally, manual aspiration was applied through the 6 French DGS, which was further advanced with triaxial support across the petrous segment into the posterior genu cavernous ICA for the GUARD technique, resulting in TICI 2b reperfusion (Fig. 17.3c).

Post-thrombectomy, the 6F DGS was retracted into the distal right common carotid artery over a safety 0.014 inch exchange microwire to maintain access across the severe cervical and petrous ICA dissection.

Although initial angiography demonstrated patency of the true lumen with near-normal antegrade opacification across the cervical dissection after successful thrombectomy and coaxial catheter revascularization, delayed serial angiography over 15–30 minutes identified interval collapse of the intimal flap due to a severely refractory, unstable dissection with flow limitation and impending reocclusion (Fig. 17.3d). Therefore, stent reconstruction across the cervical and petrous segment dissection was required for vessel salvage.

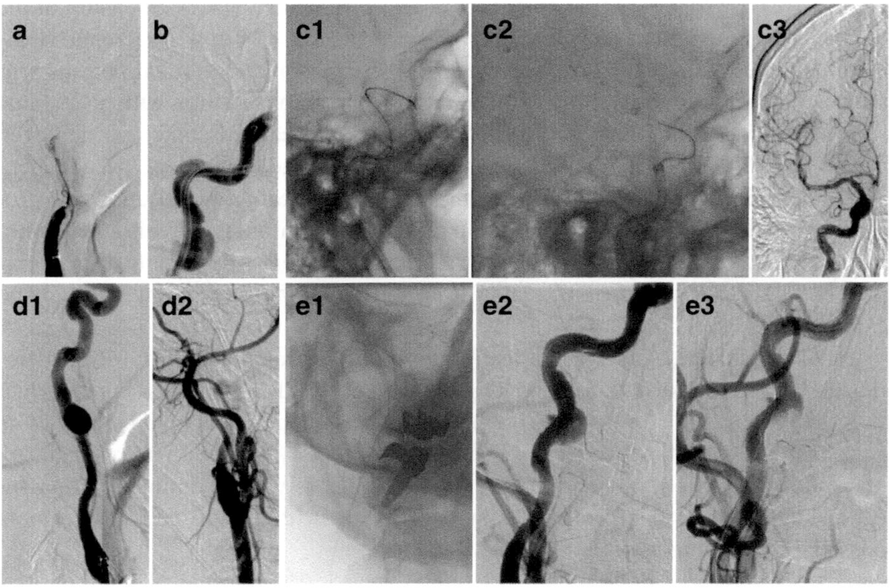

Fig. 17.3 Mechanical thrombectomy with stent reconstruction of unstable tandem cervical dissection. (**a**) Lateral DSA image of right common carotid artery injection demonstrates a severe, flow-limiting cervical right ICA dissection with tapering in the mid cervical segment and terminal occlusion in the distal cervical segment. (**b**) Lateral DSA image after coaxial catheter and DGS recanalization (with local aspiration thrombectomy) and access across the entire dissection flap into the horizontal petrous segment of the right ICA. Contrast reflux also opacifies a large fusiform dissecting pseudoaneurysm in the distal cervical ICA. However, there is persisting obstruction of antegrade flow due to intracranial thromboembolic occlusions of the cavernous/supraclinoid ICA extending into the M1–M2 MCA. (**c1–c2**) Lateral radiographs demonstrate serial mechanical thrombectomy passes with stent retriever deployment, under vacuum aspiration via proximal reperfusion catheter, and manual aspiration via the DGS that was advanced into the posterior genu/cavernous segment (GUARD technique), resulting in TICI 2b reperfusion on final post-thrombectomy AP DSA image (**c3**). (**d1, d2**) Serial cervical angiograms over 15 minutes with lateral (early) and AP (delayed) DSA images after retraction of the DGS identifies interval reocclusion of the cervical ICA dissection due to an unstable intimal flap, refractory to coxial catheter revascularization. (**e1–e3**) Oblique radiograph and final cervical DSA images demonstrate Neuroform 4.5 × 30 mm and 4.5 × 20 mm intracranial stent reconstruction across the distal extent of the dissection flap at the junction of the horizontal and vertical petrous segments, as well as cervical ICA reconstruction with self-expanding Precise 6 × 30 mm and 7 × 30 mm carotid stents. Note complete stent reconstruction of the vessel wall with no residual intimal flap or dissection related stenosis, and decreased opacification of the fusiform dissecting aneurysm due to flow remodeling

An intraoperative flat detector CT head study was performed demonstrating stable infarct volume with contrast staining, but importantly, no evidence of reperfusion hemorrhage or hemorrhagic transformation status post thrombectomy. An eptifibatide loading bolus (0.18 mg/kg) was infused intravenously in preparation for stent reconstructions across the long segment cervical ICA dissection.

Using a 0.027 inch microcatheter for access across the petrous extension of the cervical dissection, two Neuroform 4.5 × 30 mm and 4.5 × 20 mm intracranial stents were deployed with partial overlap across the horizontal and vertical petrous segments of the right ICA resulting in distal intimal flap reconstruction with no residual stenosis. Next, a Precise 6 × 30 mm self-expanding carotid stent was deployed across the tortuous distal cervical segment and associated dissecting pseudoaneurysm with minimum gap abutting the intracranial stent. Subsequently, a Precise 7 × 30 mm carotid stent was deployed with partial overlap within the Precise 6 × 30 mm carotid stent, extending across the mid cervical segment of the right ICA, completely reconstructing the intimal flap from the proximal inflow zone to the distal extent of the dissection.

Final cervical and intracranial angiograms demonstrated successful recanalization and stent reconstruction of the long segment cervical and petrous segment right ICA dissection with robust TICI 2b reperfusion of the intracranial circulation. Excellent vessel wall apposition of the stent constructs is seen with no residual stenosis, flow limitation, in-stent kinking, or thrombus, as well as diminished opacification of the large fusiform dissecting aneurysm in the distal cervical segment secondary to flow remodeling (Fig. 17.3e).

Discussion

As the above cases demonstrate, tandem occlusion due to cervical dissection and an intracranial thromboembolus is a complex pathology that requires emergent, but thoughtful preoperative planning as well as intraoperative assessment of treatment options. Technical efficacy of intracranial thrombectomy with adjunctive stent reconstruction techniques can be performed with low complication rates and translate into favorable clinical outcomes. Although not always necessary as was evident in Case 2, stent reconstruction can salvage acutely occluded or severe flow-limiting dissections refractory to coaxial catheter revascularization, and confer an ability to navigate larger guide or intermediate catheters for the management of associated distal occlusions. Moreover, re-establishing robust cervical antegrade flow can be inherently thrombolytic for small-vessel intracranial occlusions, prevent recurrent thromboemboli or reocclusion after successful cervical and intracranial recanalization, and provide hemodynamic augmentation to pial collaterals supplying any residual ischemic tissue. Even in the absence of a LVO or distal small intracranial thromboemboli, severe flow-limiting cervical dissections without adequate circle of Willis or pial collateral supply can present with profound hypoperfusion-related ischemia, requiring emergent endovascular stent reconstruction for cerebral reperfusion to salvage the ischemic penumbra, as in Case 1.

Proximal-to-distal approaches for tandem occlusions have been described with angioplasty/stent placement to re-establish antegrade flow and access to the intracranial circulation for thrombectomy, but a coaxial catheter/dilator recanalization (Dotter technique) may also be sufficient. Although severe calcified atherosclerotic carotid stenoses may require angioplasty/stenting for distal access, acute cervical dissections can usually be traversed with current guidewires/microwires and distal-access catheter/microcatheter technology for coaxial recanalization to first target the distal intracranial LVO, for rapid cerebral reperfusion with standard aspiration and/or stent-retriever thrombectomy techniques . In our experience, the use of proximal balloon-guide catheters is deferred in preference for lower-profile DGS and distal-access aspiration catheters to prevent further injury to the cervical carotid wall during thrombectomy. We prefer the GUARD technique with a 6F DGS as a valid substitute for balloon guide catheters, due to the atraumatic construction of these flexible guide sheaths and presumably less risk of further intimal injury [9].

After cerebral blood flow has been restored, the cervical dissection requires careful diagnostic assessment; delayed angiography may demonstrate that the intimal flap is stable after coaxial catheter recanalization and true lumen expansion. Furthermore, a patient may possess an adequate circle of Willis or pial collaterals to supply the affected hemisphere without ischemia, despite a residual cervical dissection-related stenosis or flow limitation. Serial angiography over 15–30 minutes must identify a stable dissection flap and vessel patency without interval reocclusion, and/or of an adequate circle of Willis (anterior/posterior communicating arteries) with <2-second venous phase delay in the affected cerebral hemisphere before concluding that vessel recanalization is sufficient and the cervical dissection will be managed medically. In the case of medical management, early transition to antiplatelets or anticoagulation is recommended after excluding intracranial hemorrhage complications, as well as early follow-up MRA/CTA imaging to monitor vessel stability and patency.

If the dissection flap is unstable with severe flow limitation, early reocclusion, and/or poor intracranial collaterals, tandem stent reconstruction of long segment cervical dissections can be performed as described above, from a distal-to-proximal approach, maintaining access across the true lumen and securing the distal extension of the intimal flap to the proximal inflow zone. Multiple groups have demonstrated the successful use of self-expanding carotid/peripheral stents and covered stent grafts in the endovascular reconstruction of cervical dissections and dissecting aneurysms. In fact, after stent realignment of the intimal flap, acute dissecting aneurysms will often undergo spontaneous thrombosis due to flow diversion and reduced inflow into the false aneurysm lumen after stent realignment of the intimal flap. Long-segment carotid dissections may extend into the distal cervical, skull base/petrocavernous, and even intracranial segments, requiring off-label applications of lower-profile balloon-expanding coronary stents or flexible/navigable self-expanding intracranial stents. Although intracranial stents are highly trackable and accommodating to the tortuous distal cervical vasculature with sufficient radial force for the treatment of cervical dissections, this application is considered an off-label use, and may need institutional review board and manufacturer notification for HDE (Humanitarian Device Exemption) devices. Flow-diverting intracranial stents are an evolving technology and may have a future role in the stent reconstruction of highly tortuous dissection flaps in large diameter distal cervical vasculature, including the simultaneous treatment of associated dissecting pseudoaneurysms.

Alternatively, balloon-expanding coronary stents can be advantageous in severe dissection-related stenoses with focal intramural hemorrhage, spiral dissections, or in the constrained osseous compartment of the petrous carotid canal, provide greater angioplasty-dependent radial force and precise placement for vessel reconstruction, albeit with increased risk of vessel injury and stent sizing mismatch.

Dual antiplatelet therapy is mandatory when deploying cervical/intracranial stents, even in the emergent acute stroke intervention setting, in order to prevent in-stent thromboembolic/vessel occlusion complications. Deployment of multiple tandem stents, as in two of the cases detailed above, results in extensive vessel wall exposure to foreign metallic material and increases the risk of platelet aggregation and thromboemboli. However, antiplatelets and anticoagulation may be contraindicated or used with trepidation in the acute stroke setting, as patients may have received intravenous r-tPA thrombolysis and/or may have just underwent mechanical thrombectomy; caution is warranted, especially if there is a high risk of intracranial hemorrhage from reperfusion or infarct transformation complications. We have used several antiplatelet strategies in this precarious setting including intravenous glycoprotein IIb/IIIA inhibitors (eptifibatide) and a novel intravenous P2Y12 inhibitor (cangrelor) during carotid stent reconstruction. Several advantages of IIb/IIIa inhibitors and cangrelor include immediate antiplatelet protection without the need for oral aspirin/clopidogrel loading and a reduced time to peak platelet inhibition (minutes versus hours depending on dose and class of oral thienopyridines). As a reversible competitive inhibitor with a short half-life, eptifibatide rapidly decays with normalizing platelet function over hours, providing time to initiate aspirin/clopidogrel loading or terminate antiplatelet therapy if hemorrhagic complications are suspected. Cangrelor is also a reversible P2Y12 inhibitor with an even shorter half-life and normalization of platelet function over 30 minutes, and a viable alternative to eptifibatide. If CT head findings are equivocal or concerning, clopidogrel loading can be delayed until repeat follow-up imaging definitively excludes evolving intracranial hemorrhage. New dual-energy CT applications may assist in the earlier diagnosis of infarct related contrast staining versus hemorrhagic complications after endovascular stroke thrombectomy, allowing confident initiation of dual-antiplatelet therapy and prophylaxis from stent-related thromboembolic complications.

In conclusion, endovascular revascularization with coaxial catheter recanalization or stent reconstruction techniques is an effective technique for restoring cerebral perfusion in the setting of tandem cervical dissections and LVO requiring acute stroke thrombectomy. If the dissection flap is stable without significant stenosis or flow-limitation, conservative catheter recanalization and medical management with antiplatelet/anticoagulation therapy can be effective to promote spontaneous vessel wall healing. Furthermore, adequate circle of Willis or pial collaterals to the affected cerebral hemisphere without persisting ischemia (clinical and/or imaging evaluation) may also warrant a trial of medical management. However, in refractory cervical dissections with long segment, severe flow-limiting stenoses, and impending occlusion on serial delayed angiography and/or in patients with a poor circle of Willis, intravenous antiplatelet loading followed by stent reconstruction should be the preferred revascularization technique.

References

1. Ansari SA, Parmar H, Ibrhaim M, et al. Cervical dissections: diagnosis, management, and endovascular treatment. Neuroimaging Clin N Am. 2009;19:257–70.
2. Hoving JW, Marquering HA, Majoie CBLM. Endovascular treatment in patients with carotid artery dissection and intracranial occlusion: a systematic review. Neuroradiology. 2017;59:641–7.
3. Stampfl S, Ringleb PA, Mohlenbruch M, et al. Emergency cervical internal carotid artery stenting in combination with intracranial thrombectomy in acute stroke. Am J Neuroradiol. 2014;35:741–6.
4. Ansari SA, Kuhn AL, Honarmand AR, et al. Emergent endovascular management of long-segment and flow-limiting carotid artery dissections in acute ischemic stroke intervention with multiple tandem stents. Am J Neuroradiol. 2017;38:97–104.
5. Marnat G, Mourand I, Eker O, Machi P, Arquizan C, Riquelme C, Ayrignac X, Bonafé A, Costalat V. Endovascular management of tandem occlusion stroke related to internal carotid artery dissection using a distal to proximal approach: insight from the RECOST study. AJNR Am J Neuroradiol. 2016;37(7):1281–8.
6. Goyal M, Menon BK, van Zwam WH, Dippel DW, Mitchell PJ, Demchuk AM, Dávalos A, Majoie CB, van der Lugt A, de Miquel MA, Donnan GA, Roos YB, Bonafe A, Jahan R, Diener HC, van den Berg LA, Levy EI, Berkhemer OA, Pereira VM, Rempel J, Millán M, Davis SM, Roy D, Thornton J, Román LS, Ribó M, Beumer D, Stouch B, Brown S, Campbell BC, van Oostenbrugge RJ, Saver JL, Hill MD, Jovin TG, HERMES Collaborators. Endovascular thrombectomy after large-vessel ischaemic stroke: a meta-analysis of individual patient data from five randomised trials. Lancet. 2016;387(10029):1723–31.
7. Albers GW, Marks MP, Kemp S, Christensen S, Tsai JP, Ortega-Gutierrez S, McTaggart RA, Torbey MT, Kim-Tenser M, Leslie-Mazwi T, Sarraj A, Kasner SE, Ansari SA, Yeatts SD, Hamilton S, Mlynash M, Heit JJ, Zaharchuk G, Kim S, Carrozzella J, Palesch YY, Demchuk AM, Bammer R, Lavori PW, Broderick JP, Lansberg MG, DEFUSE 3 Investigators. Thrombectomy for stroke at 6 to 16 hours with selection by perfusion imaging. N Engl J Med. 2018;378(8):708–18.
8. Nogueira RG, Jadhav AP, Haussen DC, Bonafe A, Budzik RF, Bhuva P, Yavagal DR, Ribo M, Cognard C, Hanel RA, Sila CA, Hassan AE, Millan M, Levy EI, Mitchell P, Chen M, English JD, Shah QA, Silver FL, Pereira VM, Mehta BP, Baxter BW, Abraham MG, Cardona P, Veznedaroglu E, Hellinger FR, Feng L, Kirmani JF, Lopes DK, Jankowitz BT, Frankel MR, Costalat V, Vora NA, Yoo AJ, Malik AM, Furlan AJ, Rubiera M, Aghaebrahim A, Olivot JM, Tekle WG, Shields R, Graves T, Lewis RJ, Smith WS, Liebeskind DS, Saver JL, Jovin TG, DAWN Trial Investigators. Thrombectomy 6 to 24 hours after stroke with a mismatch between deficit and infarct. N Engl J Med. 2018;378(1):11–21.
9. Ansari SA, Darwish M, Abdalla RN, et al. GUide sheath Advancement and aspiRation in the Distal petrocavenous internal carotid artery (GUARD) technique during thrombectomy improves reperfusion and clinical outcomes. Am J Neuroradiol. 2019;40:1356–62.
10. Ansari SA, Thompson BG, Gemmete JJ, Gandhi D. Endovascular treatment of distal cervical and intracranial dissections with the neuroform stent. Neurosurgery. 2008;62(3):636–46.

Chapter 18
Acute Stroke Following Carotid Endarterectomy: Approach and Strategy

Eleonora Francesca Spinazzi, Pavan S. Upadhyayula, Belinda Shao, and Philip M. Meyers

Introduction

Stroke is the second leading cause of mortality and the third leading cause of disability – adjusted life years (DALYs) worldwide [1]. First described in 1951 by C. Miller Fisher, internal carotid artery stenosis (ICAS) has been identified as a major cause of ischemic stroke, with atherosclerosis and thrombosis representing the most common occlusive etiologies, accounting for roughly 60% of all strokes [2]. Several large, multicenter, randomized, prospective clinical trials have demonstrated the benefits of carotid revascularization for stroke prevention in selected patients with extracranial ICAS. For prevention of ischemic stroke due to carotid bifurcation stenosis, carotid endarterectomy (CEA) remains a common procedure for the treatment of symptomatic [3, 4] and selected asymptomatic [5–7] patients with ICAS. More specifically, the North America Symptomatic Carotid Endarterectomy Trial (NASCET) and the European Carotid Surgery Trial (ESCT) proved the benefit of CEA and led to American Heart Association Class I, Level of Evidence A Recommendation for surgical intervention in patients with severe symptomatic carotid stenosis. The benefit of CEA is directly proportional to the degree of stenosis in symptomatic patients with ≥70% ICAS. By contrast, in asymptomatic patients, the size of this treatment effect is more limited. ACAS and ACST demonstrated only 5.4–5.9% absolute risk reduction of CEA; thus, maintaining a periprocedural risk less than 3.1% becomes particularly important to maximize surgical benefit [6, 7] (Table 18.1). Utilization of CEA varies significantly throughout the developed world: in the United States, about ¾ of all CEAs are performed on asymptomatic patients [8].

E. F. Spinazzi (✉) · P. S. Upadhyayula · B. Shao · P. M. Meyers
Department of Neurological Surgery, Columbia University Medical Center, New York, NY, USA
e-mail: efs2110@cumc.columbia.edu; pmm2002@cumc.columbia.edu

F. K. Hui et al. (eds.), *12 Strokes*, https://doi.org/10.1007/978-3-030-56857-3_18

Table 18.1 Natural history of carotid stenosis: medical versus surgical management

RTC	Degree of stenosis (%)	Follow-up period (years)	Long-term primary event rate: Medical management (%)	Carotid endarterectomy (%)	30-day surgical CSM (%)	ARR (%)	RRR (%)
Asymptomatic:							
ACAS	60–99	5	11.0	5.1	2.3	5.9	53
ACST	60–99	5	11.8	6.4	3.1	5.4	46
	60–99	10	17.9	13.4	3.1	4.5	25
Symptomatic:							
NASCET	50–69	5	22.2	15.7	6.7	6.5	29
	70–99	2	26.0	9.0	5.8	17	65
ESCT	*50–69*[a]	3	18.4	15.6	7.9	2.8	None
	70–99[a]	8	21.9	12.3	7.5	9.6	44

Abbreviations: *ACAS* Asymptomatic Carotid Atherosclerosis Study, *ACST* Asymptomatic Carotid Surgery Trial, *ARR* absolute risk reduction, *CSM* combined stroke and/or mortality rate, *ECST* European Carotid Surgery Trial, *NASCET* North American Symptomatic Carotid Endarterectomy Trial, *RRR* relative risk reduction

[a](%) stenosis by ECST = 0.6 × (%) stenosis by NASCET + 40% [33]

Because the purpose of carotid revascularization is stroke prevention, perioperative stroke is a serious complication. Moreover, perioperative stroke is associated with poor neurological and functional outcomes. Patients experiencing a stroke following CEA have an almost threefold increase in mortality at 4-year follow-up [5]. Even for experienced surgeons, the rate of CEA-associated perioperative stroke reportedly ranges as high as 3.24–6% [3, 4]. Stroke risk during surgery must be weighed against the risk of stroke in untreated ICAS, which ranges from 2% in asymptomatic patients to 26% in symptomatic patients at 2-year follow-up [3]. In two studies, operative factors such as intraoperative neurophysiology monitoring changes, and use of a vascular shunt were significantly associated with postoperative neurological events [9]. It is difficult to determine whether the increased operative stroke risk is due to patient or surgeon characteristics, since shunts are used more frequently in conjunction with general anesthesia. Periprocedural stroke usually occurs in symptomatic patients, who have a more tenuous neurological status [10]. This ambiguity in the data highlights one of the critical shortcomings of the literature. The rarity of postoperative stroke precludes rigorous prospective trials studying optimal management strategies. This chapter will highlight the various etiologies and management strategies available for the treatment of postoperative CEA stroke. Our goal is to bring together a previously dichotomized literature to provide the surgeon with a single action algorithm in cases where this were to present.

Etiologies and Time Course of Stroke After CEA

Effectively managing perioperative CEA stroke requires prompt determination of the pathologic cause. Broadly, postoperative CEA stroke falls into four categories: thromboembolic, hemorrhagic, clamp-related ischemia, and incidental/unrelated [10].

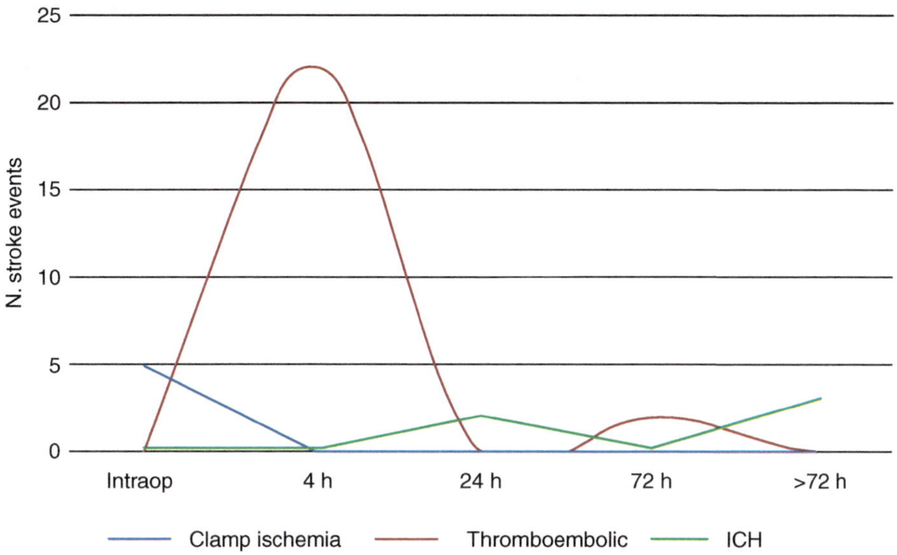

Fig. 18.1 Relationship between timing and etiology of perioperative stroke events. Intraop = intraoperative. (Figure adapted from Rockman et al. [10])

A majority of post-CEA stroke occurs within the first 24 hours after surgery (Fig. 18.1). Between 54.5% and 66.6% of postoperative neurologic events occur in this window [10–12]. Immediately postoperatively, the risk of thromboembolic strokes is the highest. Multiple studies, both using CT angiography as well as surgical re-exploration, have shown that in patients presenting with a new-onset neurological deficit within 24 hours of CEA, the rate of carotid luminal irregularities such as an intraluminal thrombus exceeds 80% [10, 13]. Other findings such as intimal flaps or step-offs of the CCA, ECA, or ICA have not been correlated with neurologic deficits and seem to be inevitable consequences of the surgical procedure [14]. Reasons for postoperative thromboembolic complications are not clear. One possibility is mechanical dislodgement of clot during surgery, leading to intraoperative emboli [9, 15]. A second possibility is a systemic inflammatory response creating a prothrombotic environment during surgery [9, 16]. In one of the largest studies to date of 2250 CEA patients, Radak et al. showed that these two pathophysiologic mechanisms may have unique temporal distributions [17]. Intraoperative strokes were associated with thromboembolic events and patent carotid arteries. Postoperative strokes were associated with carotid artery thrombosis [17]. Some authors argue that intraoperative ischemia is more likely due to clamp intolerance. As mentioned previously, clamp intolerance and use of a shunt are both independently associated with postoperative neurological outcomes, morbidity, and mortality [10]. Notably, this type of stroke affects anterior cerebral circulation in over 70% of cases [9].

A second type of post-CEA stroke is hemorrhagic. This complication occurs later during the recovery period – namely, 24–72 hours postoperation – and accounts for up to 13% of postoperative neurological deficits [9–11]. Patients usually present with signs and symptoms consistent with increased intracranial pressure or neuronal irritation. These may include headache, lethargy, obtundation, and seizures along with elevations in systolic blood pressure [10]. Based on the clinical time course and patient presentation, emergent CT is the diagnostic tool of choice. Cerebral hyperperfusion syndrome and hemorrhagic transformation of ischemic regions are two pathophysiologic mechanisms that can cause postoperative hemorrhage [18, 19].

The final group to consider are patients suffering strokes that are incidental, or unrelated, to the operation. Causes for this finding may include diffuse global hypoxia due to improper medical management, cardio-embolic stroke, or contralateral thrombo-embolic stroke. It is possible, however, for ipsilateral intraluminal defects to cross over, causing contralateral deficits [10]. These incidental neurologic events may occur any time during the operative and the postoperative period.

Existing Management Algorithms: Two Schools of Thought

Current approaches to the evaluation and treatment of perioperative stroke after CEA remain controversial. The infrequent occurrence of this perioperative complication has translated into scant literature; small case series and retrospective data diminish the quality of conclusions drawn. For this reason, no consensus has been reached regarding optimal evaluation and treatment of neurologic deficits post CEA, with recommendations varying according to the clinician's experience and discretion. Controversy mainly exists over the role for diagnostic imaging, the clinical criteria that warrant surgical reoperation, and the window of opportunity in which restitution of blood flow can still reverse ischemic damage and rescue neurologic function [10, 20]. These areas of disagreement have dichotomized management of acute stroke post-CEA into two schools of thought: the time-honored approach, which advocates for immediate surgical exploration, versus the imaging-first paradigm, which stresses the value of diagnostic imaging in guiding optimal management. Newer technology has rapidly changed the cost-benefit analysis associated with each technique. Without comparative literature, postoperative management is often based on surgeon preference rather than scientific evidence. Such an approach can be problematic in times of emergency, when acute occlusion is suspected and the surgeon has no preplanned validated strategy to guide management [10, 19].

Pearls and Pitfalls for Early Reoperation

Management of acute stroke during or immediately after CEA presents a unique neurosurgical situation; the patient's cerebral circulation has often been assessed during preoperative testing, and the new neurological defect can be ascribed to the surgical site with a high degree of certainty. Neuronal viability is tied to both the degree of collateral circulation as well as the duration of ischemia [21]. To minimize the duration of ischemia and optimize neurological outcomes, some surgeons have recommended early reoperation in the setting of new-onset neurologic deficits [17, 22].

Review of the published data, however, provides a mixed picture. Treiman et al. reported on 26 patients with acute post-CEA stroke [22]. Twelve patients underwent immediate surgical exploration. Only 7 of 12 patients had successful thrombectomy, and only 3 had symptomatic improvement. By contrast, 4 of 14 medically managed patients had symptomatic improvement. Also of note is that only 66% of reoperation patients had a thrombus at the surgical site [22]. Rockman et al. described 25 patients who developed acute post-CEA stroke. Of these, 18 were reoperated with 15 (83.3%) demonstrating CEA site thrombus; 12 had significant neurological improvement [10]. Similarly, Paty et al. found that 100% of patients with early post-CEA stroke had thrombosis of the endarterectomy site with nearly 60% good neurological outcomes [20].

The better rate of neurological improvement noted by Rockman et al. (66.6%) and Paty et al. (57.1%) may be related to the higher rates of thrombosis at the CEA surgical site [10, 20]. These findings are corroborated by the largest retrospective study of postoperative complications of CEA conducted by Radak et al. Out of 2250 CEA cases, 18 (0.80%) patients developed postoperative stroke and 11 of the 18 had CEA-site thrombosis. With prompt reoperation, 8 of the 18 patients made total recovery [17]. Beyond simply corroborating the importance for prompt reoperation, the authors also conclude most perioperative strokes are due to technical error. They advocate the use of intraoperative imaging including transcranial Doppler and EEG monitoring to help limit complications. In a range of smaller studies with fewer than ten reoperations each, the rate of symptomatic neurological improvement after urgent reoperation ranges anywhere from 25% to 100% [23–25]. Although these studies each report small case series, they all mention a correlation between neurologic recovery and time from symptom presentation to reoperation. The one case series that reported 100% (3/3) symptomatic improvement with reoperation had reoperation within 45 minutes of symptom onset [23]. When comparing reoperation to medical management for post-CEA stroke, Stewart et al. found no difference between the two treatment arms. The study is confounded by a low incidence of CEA site thrombus (25%) and a higher rate of early (<24 hours) postoperative stroke in the reoperation cohort [26].

While inconsistent in certain respects, these studies highlight *three key principles*. First, new-onset neurological deficit in the immediate postoperative window (0–24 hours) requires a high index of suspicion for CEA site thrombosis. Second, if reoperation is to be attempted, time to reoperation is critically important to long-term neurological outcome. Third, there may be a subset of patients for whom reoperation is not beneficial. For these patients, other management options including imaging should be considered.

Pearls and Pitfalls for Diagnostic Imaging

The benefits of emergent reoperation in the setting of CEA site thrombus are clear. However, this approach may oversimplify – or fail to identify – other potential causes of post-CEA stroke. In cases of intracranial ischemia/hemorrhage, intracranial tandem occlusion, and carotid artery dissection extending beyond the petrous portion of the carotid artery, reoperation is of limited utility and does not provide any diagnostic or therapeutic value [12]. A handful of recent case series – each utilizing advances in endovascular or neuroimaging techniques – explore the risks and benefits of this prompt imaging approach.

Case series that recommend emergent angiography prior to reoperation share a few characteristics. First, the rate of CEA site thrombus was lower than in the studies discussed previously, ranging between 42.8% and 55.5%, possibly due to smaller sample sizes or other selection biases. The rest of the patients demonstrated inoperable (through reexploration of surgical site) or inconclusive findings on angiography [11, 27]. Second, these studies highlight the importance of minimizing time from diagnostic imaging to potential reoperation. Recent studies of acute stroke have demonstrated that the likelihood of a good neurological outcome decreases approximately 10% every 30 minutes that effective revascularization is delayed. It is important to note that bedside ultrasound provides an additional imaging tool that can provide diagnostic information about the extracranial carotid artery in a short period of time.

An endovascular approach allows for diagnostic assessment and therapeutic intervention of CEA site thrombus along with intracranial pathologies and may represent the best current solution to this clinical conundrum. Spiotta et al. described 11 patients with post-CEA stroke, 81.8% with ipsilateral MCA stroke, and 36.4% with a tandem extracranial-intracranial occlusion [12]. These authors showed that endovascular carotid artery stenting (CAS) is a viable rescue therapy for patients with CEA site thrombus. Their findings corroborate other reports about the safety and efficacy of an endovascular approach with CAS for treatment of post-CEA stroke [28]. CAS, compared to open reoperation and thrombectomy, also facilitates mechanical thrombectomy for acute ischemic stroke with large cerebral artery occlusion, when indicated [12]. This approach may be particularly beneficial for treatment in tandem occlusions. As a technical consideration, the authors advocate a proximal-to-distal approach where the carotid artery thrombosis is stented first before mechanical thrombectomy of cerebral territories (MCA/ACA) is undertaken. Such an approach has been shown effective (56.3% with modified Rankin Score 0–2) and, using endovascular methods for cerebral artery protection, has the theoretical benefit of decreasing thromboembolism into cerebral circulation [29]. The use of catheter cerebral angiography can be performed rapidly in the context of an endovascular stroke thrombectomy program to minimize ischemic damage by reducing occlusion time.

Proposed Management Strategy

When acute stroke is suspected in a patient with previously uneventful perioperative course, including normal intraoperative monitoring and asymptomatic awakening, surgeons should be familiar with their institutional stroke protocols for rapid activation of their local acute stroke system. Because these are relatively uncommon events, reports on the utility of this postoperative complication and best treatment remain anecdotal. Hence, controversy remains mainly over the role and type of diagnostic imaging necessary to direct further intervention. The window of opportunity in which restitution of blood flow can reverse ischemic damage and rescue neurologic function was not well established until recently [10, 20]. Now, there is a burgeoning literature on image-guided stroke therapy and patient selection even in the extended time interval up to 24 hours from stroke onset or last known well [30, 31]. These areas of disagreement have dichotomized management of acute stroke post-CEA, with most authors advocating for immediate surgical exploration and stressing the delay in performing diagnostic imaging. However, a paradigm shift has emerged, with more recent acute stroke literature demonstrating the importance of imaging and mechanical thrombectomy, stressing the role of newer and faster technology in minimizing delay and guiding treatment. According to the 2018 AHA Stroke Guidelines, which address acute ischemic stroke following CEA, the usefulness of emergent surgical exploration is not well established [32].

With the foregoing recommendations in mind, we reviewed the literature and amalgamated it with our institutional experience in the attempt to propose treatment algorithm meant to guide the surgeon in the event post-CEA stroke were to be suspected (Fig. 18.2). According to our proposed protocol, unless the patient is hemodynamically unstable (i.e., has a growing neck hematoma at the arteriotomy site with impending airway compromise), a head CT without contrast should be performed immediately as soon as an acute stroke is suspected. The acute stroke team should be activated according to local hospital acute stroke protocol. The nonenhanced CT brain scan is important to distinguish between hemorrhagic and potential ischemic etiologies of stroke. In the absence of hemorrhage, timely acquisition of CT angiogram of the head and neck, and CT perfusion is important to identify large cerebral artery occlusions that require immediate intervention. Assessment for completed ischemic infarction on the nonenhanced CT scan is a guide to the use of mechanical thrombectomy within 6 hours of stroke onset or last known well. After 6 hours, CT-perfusion imaging using either DEFUSE 3 (6–16 hours) [30] or DAWN (6–24 hours) [31] criteria may be used according to the 2018 stroke guidelines [32]. If the occlusion is extracranial only, and located at the surgical site, prompt reoperation with re-exploration is the treatment of choice. If intracranial large artery occlusion is demonstrated, then endovascular mechanical thrombectomy by an experienced stroke interventionalist, according to current guidelines, is indicated as it has been proven to improve patient outcomes. If the occlusion is intracranial only, then endovascular mechanical thrombectomy is the treatment of choice (Fig. 18.2).

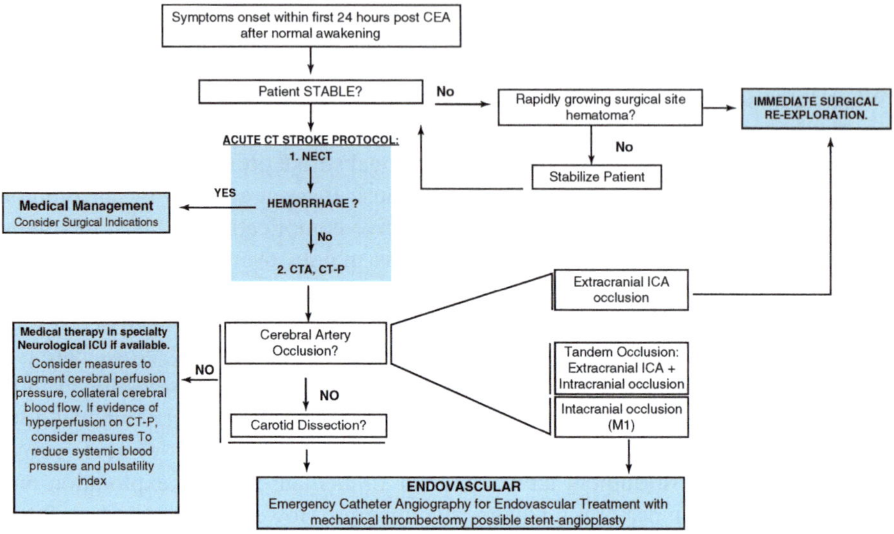

Fig. 18.2 Flow chart of the proposed treatment algorithm in case of postoperative stroke after asymptomatic normal awakening within 24 hours post CEA. Abbreviations: CT, computed tomography; CTA, computed tomography angiography; CT-P, computed tomography perfusion; ICA, internal carotid artery; NECT, nonenhancing computed tomography

Conclusion

In conclusion, optimal management of post-CEA stroke remains controversial although the modern stroke literature provides greater direction. Most postoperative strokes present within 24 hours. The majority of these neurological events are secondary to thrombus formation at the arteriotomy site, are thrombo-occlusive in etiology, extracranial, and ipsilateral to the operative site. Disagreement about treatment of these rare events historically dichotomized management of acute stroke post-CEA, with most authors advocating for immediate surgical exploration and stressing the delay in performing diagnostic imaging. However, the modern stroke literature demonstrates the importance of emergency stroke assessment, cerebral and vascular imaging to guide treatment. Endovascular mechanical thromboembolectomy has recently emerged as first-line intervention for acute stroke with large cerebral artery occlusion. For tandem intracranial-extracranial occlusion, the data is less clear although there is evidence for use of an endovascular approach. For patients with local thrombus at the operative site, questions regarding optimal management strategy remain. Because these events are relatively rare, it is unlikely that a prospective, randomized trial comparing different management strategies is feasible to address lingering questions. Multicenter registries such as the Society of Vascular Surgery (SVS) Carotid database may serve as a source of additional data over time to guide patient management in these cases. Adherence to modern stroke guidelines is important and should supersede historical disagreements.

References

1. Feigin VL, Forouzanfar MH, Krishnamurthi R, Mensah GA, Connor M, Bennett DA, et al. Global and regional burden of stroke during 1990–2010: findings from the Global Burden of Disease Study 2010. Lancet. 2014;383(9913):245.
2. Fisher M. Occlusion of the internal carotid artery. AMA Arch Neurol Psychiatry. 1951;65(3):346–77.
3. Ferguson GG, Eliasziw M, Barr HWK, Patrick Clagett G, Barnes RW, Christopher Wallace M, et al. The North American symptomatic carotid endarterectomy trial. Stroke. 1999;30(9):1751–8.
4. European Carotid Surgery Trialists' Collaborative Group. Randomised trial of endarterectomy for recently symptomatic carotid stenosis: final results of the MRC European Carotid Surgery Trial (ECST). Lancet. 1998;351(9113):1379–87.
5. Hill MD, Brooks W, Mackey A, Clark WM, Meschia JF, Morrish WF, et al. Stroke after carotid stenting and endarterectomy in the Carotid Revascularization Endarterectomy versus Stenting Trial (CREST). Circulation. 2012;126(25):3054–61.
6. Halliday A, Harrison M, Hayter E, Kong X, Mansfield A, Marro J, et al. 10-year stroke prevention after successful carotid endarterectomy for asymptomatic stenosis (ACST-1): a multicentre randomised trial. Lancet. 2010;376(9746):1074–84.
7. Endarterectomy for asymptomatic carotid artery stenosis. Executive Committee for the Asymptomatic Carotid Atherosclerosis Study. JAMA. 1995;273(18):1421–8.
8. Halm EA, Chassin MR, Tuhrim S, Hollier LH, Popp AJ, Ascher E, et al. Revisiting the appropriateness of carotid endarterectomy. Stroke. 2003;34(6):1464–71.
9. Khattar NK, Friedlander RM, Chaer RA, Avgerinos ED, Kretz ES, Balzer JR, et al. Perioperative stroke after carotid endarterectomy: etiology and implications. Acta Neurochir. 2016;158(12):2377–83.
10. Rockman CB, Jacobowitz GR, Lamparello PJ, Adelman MA, Woo D, Schanzer A, et al. Immediate reexploration for the perioperative neurologic event after carotid endarterectomy: is it worthwhile? J Vasc Surg. 2000;32(6):1062–70.
11. Pappadà G, Vergani F, Parolin M, Cesana C, Pirillo D, Pirovano M, et al. Early acute hemispheric stroke after carotid endarterectomy. Pathogenesis and management. Acta Neurochir. 2010;152(4):579–87.
12. Spiotta AM, Vargas J, Zuckerman S, Mokin M, Ahmed A, Mocco J, et al. Acute stroke after carotid endarterectomy: time for a paradigm shift? Multicenter experience with emergent carotid artery stenting with or without intracranial tandem occlusion thrombectomy. Neurosurgery. 2015;76(4):403–10.
13. Gallati CP, Jain M, Damania D, Kanthala AR, Jain AR, Koch GE, et al. 64-detector CT angiography within 24 hours after carotid endarterectomy and correlation with postoperative stroke. J Neurosurg. 2015;122(3):637–43.
14. van der Kolk AG, de Borst GJ, Jongen LM, den Hartog AG, Moll FL, Mali WPTM, et al. Prevalence and clinical consequences of carotid artery residual defects following endarterectomy: a prospective CT angiography evaluation study. Eur J Vasc Endovasc Surg. 2011;42(2):144–52.
15. Elkind MSV. Inflammatory mechanisms of stroke. Stroke. 2010;41(10 Suppl):S3–8.
16. Bastian D, Tamburstuen MV, Lyngstadaas SP, Reikerås O. Systemic and local cytokine kinetics after total hip replacement surgery. Eur Surg Res. 2008;41(4):334–40.
17. Radak D, Popovic AD, Radicević S, Nesković AN, Bojić M. Immediate reoperation for perioperative stroke after 2250 carotid endarterectomies: differences between intraoperative and early postoperative stroke. J Vasc Surg. 1999;30(2):245–51.
18. Farooq MU, Goshgarian C, Min J, Gorelick PB. Pathophysiology and management of reperfusion injury and hyperperfusion syndrome after carotid endarterectomy and carotid artery stenting. Exp Transl Stroke Med. 2016;8(1):7.

19. Yunoki M, Suzuki K, Uneda A, Hirashita K, Yoshino K. Acute internal carotid artery occlusion after carotid endarterectomy. Interdiscip Neurosurg. 2016;5:54–7.
20. Paty PS, Darling RC 3rd, Cordero JA Jr, Shah DM, Chang BB, Leather RP. Carotid artery bypass in acute postendarterectomy thrombosis. Am J Surg. 1996;172(2):181–3.
21. Gomez CR. Time is brain: the stroke theory of relativity. J Stroke Cerebrovasc Dis. 2018;27(8):2214–27.
22. Treiman RL, Cossman DV, Cohen JL, Foran RF, Levin PM. Management of postoperative stroke after carotid endarterectomy. Am J Surg. 1981;142(2):236–8.
23. Kwaan JH, Connolly JE, Sharefkin JB. Successful management of early stroke after carotid endarterectomy. Ann Surg. 1979;190(5):676–8.
24. Lindberg B. Acute carotid occlusion. Indication for surgery? J Cardiovasc Surg. 1980;21(3):315–20.
25. Najafi H, Javid H, Dye WS, Hunter JA, Wideman FE, Julian OC. Emergency carotid thromboendarterectomy. Surgical indications and results. Arch Surg. 1971;103(5):610–4.
26. Stewart AHR, McGrath CM, Cole SEA, Smith FCT, Baird RN, Lamont PM. Reoperation for neurological complications following carotid endarterectomy. Br J Surg. 2003;90(7):832–7.
27. Findlay JM, Marchak BE. Reoperation for acute hemispheric stroke after carotid endarterectomy: is there any value? Neurosurgery. 2002;50(3):486–92; discussion 92–3.
28. Anzuini A, Briguori C, Roubin GS, Pagnotta P, Rosanio S, Airoldi F, et al. Emergency stenting to treat neurological complications occurring after carotid endarterectomy. J Am Coll Cardiol. 2001;37(8):2074–9.
29. Spiotta AM, Lena J, Vargas J, Hawk H, Turner RD, Chaudry MI, et al. Proximal to distal approach in the treatment of tandem occlusions causing an acute stroke. J Neurointerv Surg. 2015;7(3):164–9.
30. Albers GW, Marks MP, Kemp S, Christensen S, Tsai JP, Ortega-Gutierrez S, et al. Thrombectomy for stroke at 6 to 16 hours with selection by perfusion imaging. N Engl J Med. 2018;378(8):708–18.
31. Nogueira RG, Jadhav AP, Haussen DC, Bonafe A, Budzik RF, Bhuva P, et al. Thrombectomy 6 to 24 hours after stroke with a mismatch between deficit and infarct. N Engl J Med. 2018;378(1):11–21.
32. Powers WJ, Rabinstein AA, Ackerson T, Adeoye OM, Bambakidis NC, Becker K, et al. 2018 guidelines for the early management of patients with acute ischemic stroke: a guideline for healthcare professionals from the American Heart Association/American Stroke Association. Stroke. 2018;49(3):e46–e110.
33. Rothwell PM, Gibson RJ, Slattery J, Sellar RJ, Warlow CP. Equivalence of measurements of carotid stenosis. A comparison of three methods on 1001 angiograms. European Carotid Surgery Trialists' Collaborative Group. Stroke. 1994;25(12):2435–9.

Chapter 19
Large Vessel Occlusion with Underlying Atherosclerosis: Approach and Strategy

Zachary R. Barnard and Michael J. Alexander

Introduction

The majority of acute large vessel occlusions (LVOs) of the cerebral arteries are due to embolic clots from the heart; however, a distinct subset of LVOs have an underlying stenosis, which is the likely cause of in situ vessel thrombosis. An underlying stenosis in LVO may be secondary to an intracranial atherosclerotic stenosis (ICAS) or other etiologies such as intracranial arterial dissection. In the case of ICAS, the vessel lumen may become so constricted with atherosclerotic plaque that slow intravascular flow may lead to thrombosis. Similarly, arterial plaques may rupture, exposing an intramural thrombus or thrombogenic disrupted fibrous cap, which leads to local in situ thrombosis of the vessel [1]. However, even after the vessel is revascularized with a thrombectomy procedure, the relatively slower blood flow through the highly stenotic ICAS vessel and the hyperthrombotic local environment may lead to immediate or early rethrombosis of the vessel. Consequently, postthrombectomy adjunctive angioplasty or angioplasty and stenting to ensure persistent vessel patency may be considered. There are certainly regional variations in the incidence of underlying ICAS following thrombectomy for LVO. Underlying ICAS lesions are reported to be about 8–10% in patients in the United States [2, 3] and 15–30% in Asian countries [4].

Prior Studies

Some early studies utilizing angioplasty and stenting indiscriminately for all large vessel occlusions, regarding of underlying ICAS lesion or embolic clot only, demonstrated the feasibility of using intracranial stents acutely in large artery occlusive

Z. R. Barnard · M. J. Alexander (✉)
Department of Neurosurgery, Neurovascular Center, Cedars-Sinai Medical Center, Los Angeles, CA, USA
e-mail: michael.alexander@cshs.org

F. K. Hui et al. (eds.), *12 Strokes*, https://doi.org/10.1007/978-3-030-56857-3_19

stroke. Zaidat et al. [5] reported nine cases of nitinol self-expanding stents used in patients with acute ischemic stroke from large vessel occlusions in the anterior and posterior circulation with a mean time to revascularization from last known well time of 5.1 hours. They achieved a TICI 3 revascularization score in 67% of the patients and TICI 2 or TICI 3 in 89% of the patients. They had one hemorrhage (11%) and one acute in-stent thrombosis.

Levy et al. [6] performed a 20-patient prospective single arm trial utilizing self-expanding stent placement in large vessel occlusions, again, in consecutive patients, whether they had underlying ICAS or not. In their series, they achieved a TICI 3 revascularization in 60% of the patients and TICI 2 in the remaining 40%. Following the procedure, 5% of patients had symptomatic hemorrhages and an additional 10% of patients had asymptomatic hemorrhages.

These early attempts to use intracranial stenting in large vessel occlusion, however, predate the availability of stent retrievers for thrombectomy. Prior to the development of stent retrievers, the successful revascularization rates with endovascular therapies were not as effective [7]. Once primary thrombectomy with stent retrievers and advanced aspiration techniques became widespread, the success rate of the intervention did not necessitate angioplasty and stenting for successful revascularization in the majority of cases. Primary stenting in large vessel occlusion for embolic clot alone fell by the way side, and the concept of angioplasty and stenting as a rescue therapy for failed thrombectomy or recalcitrant underlying stenosis became more common.

When comparing patients with and without underlying ICAS in a series of 172 thrombectomy patients for LVO, Yoon et al. [8] found a significantly higher rate of effective revascularization (TICI 2b or 3) in patients stented for underlying ICAS than those who underwent thrombectomy alone without underlying ICAS (95.0% vs. 81.8%, $p = 0.04$). They did not see any significant differences in the symptomatic hemorrhages or mortality, but did see better clinical outcomes in the stented patients with underlying ICAS (65% favorable outcome) compared to the 132 patients who underwent thrombectomy alone (40.2% favorable outcome), which was statistically significant ($p = 0.01$). They speculated that patients who had underlying ICAD may have had better outcomes, since with gradual vessel narrowing over time, they may have had better development of collaterals compared to the acute total occlusions with no underlying ICAS.

Similarly, Jia et al. [9] reported prospective data from the EAST trial (Endovascular therapy for Acute ischemic Stroke Trial) in which 140 patients with LVO who underwent thrombectomy were found to have an underlying ICAS lesion in 34% of the patients. Of the 30 patients with ICAS, 27 were stented acutely after thrombectomy. When they compared the thrombectomy plus stenting group to the thrombectomy group with no underlying ICAS, they saw no significant difference in recanalization rate, symptomatic hemorrhage, functional outcome, or death between the two groups.

In a consecutive series by Baek et al. [10], 208 patients who underwent anterior circulation thrombectomy with a stent retriever or aspiration were analyzed. Of this group, 163 patients achieved revascularization. Within the 45 remaining patients, 17 underwent angioplasty and stenting acutely and 28 did not. Follow-up assessment found that the patients in the stenting group clinically did better, with better postprocedure modified Rankin scores, and a lower rate of cerebral herniation, although similar hemorrhage rates compared to the patients not stented.

A retrospective study from the United States of 435 thrombectomy patients by Al Kasab et al. [2] found 36 patients (8.3%) had underlying atherosclerotic stenoses. Patients were treated for their LVO with either direct aspiration or stent retriever and aspiration. Subsequently, directly following the thrombectomy procedure, two patients had balloon angioplasty alone and 34 patients had acute angioplasty and stenting. Patients were loaded with abciximab intravenously prior to the stent placement and had subsequent treatment with aspirin and clopidogrel. They had four periprocedural hemorrhages and their inpatient mortality was 22%.

A multicenter experience reported by Chang et al. [11] evaluated rescue stenting in patients who failed thrombectomy for large vessel occlusion. In a combined series of 591 thrombectomy patients, 148 (25%) could not be revascularized. Within this group, 48 patients underwent angioplasty and stenting and 100 patients had no further intervention. Within the stenting group, the successful revascularization rate was 64.6%. The patients who underwent successful stenting had a similar rate of good outcomes as the patients who were successfully revascularized with thrombectomy only, and superior outcomes to patients in whom revascularization was not achieved. There was a delayed stent thrombosis rate of 13% in the study. Clinically, however, in the patients who failed thrombectomy, patients with stenting did better than those without stenting (mRS 0–2, 39.6% in the stenting group, 22.0% in the nonstenting group, $p = 0.031$). It is unclear from this study if all the patients who underwent angioplasty and stenting actually had an underlying atherosclerotic lesion or alternatively a very firm or tenacious embolic clot. The medical comorbidity assessment of patients in the stenting group indicated that 35.4% of the patients had a history of atrial fibrillation. Therefore, it is likely that an indeterminate percentage of these patients' stroke etiology was embolic, and not in situ thrombosis of an ICAS lesion.

Wu et al. [12] reviewed a consecutive series of 113 patients who had underlying ICAS following thrombectomy for large vessel occlusion in the anterior circulation who had an underlying intracranial atherosclerotic stenosis of greater than 70%. Of those patients, they performed angioplasty and/or stenting in 81 of these patients (71.7%) at the time of the thrombectomy procedure, and 32 patients had no further intervention. In the cohort that underwent angioplasty and/or stenting, patients were significantly more likely to have persistent vessel recanalization at 24 hours post procedure than those patients who underwent thrombectomy alone (adjusted odds ratio 3.782, 95% confidence interval 1.821–9.125, $p = 0.02$) and less likely to have early neurologic deterioration (OR 0.299; 95% CI 0.110–0.821, $p = 0.01$). In addition, the emergent angioplasty and/or stenting group did not have a significant difference in the incidence of symptomatic or asymptomatic postprocedural intracranial hemorrhages compared to the thrombectomy-only group.

Feng et al. [13] performed a retrospective review of a single-center consecutive series of 458 thrombectomy procedures in patients with anterior or posterior circulation large vessel occlusion, and reported that 55 of these patients underwent angioplasty and stenting as a salvage treatment for unsuccessful primary thrombectomy due to underlying atherosclerotic stenosis. In the study, 65.5% of the patients had anterior circulation occlusions, and 34.5% had posterior circulation occlusions. In the cohort who underwent angioplasty and stenting, 98.2% of patients achieved a TICI grade 2b or 3 revascularization. The posttreatment intracranial hemorrhage rate was 12.7%, with symptomatic hemorrhage occurring in only 2 patients (3.6% of the cohort). The persistence of revascularization was assessed by CT perfusion 3–5 days post stenting in 39 patients. Within this subgroup, 84.6% of patients demonstrated stent patency, 5.1% had moderate stenosis of the target artery, and 10.3% demonstrated early stent thrombosis. The 90-day prognosis was good (modified Rankin scale score 0–2) in 79.1% of the patients and 20.9% of the patients died.

Although these major studies had slightly dissimilar inclusion criteria, techniques, and periprocedural medical therapy, they all had the intention of revascularization during the thrombectomy procedure and not staged for a later date. The summary data for these trials are summarized in Table 19.1. In total, these trials treated 372 patients with LVO and underlying ICAS acutely and achieved an 86.1% successful revascularization rate. The symptomatic intracranial hemorrhage rate was 8.3%, and all-cause mortality was 16.0%. Overall, these results, in very complex patients with LVO and ICAS, are favorable when compared to acute LVO patient angiographic results and clinical outcomes, suggesting that early and complete revascularization is the key to better patient outcomes, despite any potential risks of stent placement or the concomitant medical therapy necessary to prevent acute stent thrombosis.

Table 19.1 Major studies of underlying atherosclerosis in large vessel occlusion

	Publication	Number of patients stented	Successful revascularization rate (%)	Symptomatic hemorrhage rate (%)	Mortality (%)
Yoon	Neurosurgery 2015	40	95.0	7.5	15
Baek	Stroke 2016	17	83.3	11.8	23.5
Al Kasab	JNIS 2017	32	64.7	12.5	22
Chang	Stroke 2018	48	64.6	16.7	12.5
Jia	JNIS 2018	27	95.7	4.3	12.8
Wu	Neuroradiology 2019	81	91.1	8.6	11.1
Kang	J of Neurosurgery 2018	72	95.8	1.4	9.7
Feng	World Neurosurgery 2019	55	98.2	3.6	20.9
Total		**372**	**86.1**	**8.3**	**16.0**

Techniques

It may be difficult to determine, prior to thrombectomy, that there is an underlying severe atherosclerotic stenosis in the target artery of revascularization. While high-resolution (HR) MRI, vessel wall imaging may be able to determine this, HR MRI is not commonly used as a rapid screening study in acute large vessel occlusion [14]. Some of the factors that many indicate a higher likelihood of an underlying atherosclerotic lesion may include multivessel atherosclerotic disease in other intracranial arteries on the prethrombectomy CT angiogram, calcific density at the target artery on the noncontrast head CT, and a lack of other significant risk factors such as atrial fibrillation, patent foramen ovale, atrial appendage, and hypercoagulable state.

During the endovascular thrombectomy procedure itself, there may be some indication early that the large vessel occlusion may have underlying ICAS. An initial angiogram indicating an occlusion more proximal than would be expected for a soft red clot may indicate underlying ICAS. Embolic clot, particularly soft clot, tends to travel forward in the circulation until it engages the luminal artery diameter that matches its size, and at that point it corks into the vessel, or it may stop at arterial branch points, such as the middle cerebral artery bifurcation or the basilar apex. Occlusions at the proximal basilar artery, for example, may be more characteristic of ICAS lesions with in situ thrombosis. Similarly, difficulty in passing the occlusion with a microwire and microcatheter may be more indicative of underlying ICAS, or, in some more rare cases, an underlying arterial dissection. Some interventionalists prefer to pass an LVO with either a 0.010 inch or 0.014 inch microwire in a J-shape position to avoid entering perforators or smaller arteries, since they are blindly passing into an area in which the arterial anatomy is not seen. In this J-shape configuration of the wire, the microwire will not pass a significant ICAS lesion. Similarly, even with the microwire with a 45° angulated curve, it may be difficult to pass a severely atherosclerotic lesion. In contrast, it is not difficult to pass a red clot with either technique.

Given the uncertainty of whether there is an underlying ICAS lesion in large vessel occlusion, Kang et al. [15] performed an analysis of 130 thrombectomy patients with underlying ICAS, comparing thrombectomy with a stent retriever with thrombectomy with contact aspiration of clot. In their series, 70 patients had first-line thrombectomy with a stent retriever and 60 patients had first-line therapy with direct aspiration. The femoral access to initial revascularization time was shorter in the stent retriever group compared to the aspiration-only group (17 minutes vs. 31 minutes, $p < 0.001$). Likewise, the probability of the first-line treatment not being successful was higher in the aspiration group compared to stent retriever (40% vs 4.3%; OR 2.543, 95% CI 1.893–3.417, $p < 0.001$). Based on these data, the authors conclude that stent retrievers should be used as a first-line therapy with large vessel occlusion, since its success in revascularization was superior to aspiration in patients with underlying ICAS lesions. Having noted this, however, the clot burden within a stenotic ICAS lesion that has thrombosed is typically lower than those of embolic nature, and aspiration often is quickly effective, particularly with the most recent generation of larger, more effective primary aspiration catheters designed for thrombectomy, and more powerful aspiration pumps.

Once successful thrombectomy is performed and an underlying atherosclerotic lesion is diagnosed, the decision to move forward with angioplasty or angioplasty and stenting may be based on several factors. It is certainly possible, though less common, that an intracranial artery plaque may rupture and cause in situ thrombosis when the ICAS lesion is less than 50% of the true luminal diameter. This lesion may still be highly thrombogenic and may lead to reocclusion of the vessel, but none of the single- or multi-center reports to date appear to have advocated stenting of these subcritical stenoses. Underlying ICAS lesions in the 50–69% range have been treated by stenting and medical therapy, and although these are less hemodynamically significant lesions, they still can have a propensity for early recurrent thrombosis. In study cohorts that have compared stenting and medical therapy in these types of lesions, there is data to suggest better imaging and clinical outcomes in the stenting group. This difference becomes more significant in favor of stenting in the 70% or higher stenosis group.

In patients undergoing thrombectomy for LVO with underlying ICAS, there has been noted a higher risk for immediate rethrombosis, compared to thrombectomy in which there is no underlying ICAD [16]. In a study of 40 consecutive patients with thrombectomy for LVO with underlying ICAS, Kang et al., found an early rethrombosis in 65% of patients who underwent thrombectomy only with no subsequent angioplasty and/or stenting versus a 3% early rethrombosis rate in thrombectomy patients who did not have an underlying stenosis ($p < 0.001$). In the cohort of patients who had underlying ICAS, their group began using low dose tirofiban infusion, which resulted in an 85.7% successful revascularization rate, with no cases of symptomatic intracranial hemorrhage.

While angioplasty alone has not been extensively studied separately in LVO patients with underlying ICAS, several studies have included angioplasty-alone subgroups. Many interventionalists will not place a stent acutely after LVO thrombectomy if the angioplasty procedure results in excellent luminal improvement, with no evidence of dissection, and markedly improved distal blood flow. The clinical example in Fig. 19.1 demonstrates a patient with an acute basilar artery occlusion with CT evidence of hyperdense basilar artery. Following stent retriever and aspiration thrombectomy, there was a Mori A underlying ICAS lesion, which was treated with angioplasty alone with excellent revascularization and no subsequent restenosis or need for stent placement. The important factor in this type of decision making is to wait for at least 10–15 minutes after angioplasty and repeat angiographic imaging to assess for potential artery recoil or intraluminal thrombus accumulation. Vessels that demonstrate these delayed findings may require stenting to preserve luminal patency with the assistance of antiplatelet therapy. Figure 19.2 demonstrates a patient with an acute left middle cerebral artery occlusion who underwent direct aspiration thrombectomy revealing a severe underlying ICAS lesion. Balloon angioplasty alone did not yield satisfactory luminal diameter due to recoil, and stenting was performed acutely with a TICI3 revascularization result and mRS of 0 at 30 days.

Finally, there are more rare situations in which a firm embolus may mimic an underlying ICAS lesion. While red clots are easily passed with a microwire and microcatheter (Fig. 19.3a), white clots may be more firm in nature (Fig. 19.3b).

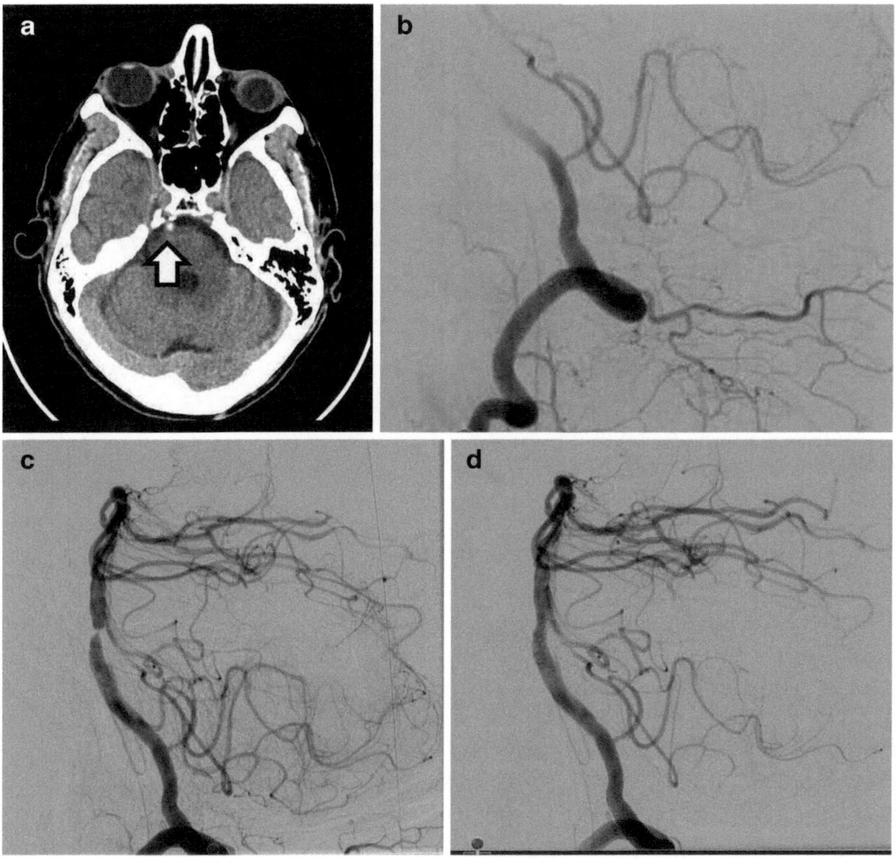

Fig. 19.1 (**a**) Noncontrast head CT demonstrating basilar artery occlusion. (**b**) Initial cerebral angiogram with patency of vertebral and proximal basilar artery. (**c**) Following thrombectomy with stent retriever and aspiration, a Mori A atherosclerotic stenosis was seen. (**d**) Following angioplasty alone, excellent luminal diameter of the basilar and no clear evidence of dissection with robust distal flow

They may be more difficult to pass with a wire or microcatheter and may deform the stent retriever to make it appear that there is an underlying ICAS lesion. The key differentiating feature is that with subsequent passes of a thrombectomy device, the firm fibrous clots may either move or change shape on the follow-up angiographic run. This does not occur with an underlying ICAS lesion. Therefore, if these changes are seen, it would be best to attempt further embolus removal as opposed to stenting it in place. Similarly, embolic plaque from extracranial origin, as seen in the case shown in Fig. 19.3b, should be removed by thrombectomy procedure instead of stented. This was a patient who had just undergone a percutaneous artificial heart valve placement in which atherosclerotic plaque may break off from the old valve and embolize, so we were prepared for possible atherosclerotic embolus. It was retrieved with a large bore aspiration catheter in a single pass.

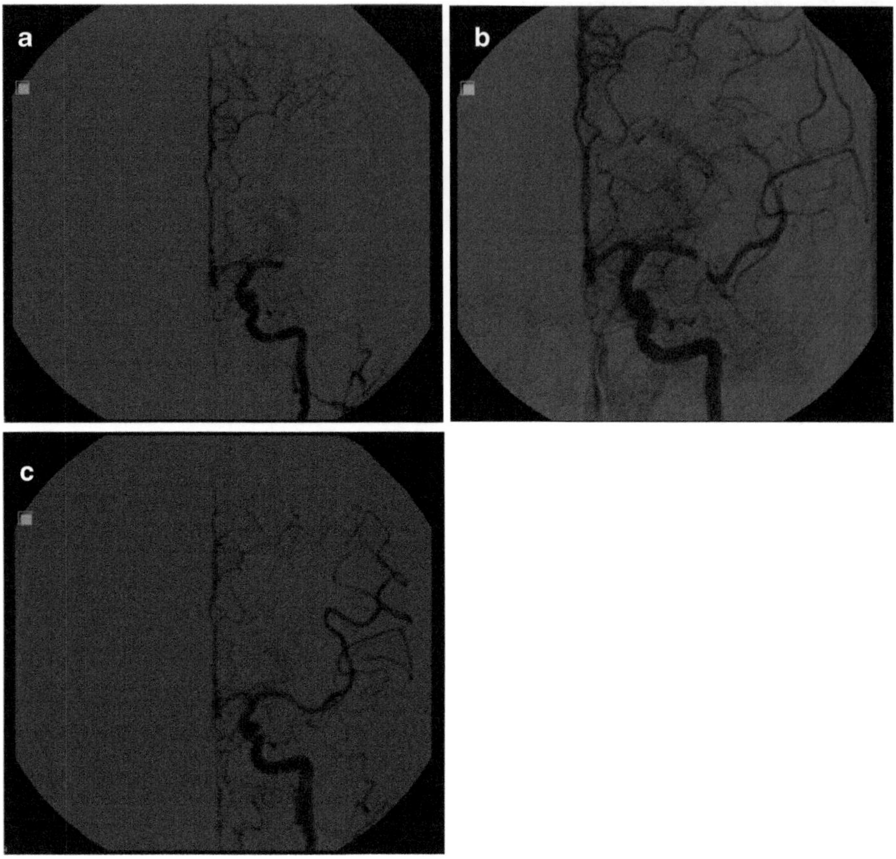

Fig. 19.2 (**a**) Acute large vessel occlusion of left middle cerebral artery baseline angiogram. (**b**) Following aspiration thrombectomy, and underlying atherosclerotic lesion seen. (**c**) Following angioplasty and stenting a TICI 3 revascularization result

Periprocedural and Postoperative Management

As opposed to thrombectomy in an otherwise normal target artery, in which we typically would avoid anticoagulant and antiplatelet therapy for 24 hours, thrombectomy with an underlying atherosclerotic stenosis may necessitate acute management with antithrombotic therapy. Not only are ruptured plaques hyperthrombotic due to the irregular luminal surface and inflammatory local environment, but the performance of angioplasty can incur further intimal injury and the placement of a stent, which is a foreign body, makes the artery more likely to thrombose or cause distal emboli in the immediate periprocedural period if appropriate therapeutic antiplatelet therapy is not initiated.

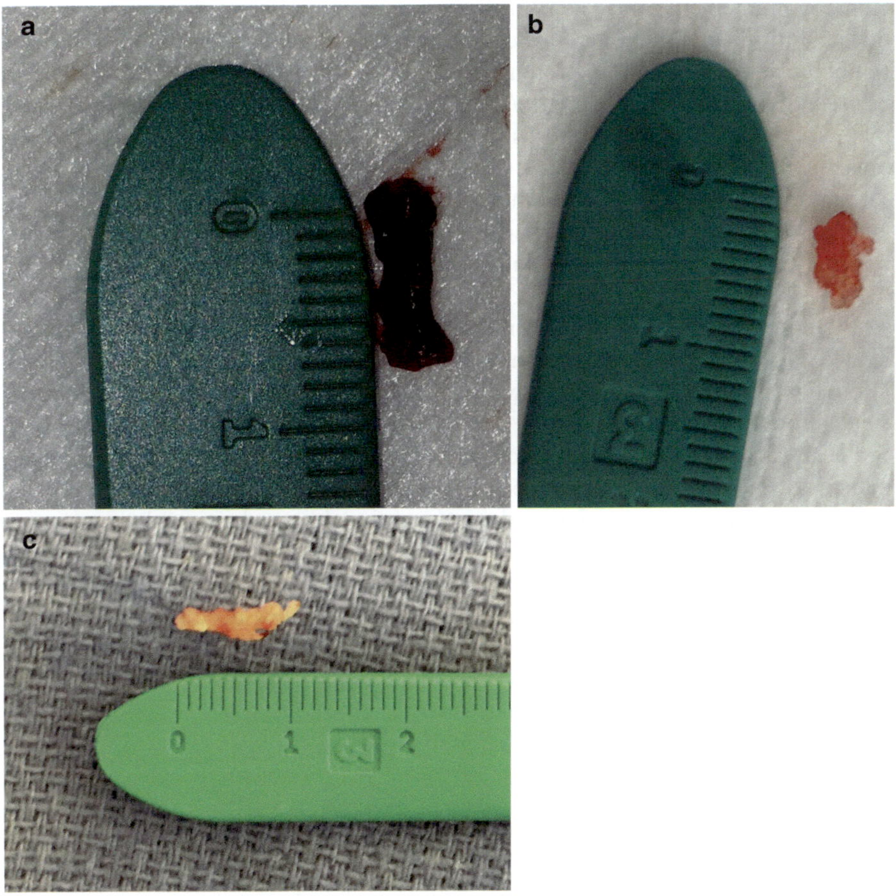

Fig. 19.3 (**a**) Soft red clot aspirated during thrombectomy of large vessel occlusion. (**b**) Fibrin-rich firm white clot aspirated with ADAPT technique. (**c**) Atherosclerotic plaque embolus retrieved from the middle cerebral artery with a stent retriever following a percutaneous aortic valve replacement procedure

An oral load, or bolus per nasogastric tube, of clopidogrel with 600 mg may take approximately 6 hours to reach therapeutic effect. Therefore, in the acute stenting scenario, oral loading alone is insufficient immediate antiplatelet therapy and intravenous medications must be considered [17, 18]. Intravenous aspirin is available in Europe but not commercially distributed in the United States. This leaves the options of intravenous IIb/IIIa inhibitors or intravenous P2Y12 inhibitors. Both options can result in rapid therapeutic antiplatelet effects and following a bolus, a continuous drip may be initiated to provide intravenous coverage until oral agents take effect. Intravenous cangrelor provides antiplatelet action at the same receptor, P2Y12, that clopidogrel interacts with. The IIb/IIIa glycoprotein inhibitors, abciximab, eptifibatide, and tirofiban, inhibit the final common pathway receptor IIb/IIIa glycoprotein. Inhibition at this level is very profound and these medications actually possess a type of pseudolytic effect. While the IIb/IIIa inhibitors are not a lytic in the same respect that tissue plasminogen activator is, they are tightly bound inhibitors, so they may break up platelet aggregations [19]. Since a fresh clot is in a dynamic process of clot formation and dissolution, when these agents bind to the receptors, clot dissolutes but does not have the ability to re-form, since the receptors are so competitively bound by the inhibitor. However, with such strong antiplatelet aggregation blockade, there is also a potentially higher risk for periprocedural intracranial hemorrhage [20].

Preliminary reports on cangrelor, an intravenous P2Y12 inhibitor, have demonstrated safety for neurovascular patients requiring acute stenting. A single-center pilot study of eight patients by Aguilar-Salinas et al. showed no hemorrhages or stent thromboses in a consecutive series of carotid and intracranial stents [21]. Similarly, an early multicenter study by Godier et al. [22] demonstrated safety in patients undergoing intracranial stenting for cerebral aneurysms who were bridged with intravenous cangrelor during the interventional procedure and later managed with oral antiplatelet agents with no patients experiencing in-stent thrombosis or intracranial hemorrhage.

It appears from these studies that either intravenous low-dose IIb/IIIa inhibitors or intravenous P2Y12 inhibitors may be effective and safe at maintaining stent patency acutely with low incipient intracranial hemorrhage rate.

Summary

The incidence of underlying ICAS following thrombectomy for LVO is reported to be about 8–10% in patients in the United States and 15–30% in some Asian countries. Although there may be some indications prior to thrombectomy that there may be a higher likelihood of underlying ICAS, these determinations are imperfect and the discovery of the ICAS may not occur until after the thrombectomy is performed. Both direct clot aspiration and stent retriever with aspiration techniques may revascularize the LVO with underlying ICAS. Balloon angioplasty alone or angioplasty and stenting may be indicated in underlying lesions 50–99% or in reoccluded arteries within a few minutes of thrombectomy. Some interventionalists prefer a staged process in which angioplasty alone is performed after thrombectomy, and if satisfactory results are not obtained with the balloon alone, then to place a stent. Others prefer nonstaged angioplasty and stenting, believing there is a better chance of short- and long-term patency of the vessel with stenting, if proper medical therapy, such as an intravenous P2Y12 inhibitor or IIb/IIIa inhibitor, is initiated during the procedure [22]. Postprocedural blood pressure control is critical in any of these treatment pathways in an effort to reduce the postprocedural intracerebral hemorrhage rate. Even with these techniques and management protocols, however, it is important to remember that the periprocedural thrombotic and hemorrhagic complication rates and outcomes in patients who are stented in LVO with associated ICAS should be compared to complications and outcomes in LVO patients and not compared to angioplasty and stenting data from studies, such as the WEAVE intracranial stenting trial for ICAS [23], which demonstrated a 2.6% complication rate and 1.3% intracranial hemorrhage rate, since these stenting trials excluded patients with complete occlusion. As is the theme in thrombectomy trials without ICAS, the principle in the management of LVO with underlying ICAS is that patients have better outcomes with early and complete revascularization.

References

1. Shah PK. Inflammation and plaque vulnerability. Cardiovasc Drugs Ther. 2009;23(1):31–40. https://doi.org/10.1007/s10557-008-6147-2.
2. Al Kasab S, Almadidy Z, Spiotta AM, et al. Endovascular treatment for AIS with underlying ICAD. J Neurointerv Surg. 2017;9(10):948–51. https://doi.org/10.1136/neurintsurg-2016-012529.
3. Sacco RL, Kargman DE, Gu Q, et al. Race-ethnicity and determinants of intracranial atherosclerotic cerebral infarction. The Northern Manhattan Stroke Study. Stroke. 1995;26(1):14–20. https://doi.org/10.1161/01.str.26.1.14.
4. Kang DH, Yoon W. Current opinion on endovascular therapy for emergent large vessel occlusion due to underlying intracranial atherosclerotic stenosis. Korean J Radiol. 2019;20(5):739–48. https://doi.org/10.3348/krr.2018.0809.
5. Zaidat OO, Wolfe T, Hussain SI, et al. Interventional acute ischemic stroke therapy with intracranial self-expanding stent. Stroke. 2008;39(8):2392–5. https://doi.org/10.1161/STROKEAHA.1o7.510966.
6. Levy EI, Siddiqui AH, Crumlish A, et al. First Food and Drug Administration-approved prospective trial of primary intracranial stenting for acute stroke: SARIS (stent-assisted recanalization in acute ischemic stroke). Stroke. 2009;40(11):3552–6. https://doi.org/10.1161/STROKEAHA.109.561274.
7. Broderick JP, Palesch YY, Demchuk AM, et al. Interventional Management of Stroke (IMS) III Investigators. Endovascular therapy after intravenous t-PA versus t-PA alone for stroke. N Engl J Med. 2013;368:893–903. https://doi.org/10.1056/NEJMoa1214300.
8. Yoon W, Kim SK, Park MS, et al. Endovascular treatment and the outcomes of atherosclerotic intracranial stenosis in patients with hyperacute stroke. Neurosurgery. 2015;76(6):680–6. https://doi.org/10.1227/neu.0000000000000694.
9. Jia B, Feng L, Liebeskind DS, et al. Mechanical thrombectomy and rescue therapy for intracranial large artery occlusion with underlying atherosclerosis. J Neurointerv Surg. 2018;10(8):746–50. https://doi.org/10.1136/neurintsurg-2017-013489.
10. Baek JH, Kim BM, Kim DJ, et al. Stenting as a rescue treatment after failure of mechanical thrombectomy for anterior circulation large artery occlusion. Stroke. 2016;47(9):2360–3. https://doi.org/10.1161/STROKEAHA.116.014073.
11. Chang Y, Kim BM, Bang OY, et al. Rescue stenting for failed mechanical thrombectomy in acute ischemic stroke: a multi-center experience. Stroke. 2018;49:958–64. https://doi.org/10.1161/STROKEAHA.117.020072.
12. Wu C, Chang W, Wu D, et al. Angioplasty and/or stenting after thrombectomy in patients with underlying intracranial atherosclerotic stenosis. Neuroradiology. 2019;61(9):1073–81. https://doi.org/10.1007/s00234-019-02262-5.

13. Feng M, Zhang H, Zhang Y, et al. Stent angioplasty for acute intracranial atherosclerotic occlusion after failed thrombectomy: a single-institution series of 55 patients. World Neurosurg. 2019;130:e444–8. https://doi.org/10.1016/j.wneu.2019.06.112.
14. Zhao DL, Li C, Chen XH, et al. Reproducibility of 3.0T high-resolution magnetic resonance imaging for the identification and quantification of middle cerebral arterial atherosclerotic plaques. J Stroke Cerebrovasc Dis. 2019;28(7):1824–31. https://doi.org/10.1016/j.jstrokecerebrovasdis.2019.04.020.
15. Kang DH, Yoon W, Baek BH, et al. Front-line thrombectomy for acute large-vessel occlusion with underlying severe intracranial stenosis: stent retriever versus contact aspiration. J Neurosurg. 2019:1–7. https://doi.org/10.3171/2019.1.JNS182905.
16. Kang DH, Kim YW, Hwang YH, et al. Instant reocclusion following mechanical thrombectomy of in situ thromboocclusion and the role of low-dose intra-arterial tirofiban. Cerebrovasc Dis. 2014;37(5):350–5. https://doi.org/10.1159/000362435.
17. Alexander MJ. Intracranial stenting for intracranial atherosclerotic disease: still much to learn. J Neurointerv Surg. 2012;4(2):85–6. https://doi.org/10.1136/neurintsurg-2012-010269.
18. Alexander MJ. Patient selection, physician experience and antiplatelet testing are critical. J Neurointerv Surg. 2016;8(e1):e5. https://doi.org/10.1136/neurintsurg-2012-010492.
19. Alexander MJ, Duckwiler GR, Gobin YP, et al. Management of intraprocedural arterial thrombus in cerebral aneurysm embolization with abciximab: technical case report. Neurosurgery. 2002;50(4):899–901. https://doi.org/10.1097/00006123-200204000-00045.
20. Qureshi A, Saad M, Zaidat OO, et al. Intracerebral hemorrhages associated with neurointerventional procedures using a combination of antithrombotic agents including abciximab. Stroke. 2002;33(7):1916–9. https://doi.org/10.1161/01.str.0000019423.08947.43.
21. Aguilar-Salinas P, Agnoletto GJ, Brasiliense LBC, et al. Safety and efficacy of cangrelor in acute stenting for the treatment of cerebrovascular pathology: preliminary experience in a single-center pilot study. J Neurointerv Surg. 2019;11(4):347–51. https://doi.org/10.1136/neurintsurg-2018-014396.
22. Godier A, Mesnil M, DeMesmay M, et al. Bridging antiplatelet therapy with cangrelor in patients with recent intracranial stenting undergoing invasive procedures: a prospective case series. Br J Anaesth. 2019;123(1):e2–5. https://doi.org/10.1016/j.bja.2019.03.019.
23. Alexander MJ, Zauner A, Chaloupka JC, et al. WEAVE trial: results in 152 on-label patients. Stroke. 2019;50:889–94. https://doi.org/10.1161/STROKEAHA.118.023996.

Chapter 20
Large Vessel Occlusion with Low NIHSS: Approach and Strategy

Russell Cerejo and Gabor Toth

Case Presentation/Clinical Vignette

A healthy nonagenarian male woke up with left-sided hemiplegia, facial droop, and dysarthria. On arrival to the hospital, his symptoms completely resolved with an initial National Institute of Health Stroke Scale (NIHSS) of 0. His blood pressure was 167/82, and he was hemodynamically stable. His noncontrast CT scan of the head was unremarkable for any intracranial hemorrhage, and he had an Alberta stroke program early CT (ASPECT) score of 10. He was not a candidate for intravenous (IV) thrombolysis as he was out of the approved time window. CT angiogram showed a right middle cerebral artery (MCA) M1 segment occlusion. He also underwent CT-perfusion imaging, which showed a large penumbra and no ischemic core in the right MCA territory (Fig. 20.1). The patient was able to walk without any assistance in the emergency department. However, after ambulation, he developed worsening and fluctuation of his symptoms with left arm drift and mild facial droop, corresponding with an NIHSS of 2. After discussion with the patient and family about medical management versus off-label endovascular therapy, the patient elected early intervention. He underwent successful mechanical thrombectomy (MT) with complete recanalization of the occluded M1 segment (Fig. 20.2). The patient had no neurological deficits after the procedure, and was discharged home the following day. His 24-hour postprocedure MRI brain showed only a very small ischemic stroke in the deep right MCA territory (Fig. 20.3).

R. Cerejo
Cerebrovascular Center, Allegheny Health Network, Pittsburgh, PA, USA

G. Toth (✉)
Cerebrovascular Center, Cleveland Clinic, Cleveland, OH, USA
e-mail: tothg@ccf.org

F. K. Hui et al. (eds.), *12 Strokes*, https://doi.org/10.1007/978-3-030-56857-3_20

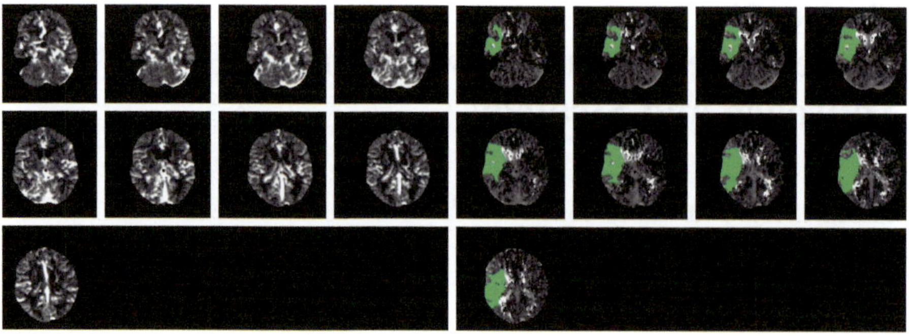

Fig. 20.1 CT-perfusion imaging showing no visible ischemic core (left panel, cerebral blood flow <30%), and a large penumbra (right panel, $T_{max} > 6$ seconds)

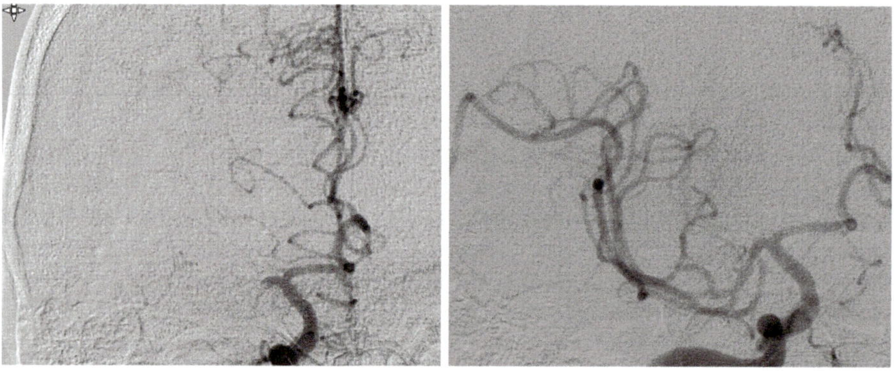

Fig. 20.2 Cerebral angiogram showing occlusion of the right M1 segment of the middle cerebral artery, anteroposterior view (left panel). Cerebral angiogram showing complete recanalization of the occluded segment, oblique view (right panel)

Fig. 20.3 MRI brain (axial, diffusion weighted imaging) 24 hours post procedure showing a small area of restricted diffusion in the right basal ganglia (arrow)

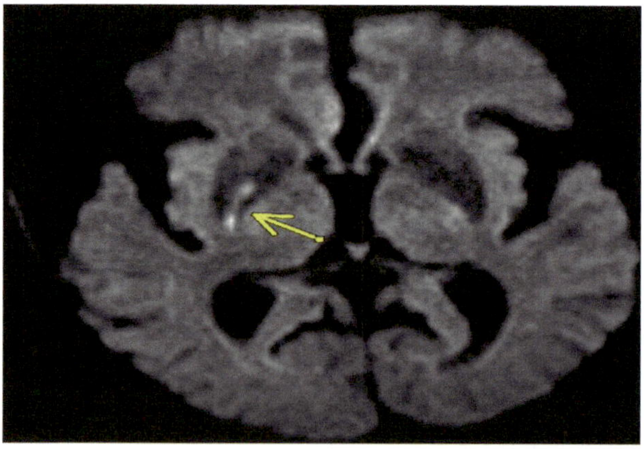

Introduction

Acute stroke therapy has come a long way since the approval of recombinant tissue plasminogen activator (t-PA) for acute ischemic stroke in the mid-1990s. The successful mechanical thrombectomy (MT) trials for large vessel occlusions (LVOs) in 2014–15 cemented the role of endovascular therapy for moderate-to-severe strokes. The landscape has changed further with the addition of extended time window studies in late 2017 and early 2018, reaffirming MT as the standard of care for patients with LVO and disabling deficits [1–3]. However, acute stroke therapy in patients presenting with low NIHSS and LVO has been a clinical conundrum. These patients are usually referred to as "too good to treat" or "mild stroke." However, the natural outcomes of this population may not be as benign as their initial presentation. The exact definition of "low NIHSS" or "mild stroke" has changed over time. Some earlier studies classified "mild" ischemic stroke as NIHSS of 8 or less [4–7], while others used NIHSS of 6 as a cutoff [8–13]. The majority of the landmark MT studies only included patients with an NIHSS of ≥6, which serves as the cutoff score in most current stroke treatment guidelines by major neurovascular societies [1]. In addition, it has been well known that the NIHSS has a poor representation for posterior circulation ischemia, even though these strokes can be associated with significant morbidity and mortality [14]. A possible explanation for mild symptoms despite LVO is temporary blood supply to the affected territory from robust collateral vessels, the failure of which over time has been associated with infarct growth and clinical worsening [15].

Incidence and Natural Outcomes

The exact incidence of patients presenting with low NIHSS and LVO is difficult to ascertain, as there may be delay in or lack of intracranial vessel imaging given the minimal symptoms. There may be a clinical and/or diagnostic challenge clarifying if the patient's vessel occlusion is chronic or acute, and if it is the actual cause of the presenting stroke symptoms. Mimics may include chronic asymptomatic occlusions with unrelated stroke-like deficits due to seizure, Todd's paralysis, migrainous phenomenon, transient ischemic attack, metabolic derangement, or malingering [16]. Data from large thrombolysis databases from Europe and USA suggest that, in patients undergoing intravenous (IV) thrombolysis, the incidence of low NIHSS (<6) is around 21–22% [17, 18]. In a European database, about 25% of these low NIHSS patients had visible arterial occlusion on baseline imaging [18]. The incidence of large vessel occlusion and low NIHSS varied from 14% to 54% in other smaller cohort studies, which is likely due to variability in the definition of low NIHSS and the vascular territory involved [18–22]. The natural course of the disease is unfavorable in several studies. A Swiss study showed that 22.7% mild stroke-LVO patients deteriorated within 24 hours, 33.3% during hospital stay, 41.4% within 3 months, and death occurred in 6.7% [9]. Patients with mild ischemic symptoms or rapidly improving symptoms, when IV thrombolysis was withheld, showed significant deterioration and poor 3-month outcomes despite their low initial NIHSS [23]. This effect was amplified in patients with LVO, leading to an early neurological deterioration and a sevenfold increase in poor outcomes [7, 24, 25]. Other studies found that about half of the patients who received no treatment for low NIHSS and LVO had an unfavorable outcome [4], while only 66.7% patients reached modified Rankin scale (mRS) 0–2 with conservative management [9], and only two-thirds of LVO patients who were excluded from thrombolysis could walk independently at discharge [7]. A large European observational cohort demonstrated that one-third of low NIHSS stroke patients with LVO did not have a successful recovery [8].

Acute Stroke Therapy

Basic Management and Intravenous Thrombolysis

Due to lack of randomized clinical trials, there is a clinical equipoise regarding acute stroke therapy in patients with low NIHSS and LVO. Most centers admit patients with low NIHSS and LVO for close neurological monitoring, preferably in the intensive care unit. The most recent American stroke association guidelines do not definitely recommend IV thrombolysis in patients with mild nondisabling ischemic symptoms [1]. This guideline was revised after the Potential of t-PA for Ischemic Strokes With Mild Symptoms (PRISMS) trial was prematurely terminated due to slow recruitment, and failed to show benefit of IV thrombolysis over aspirin [26]. The identification of large vessel status was not required for PRISMS enrollment. Intravenous t-PA has been shown to have decreased efficacy for proximal large vessel occlusions [27], which may discourage the use of the drug in LVO patients in some institutions. If IV thrombolysis is not administered, these patients are expected to be started on antiplatelet therapy. Methods to increase the cerebral perfusion pressure, including permissive hypertension, intravenous fluids, holding antihypertensive medications, keeping the head of bed flat, and bed rest, are usually considered, although there is no clear evidence to prove the efficacy of these measures. In a retrospective cohort comparing acute stroke therapy (mostly IV thrombolysis) versus conservative management, the odds of a favorable outcome (mRS 0–2) was 4.5 times higher in patients undergoing acute therapy [4]. In an Austrian stroke unit registry, there was a shift toward improved outcome in patients with IV thrombolysis (OR, 1.49; CI, 1.17–1.89; $p < 0.001$) [28]. Thrombolysis therapy has been shown to be a predictor of favorable outcome (mRS 0–2; OR, 3.103; CI, 1.021–9.428; $p = 0.03$) in another study where about 50% of the patients received IV thrombolysis [9]. In the largest observational study of low NIHSS and LVO, patients with internal carotid artery (ICA) terminus and tandem occlusion (ICA + MCA) had a tenfold increase in early neurological deterioration compared with patients without visible occlusion, despite IV thrombolysis. At 3 months, 77% of these patients with deterioration had an mRS of 3–6 [18]. The rate of parenchymal hemorrhage post IV thrombolysis was similar to patients without LVO (3%).

Endovascular Therapy

Randomized data is lacking, but many tertiary care centers consider endovascular therapy in low NIHSS patients with acute stroke symptoms and documented LVO. While some advocate for immediate intervention, others recommend close monitoring and MT only if there is worsening of the neurological status. A smaller study looking at early MT versus late MT (at the time of neurologic deterioration) found excellent outcomes (mRS 0–1) in the early versus late group (75% vs. 33%), with no symptomatic intracranial hemorrhage (sICH) in either group [12]. Another study reported that patients who deteriorated early (within 3 hours) had better outcomes with MT compared with patients who deteriorated after 3 hours from arrival [11]. A retrospective analysis of six international comprehensive stroke center databases investigated immediate or delayed (rescue therapy after neurologic deterioration) MT versus best medical management for patients with mild stroke and LVO. The odds of good outcome were increased with immediate MT (adjusted OR, 3.1; 95% CI, 1.4–6.9). At 90 days, in the matched analysis, there was a 14.3% absolute difference in good outcome favoring immediate MT (84.4% vs. 70.1%; $p = 0.03$). There were no safety concerns in the study.

Retrospective data from multicenter cohort studies comparing MT to standard medical therapy has shown mixed results. In two European studies, there was no significant difference in excellent outcome at 90 days (mRS 0–1) between MT versus standard medical therapy [6, 8]. Both of these studies had a higher rate of sICH in the MT arm (11.8% and 16.5%). However, in one of these studies, 18.3% of the patients in the medical arm had early deterioration and underwent MT, but were still analyzed in the medical arm [6]. In a univariate analysis, patients with no early deterioration were noted to have a lower mRS score at 90 days, and outcomes were unrelated to initial collateral scores, likely due to the fact that both arms had good collateral scores [8]. In a North American multicenter study evaluating MT versus standard medical therapy, the authors noted favorable outcome (mRS 0–2) at 3–6 months in patients undergoing MT versus medical management, which was significant after matched analysis (93% vs. 69.2%; $p = 0.04$) [29]. Endovascular therapy was statistically associated with a lower NIHSS score at discharge, a favorable NIHSS score shift, and independence rates increased at discharge. Parenchymal hemorrhage rate was 7.7% in the endovascular arm in the matched analysis.

In terms of safety, single arm cohort studies evaluating MT in this population found that the rates of symptomatic intracranial hemorrhage (sICH) ranged from 0% to 6% [5, 10, 11, 13]. Data from the Multicenter Clinical Registry of Endovascular Treatment of Acute Ischemic Stroke in the Netherlands (MR CLEAN) registry evaluating 71 patients with low NIHSS and MT showed that almost half of the patients reached excellent functional outcome (mRS 0–1), 75% had good functional outcome (mRS 0–2), and the peri-interventional complication rate was low (4%) [30]. A similar trend was seen in a north American study comparing acute stroke therapy in patients with NIHSS ≤ 5 and NIHSS > 5 [31]. One of the first prospective single-arm studies in this particular population showed excellent safety and feasibility of MT in the enrolled patients, with no evidence of symptomatic intracranial hemorrhage or other periprocedural complications, and a low incidence (5%) of postprocedural neurologic worsening [32]. This study enrolled patients with a median initial NIHSS of 3, with significant improvement of the last follow-up median NIHSS to 0 ($p < 0.001$). Excellent outcome (mRS 0–1) on last follow-up was seen in 95% of patients. In a small retrospective cohort, endovascular thrombectomy patients demonstrated an increased overall rate of intracranial hemorrhage (35.3% vs. 10.0%; $p = 0.04$), but symptomatic intracranial hemorrhage was similar between groups ($p = 0.25$) [33].

In a meta-analysis of five studies evaluating acute stroke therapy in this population, the odds of a favorable outcome (mRS 0–2) at 90 days were 4 times higher with MT + IV thrombolysis compared with no acute stroke therapy (95% CI 1.82–10.48, $p = 0.001$), and the odds of excellent outcome (mRS 0–1) was nearly two times higher with acute stroke therapy [34]. There was no significant difference in complication rates between the two arms, but there was substantial heterogeneity between the individual studies [34]. In the HERMES meta-analysis of the major MT trials, a subgroup analysis of patients presenting with NIHSS ≤ 10 favored a trend toward MT; however, this was not statistically significant [35]. In a more recent meta-analysis, there was no difference in outcomes with MT compared with medical management, and an increased risk of asymptomatic ICH with MT was demonstrated [36].

Future Directions

There is an urgent need for randomized trials of MT in this population to establish efficacy and safety of this treatment approach. Two ongoing studies include the MOSTE, part of the IN EXTREMIS trial (https://www.inextremis-study.com/), and the ENDOLOW (https://med.emory.edu/departments/emergency-medicine/innovation-discovery/academic-research-clinical-coordinating-center/index.html). Potential difficulties with such trials include expected slow enrollment rate owing to the small number of patients with both low NIHSS and LVO, the reluctance of patients and families to participate due to overwhelming evidence of MT benefit for more severe strokes, and the fact that many centers are already offering MT to these patients off-label.

Identifying LVO in patients with low NIHSS is often delayed, because symptoms are not concerning enough for rapid workup that includes vessel status. Inclusion of early vascular imaging in acute stroke protocols is increasing in many centers, and will undoubtedly help better identify and triage these patients. Determining if the occlusion is acute or chronic can be very challenging at times, especially given the mild symptoms. Advanced MRI techniques, like intra-arterial signal on arterial spin imaging and susceptibility vessel sign, may be beneficial in determining the characteristics and chronicity of the thrombus and vessel occlusion [37]. However, some of these imaging modalities may not be currently practical in the acute setting in most institutions. Quantifying the collateral blood supply, and the ability to determine patients susceptible to collateral failure and need for early intervention, is another important area of research.

Lastly, newer intravenous agents and more advanced endovascular devices may potentially offer faster and safer thrombolysis, and may improve the efficacy of interventional therapy. A recent study showed that IV Tenecteplase resulted in higher incidence of reperfusion compared to IV tPA in patients with LVO [38]. An ongoing study is looking at the efficacy of IV Tenecteplase compared to antiplatelet therapy in this population after establishing safety and feasibility in a phase II study [39].

Conclusions

Patients with mild acute stroke and associated large vessel occlusion may have non-disabling symptoms on presentation, but they have an elevated risk of deterioration and long-term disability. On the other hand, there is a concern for offering invasive MT for patients with only mild deficits. In the absence of any dedicated randomized trial data, acute stroke therapy, especially MT, needs to be individualized and tailored to each patient based on the clinical scenario, comorbidities, collateral flow, operator experience, and patient preference. Randomized clinical trials will be necessary to fully validate acute stroke therapy in this special patient population.

References

1. Powers WJ, Rabinstein AA, Ackerson T, Adeoye OM, Bambakidis NC, Becker K, Biller J, Brown M, Demaerschalk BM, Hoh B, Jauch EC, Kidwell CS, Leslie-Mazwi TM, Ovbiagele B, Scott PA, Sheth KN, Southerland AM, Summers DV, Tirschwell DL, American Heart Association Stroke Council. Guidelines for the early management of patients with acute ischemic stroke: 2019 update to the 2018 guidelines for the early management of acute ischemic stroke: a guideline for healthcare professionals from the American Heart Association/American Stroke Association. Stroke. 2019;50(12):e344–418. https://doi.org/10.1161/STR.0000000000000211.
2. Nogueira RG, Jadhav AP, Haussen DC, Bonafe A, Budzik RF, Bhuva P, et al. Thrombectomy 6 to 24 hours after stroke with a mismatch between deficit and infarct. N Engl J Med. 2018;378(1):11–21.
3. Albers GW, Marks MP, Kemp S, Christensen S, Tsai JP, Ortega-Gutierrez S, et al. Thrombectomy for stroke at 6 to 16 hours with selection by perfusion imaging. N Engl J Med. 2018;378(8):708–18.
4. Cerejo R, Cheng-Ching E, Hui F, Hussain MS, Uchino K, Bullen J, et al. Treatment of patients with mild acute ischemic stroke and associated large vessel occlusion. J Clin Neurosci. 2016;30:60–4.

5. Pfaff J, Herweh C, Pham M, Schönenberger S, Nagel S, Ringleb PA, et al. Mechanical thrombectomy in patients with acute ischemic stroke and lower NIHSS scores: recanalization rates, periprocedural complications, and clinical outcome. AJNR Am J Neuroradiol. 2016;37(11):2066–71.
6. Dargazanli C, Arquizan C, Gory B, Consoli A, Labreuche J, Redjem H, et al. Mechanical thrombectomy for minor and mild stroke patients harboring large vessel occlusion in the anterior circulation: a multicenter cohort study. Stroke. 2017;48(12):3274–81.
7. Mokin M, Masud MW, Dumont TM, Ahmad G, Kass-Hout T, Snyder KV, et al. Outcomes in patients with acute ischemic stroke from proximal intracranial vessel occlusion and NIHSS score below 8. J Neurointerv Surg. 2014;6(6):413–7.
8. Urra X, San Román L, Gil F, Millán M, Cánovas D, Roquer J, et al. Medical and endovascular treatment of patients with large vessel occlusion presenting with mild symptoms: an observational multicenter study. Cerebrovasc Dis. 2014;38(6):418–24.
9. Heldner MR, Jung S, Zubler C, Mordasini P, Weck A, Mono ML, et al. Outcome of patients with occlusions of the internal carotid artery or the main stem of the middle cerebral artery with NIHSS score of less than 5: comparison between thrombolysed and non-thrombolysed patients. J Neurol Neurosurg Psychiatry. 2015;86(7):755–60.
10. Bhogal P, Bücke P, Ganslandt O, Bäzner H, Henkes H, Pérez MA. Mechanical thrombectomy in patients with M1 occlusion and NIHSS score $\leq$5: a single-centre experience. Stroke Vasc Neurol. 2016;1(4):165–71.
11. Haussen DC, Bouslama M, Grossberg JA, Anderson A, Belagage S, Frankel M, et al. Too good to intervene? Thrombectomy for large vessel occlusion strokes with minimal symptoms: an intention-to-treat analysis. J Neurointerv Surg. 2017;9(10):917–21.
12. Messer MP, Schönenberger S, Möhlenbruch MA, Pfaff J, Herweh C, Ringleb PA, et al. Minor stroke syndromes in large-vessel occlusions: mechanical thrombectomy or thrombolysis only? AJNR Am J Neuroradiol. 2017;38(6):1177–9.
13. Kaschner MG, Caspers J, Rubbert C, Lande R, Kraus B, Lee J-I, et al. Mechanical thrombectomy in MCA-mainstem occlusion in patients with low NIHSS scores. Interv Neuroradiol. 2018;24(4):398–404.
14. De Marchis GM, Kohler A, Renz N, Arnold M, Mono M-L, Jung S, et al. Posterior versus anterior circulation strokes: comparison of clinical, radiological and outcome characteristics. J Neurol Neurosurg Psychiatry. 2011;82(1):33–7.
15. Campbell BCV, Christensen S, Tress BM, Churilov L, Desmond PM, Parsons MW, et al. Failure of collateral blood flow is associated with infarct growth in ischemic stroke. J Cereb Blood Flow Metab. 2013;33(8):1168–72.
16. Nguyen PL, Chang JJ. Stroke mimics and acute stroke evaluation: clinical differentiation and complications after intravenous tissue plasminogen activator. J Emerg Med. 2015;49(2):244–52.
17. Romano JG, Smith EE, Liang L, Gardener H, Camp S, Shuey L, et al. Outcomes in mild acute ischemic stroke treated with intravenous thrombolysis: a retrospective analysis of the Get With the Guidelines-Stroke registry. JAMA Neurol. 2015;72(4):423–31.
18. Mazya MV, Cooray C, Lees KR, Toni D, Ford GA, Bar M, et al. Minor stroke due to large artery occlusion. When is intravenous thrombolysis not enough? Results from the SITS International Stroke Thrombolysis Register. Eur Stroke J. 2018;3(1):29–38.
19. Köhrmann M, Nowe T, Huttner HB, et al. Safety and outcome after thrombolysis in stroke patients with mild symptoms. Cerebrovasc Dis. 2009;27:160–6.
20. Zhu W, Churilov L, Campbell BC, et al. Does large vessel occlusion affect clinical outcome in stroke with mild neurologic deficits after intravenous thrombolysis? J Stroke Cerebrovasc Dis. 2014;23:2888–93.
21. Laurencin C, Philippeau F, Blanc-Lasserre K, et al. Thrombolysis for acute minor stroke: outcome and barriers to management. Results from the RESUVAL stroke network. Cerebrovasc Dis. 2015;40:3–9.
22. Choi JC, Jang MU, Kang K, et al. Comparative effectiveness of standard care with IV thrombolysis versus without IV thrombolysis for mild ischemic stroke. J Am Heart Assoc. 2015;4:e001306. ug;50(8):2101–7.

23. Barber PA, Zhang J, Demchuk AM, Hill MD, Buchan AM. Why are stroke patients excluded from TPA therapy? An analysis of patient eligibility. Neurology. 2001;56(8):1015–20.
24. Kim JT, Park MS, Chang J, Lee JS, Choi KH, Cho KH. Proximal arterial occlusion in acute ischemic stroke with low NIHSS scores should not be considered as mild stroke. PLoS One. 2013;8(8):e70996.
25. Nedeltchev K, Schwegler B, Haefeli T, Brekenfeld C, Gralla J, Fischer U, et al. Outcome of stroke with mild or rapidly improving symptoms. Stroke. 2007;38(9):2531–5.
26. Khatri P, Kleindorfer DO, Devlin T, et al. Effect of alteplase vs aspirin on functional outcome for patients with acute ischemic stroke and minor nondisabling neurologic deficits: the PRISMS randomized clinical trial. JAMA. 2018;320(2):156–66. https://doi.org/10.1001/jama.2018.8496.
27. Saqqur M, Uchino K, Demchuk AM, et al. Site of arterial occlusion identified by transcranial Doppler predicts the response to intravenous thrombolysis for stroke. Stroke. 2007;38:948–54.
28. Greisenegger S, Seyfang L, Kiechl S, Lang W, Ferrari J, Austrian Stroke Unit Registry Collaborators. Thrombolysis in patients with mild stroke: results from the Austrian Stroke Unit Registry. Stroke. 2014;45(3):765–9.
29. Haussen DC, Lima FO, Bouslama M, Grossberg JA, Silva GS, Lev MH, et al. Thrombectomy versus medical management for large vessel occlusion strokes with minimal symptoms: an analysis from STOPStroke and GESTOR cohorts. J Neurointerv Surg. 2018;10(4):325–9.
30. Goldhoorn RB, Mulder MJHL, Jansen IGH, van Zwam WH, Staals J, van der Lugt A, et al. Safety and outcome of endovascular treatment for minor ischemic stroke: results from the multicenter clinical registry of endovascular treatment of acute ischemic stroke in the Netherlands. J Stroke Cerebrovasc Dis. 2019;28(3):542–9. https://doi.org/10.1016/j.jstrokecerebrovasdis.2018.10.029. Epub 2018 Dec 6.
31. Asdaghi N, Yavagal DR, Wang K, Mueller-Kronast N, Bhatt N, Gardener HE, Gutierrez CM, Marulanda-Londoño E, Koch S, Dong C, Oluwole SA. Patterns and outcomes of endovascular therapy in mild stroke: a Florida-Puerto Rico collaboration. Stroke. 2019;50(8):2101–7. Kim JT, Park MS, Chang J, et al. Proximal arterial occlusion in acute ischemic stroke with low NIHSS scores should not be considered as mild stroke. PLoS One. 2013;8(8):e70996.
32. Toth G, Ortega-Gutierrez S, Tsai JP, Cerejo R, Al Kasab S, Uchino K, Hussain M, Bain M, Bullen J, Samaniego EA. The safety and feasibility of mechanical thrombectomy for mild acute ischemic stroke with large vessel occlusion. Neurosurgery. 2020;86(6):802–7.
33. Wolman DN, Marcellus DG, Lansberg MG, Albers G, Guenego A, Marks MP, Dodd RL, Do HM, Wintermark M, Martin BW, Heit JJ. Endovascular versus medical therapy for large-vessel anterior occlusive stroke presenting with mild symptoms. Int J Stroke. 2020;15(3):324–31. https://doi.org/10.1177/1747493019873510. [Epub ahead of print].
34. Griessenauer CJ, Medin C, Maingard J, Chandra RV, Ng W, Brooks DM, et al. Endovascular mechanical thrombectomy in large-vessel occlusion ischemic stroke presenting with low National Institutes of Health Stroke Scale: systematic review and meta-analysis. World Neurosurg. 2018;110:263–9.
35. Goyal M, Menon BK, van Zwam WH, Dippel DWJ, Mitchell PJ, Demchuk AM, et al. Endovascular thrombectomy after large-vessel ischaemic stroke: a meta-analysis of individual patient data from five randomised trials. Lancet. 2016;387(10029):1723–31.
36. Goyal N, Tsivgoulis G, Malhotra K, et al. Medical management vs mechanical thrombectomy for mild strokes: an international multicenter study and systematic review and meta-analysis. JAMA Neurol. 2019;77(1):16–24.
37. Horie N, Tateishi Y, Morikawa M, Morofuji Y, Hayashi K, Izumo T, et al. Acute stroke with major intracranial vessel occlusion: characteristics of cardioembolism and atherosclerosis-related in situ stenosis/occlusion. J Clin Neurosci. 2016;32:24–9.
38. Campbell BCV, Mitchell PJ, Churilov L, Yassi N, Kleinig TJ, Dowling RJ, et al. Tenecteplase versus alteplase before thrombectomy for ischemic stroke. N Engl J Med. 2018;378(17):1573–82.
39. Coutts SB, Dubuc V, Mandzia J, Kenney C, Demchuk AM, Smith EE, et al. Tenecteplase-tissue-type plasminogen activator evaluation for minor ischemic stroke with proven occlusion. Stroke. 2015;46(3):769–74.

Chapter 21
Challenges in Thrombectomy: Mega Clots

Monica Scarsella, Julian Hardman, Mark Bain, and Muhammad Shazam Hussain

Background

Emergent large vessel occlusion (ELVO) strokes are among the most devastating stroke types seen. Fortunately, new device technology for mechanical thrombectomy and better selection methods have led to more effective treatment and better outcomes from this devastating condition [1–8]. *Mega clots* with severe thrombus burden or continuous thrombus reaccumulation are among the most difficult types of clots to treat in the setting of ELVO, often resulting in unsuccessful recanalization and poor patient outcome. In this chapter, we seek to share methods of mega clot management found successful in our clinical practice.

Pathophysiology

Mega clots can result from a variety of factors. Large thrombus burden can accumulate with occlusion of a very large vessel such as the cervical or intracranial portion of the internal carotid artery or the basilar artery. Whether by embolism or in situ thrombosis, further thrombosis of other portions of the vessel can lead to propagation and new thrombus formation, and these same processes can also cause rapid thrombus reaccumulation despite transient recanalization. Thus, understanding the process of thrombosis is important in facilitating the development of strategies to assist with recanalization.

M. Scarsella · J. Hardman · M. Bain · M. S. Hussain (✉)
Cerebrovascular Center, Neurological Institute, Cleveland Clinic, Cleveland, OH, USA
e-mail: hussais4@ccf.org

F. K. Hui et al. (eds.), *12 Strokes*, https://doi.org/10.1007/978-3-030-56857-3_21

Predisposing Factors

Thrombosis is a pathologic state characterized by inappropriate activation of hemostatic processes.

Multiple factors predispose to the development of a mega clot. Virchow's triad presents the three main factors contributing thrombosis in general – endothelial injury, hypercoagulability, and stasis of flow [9, 10]. Endothelial injury is often the primary inciting factor in arterial thrombus development. Causes of endothelial injury include alterations in shear stress associated with hypertension, hyperlipidemia, hyperglycemia, traumatic vascular injuries (e.g., dissection), and turbulent flow [9, 10]. Following endothelial injury, clot formation occurs in four stages. First, localized vasoconstriction occurs in response to both reflex neurogenic mechanisms and endothelin release. Primary hemostasis then takes place, where platelets are activated and adhere to the exposed subendothelial matrix via von Willebrand factor (VWF) and collagen interacting with the glycoprotein receptors on the platelets [11]. These two steps form the primary hemostatic plug. The interaction of factor VII with tissue factor released from the endothelium initiates the coagulation cascade, thereby activating thrombin. Thrombin converts fibrinogen into a fibrin polymer, which forms the clot matrix [12]. Finally, platelet aggregation, via the GP IIb/IIIa receptor, and fibrin polymerization lead to the formation of a stable clot, or "permanent plug" [11, 12]. Natural antithrombotic mechanisms, including prostacyclin, antithrombin III, protein C, tissue factor pathway inhibitor, and plasmin, whose function is catalyzed by tissue plasminogen activator (tPA), exist in order to restrict clot formation to the site of vessel injury [12]. Injured endothelium prevents naturally produced antithrombotic agents from functioning appropriately [12]. The combination of endothelial injury in the location of a large vessel plays a large role in the development of a mega clot. In addition, this is likely the primary reason for rapid reaccumulation of clot after transient recanalization during mechanical thrombectomy.

Stasis within larger vessels can also contribute to rapid development of large thrombus burden. Stasis causes thromboses in that it allows platelets to come closer to vessel walls for longer amounts of time, as well as limits flow of new blood, so activated coagulation factors are not removed [12]. Particularly in the carotid artery, a long column of stagnant blood can begin to thrombose, though the consistency is often softer than the primary thrombus. However, if given enough time, fibrin begins to form. Fibrin-rich thrombi, defined as <20% red cell content, possess an elevated coefficient of static friction and have been shown to have decreased rates of revascularization [13]. Increased thrombus length also retains increased friction, which may shed light on the worse outcomes with aspiration thrombectomy seen in the THERAPY trial [14].

Hypercoagulability contributes to 5–10% of ischemic strokes [15]. A hypercoagulable state is an abnormally high coagulation response to vascular injury. The main genetic causes of arterial thrombosis are factor V Leiden mutation, ATIII deficiency, protein C or S deficiency, prothrombin G20210A mutation, and MTHFR gene mutation, due to the accumulation of homocysteine, causing endothelial damage [15]. Acquired causes of hypercoagulability include malignancy, heparin-induced thrombocytopenia, oral contraceptive pill/estrogen replacement therapy, postpartum state, paroxysmal nocturnal hemoglobinuria, the presence of antiphospholipid antibodies, polycythemia, hyperviscosity syndromes, increased lipoprotein (a), dysfibrinogenemia, nephrotic syndrome, subtherapeutic INR, obesity, smoking, surgery, and trauma [15]. Of note, two risk factors for venous thrombosis increases risk for arterial thrombosis [15, 16]. In our experience, mega clots are often associated with underlying occult malignancy, and should prompt age-appropriate cancer screening following the intervention.

Review of Endovascular Management

Despite the challenges mega clots pose to neurointerventionalists, thrombectomy remains a viable option for successful recanalization. Due to the large thrombus burden, there is poor outcome in these cases with medical management, including with recombinant IV tissue plasminogen activator (tPA). In fact, recanalization rates with IV tPA are very poor for mega clots, with only 10% recanalization reported for ICA terminus clots [17]. Thus, endovascular therapy (EVT) is the treatment of choice for these most severe ELVO situations.

The approach for mega clots is similar to other EVTs, though the choice of devices should be made to accommodate the need for extraction of large thrombi. We will typically utilize a large groin sheath (8F or 9F), in case the guide sheath becomes occluded with thrombus and needs to be removed. In cases where we have utilized a shuttle sheath, removal like this is not an option. In this case, removing the thrombus from the intracranial circulation and out of the internal carotid artery, and placing in a nonessential vessel, such as the external carotid artery, may be the only option [18]. A balloon guide sheath may be helpful to arrest flow during aspiration or during withdrawal of the stent-retriever to prevent distal embolization. The advent of new larger lumen balloon guide catheters may improve their utilization on mega clot cases. Due to the very large inner diameters, large bore sheath should be placed as close to the thrombus/occlusion as possible, and aspiration performed through the guide sheath will often remove large amounts of thrombus. Large bore intermediate catheters, now with up to 74 inner lumen, can also be attempted, but often, these large mega clots will be too large for even these catheters. However, if a good seal is obtained, they may be helpful in acting as a mechanical thrombectomy device. Stent-retrievers may also prove useful to pull from distal to proximal in the vessel under constant aspiration to pull clot through the vessel/guide sheath and may also mechanically disrupt the clot. Another beneficial strategy is to place a microcatheter with the thrombus and slowly infuse intra-arterial tPA into the thrombus along its length. This can also be effective in cases of rapid reaccumulation of the thrombus after recanalization. If suspected to have underlying arterial injury and denuding of the endothelium, platelet activation may be occurring and infusion of glycoprotein IIb/IIIa inhibitor can rapidly cause dissolution of the platelet-rich occlusion.

For large thrombus burden in the carotid artery, we have also employed emergent surgical opening of the carotid artery. The surgeon, following exposure of the carotid in which care is taken to avoid significant manipulation of the carotid artery, obtains distal control with a temporary clip placed on the distal internal carotid artery, to lessen the risk of distal embolization. An incision is made in the carotid bulb/proximal internal carotid artery with the common carotid artery (CCA) and external carotid artery (ECA) clamped. Once the CCA and ECA are clamped, the ICA clip can be opened and back-pressure from the collaterals around the circle of Willis will often push the thrombus through the arteriotomy and clear the vessel. This can also be achieved by placing a Fogarty balloon distal in the vessel through the arteriotomy and with the balloon inflated pulling the balloon proximally to remove large thrombi.

It must be kept in mind, however, that with each attempt at thrombectomy, the chance of successful retrieval decreases due to thrombus compression [14]. Complicated techniques may also take longer and ultimately pose more negative consequences. Therefore, the primary goal should be a straight-forward approach with the goal of first-pass revascularization.

Case Illustrations:

Case 1: A 63-year-old right-handed male presented with transient vision changes of right eye. Initial National Institutes of Health Stroke Scale (NIHSS) in the emergency room was 2 for left homonymous hemianopia, but shortly after arrival, the patient deteriorated, developing dysarthria, expressive aphasia, left facial droop, and left arm weakness (NIHSS 10). CT head revealed a hyperdense MCA in the right M1 segment. tPA was then administered. CTA displayed complete right ICA occlusion beginning 1 cm from its origin, as well as right M1 occlusion. The patient was taken for emergent thrombectomy. Initial angiographic runs (Fig. 21.1a and b) showed complete right ICA occlusion.

A 7F shuttle sheath was navigated into the right proximal ICA. Upon back-bleeding, a large thrombus came out of the guide sheath. Several additional aspiration attempts were made on guide sheath with additional thrombus removed. Due to a curve in the cervical internal carotid artery, which prevented further advancement of the guide sheath, a large bore intermediate catheter was introduced, with additional thrombus removed resulting in partial recanalization with a dissection seen in the mid cervical portion of the ICA (Fig. 21.1c). The intermediate catheter was advanced to the supraclinoid ICA and intracranial imaging showed the right M2 thrombus had moved distally to the M3 segment (Fig. 21.1d). Due to its distal location, it was felt that the risk outweighed benefit of thrombus removal; therefore, this was not undertaken. Upon withdrawal of the intermediate catheter, good flow was seen throughout the ICA including in the area of dissection (Fig. 21.1e). Patient was ultimately discharged home with NIH 0 and no focal neurological deficit.

This case illustrates the benefit of initial aspiration on the guide catheter or sheath in cases of ICA occlusion, as the large bore of these catheter can often result in large thrombus removal.

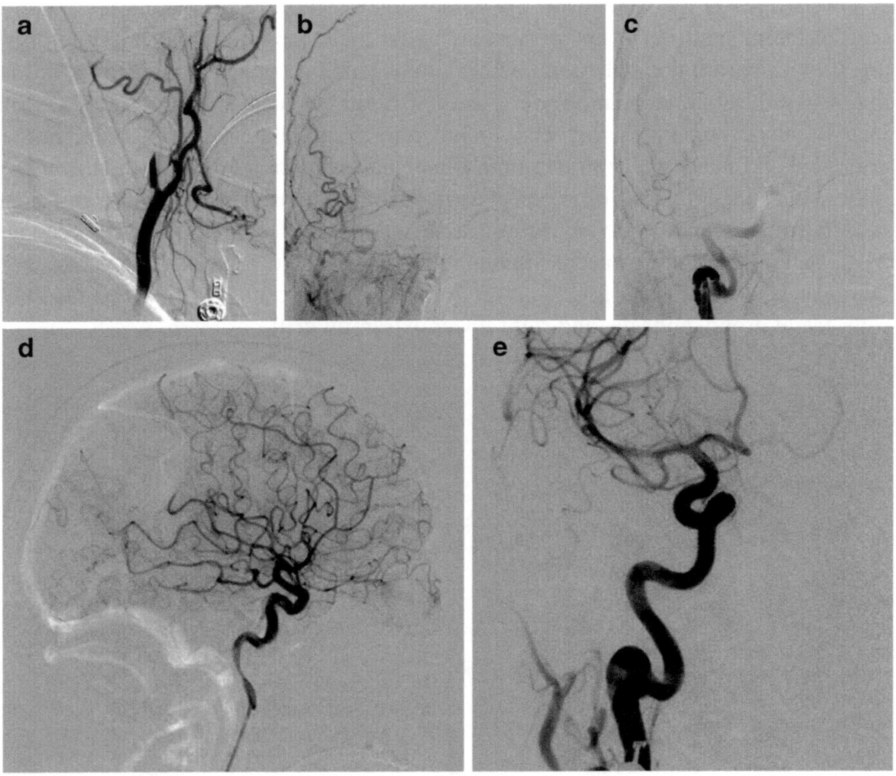

Fig. 21.1 (**a**) Right internal artery occlusion with minimal contrast penetration past the origin. (**b**) Intracranial runs show no opacification of the intracranial carotid artery. (**c**) Following placement of the guide sheath, which resulted in significant thrombus removal, slow opacification is seen in the supraclinoid segment. (**d**) After advancement of the intermediate catheter through the area of dissection, intracranial runs showed improvement in the intracranial circulation, with a parietal M3 thrombus remaining. (**e**) Final runs of the right internal carotid artery show restoration of flow in the artery, with good intracranial filling

Case 2: A 69-year-old left-handed female, with a past medical history significant for hypertension, hyperlipidemia, tobacco abuse, and prediabetes, woke up in the morning with sudden-onset expressive aphasia, dysarthria, and confusion (initial NIHSS 3.) CT head was notable for hypoattenuation within the left frontal centrum semiovale and dorsal insula. CTA demonstrated cutoff of the left M1 middle cerebral artery (MCA). MRI brain displayed restricted diffusion in the same regions of hypoattenuation seen on CT. Overnight patient progressed, developing right facial droop, right upper extremity and right lower extremity weakness, as well as worsening aphasia and confusion (NIH 11.) Hyperacute MRI showed minimal increase in infarct but large penumbra in the left MCA territory. Patient was then taken for endovascular recanalization. Initial angiographic runs confirmed the left M1 MCA occlusion with good collaterals (Fig. 21.2a). A balloon guide catheter was initially used with large bore intermediate catheter, with thrombus removed and TICI 3 flow achieved (Fig. 21.2b). However, the vessel quickly reoccluded. Multiple attempts with different stent retrievers were made under local aspiration and proximal flow arrest, with partial recanalization achieved but quick reocclusion occurring within minutes of recanalization and underlying new thrombus formation seen (Fig. 21.2c). Due to suspected underlying endothelial injury and platelet aggregation, intra-arterial abciximab was administration. This resulted in dissolution of the thrombus with TICI 3 perfusion ultimately achieved (Fig. 21.2d). Resulting transient vasospasm was managed with intra-arterial infusion of verapamil. Postprocedure MRI was notable for new acute infarcts in the left caudate, temporal pole, and parietal lobe. She was discharged to an acute rehabilitation center with NIH 3 for mild right facial droop, aphasia, and right lower extremity drift.

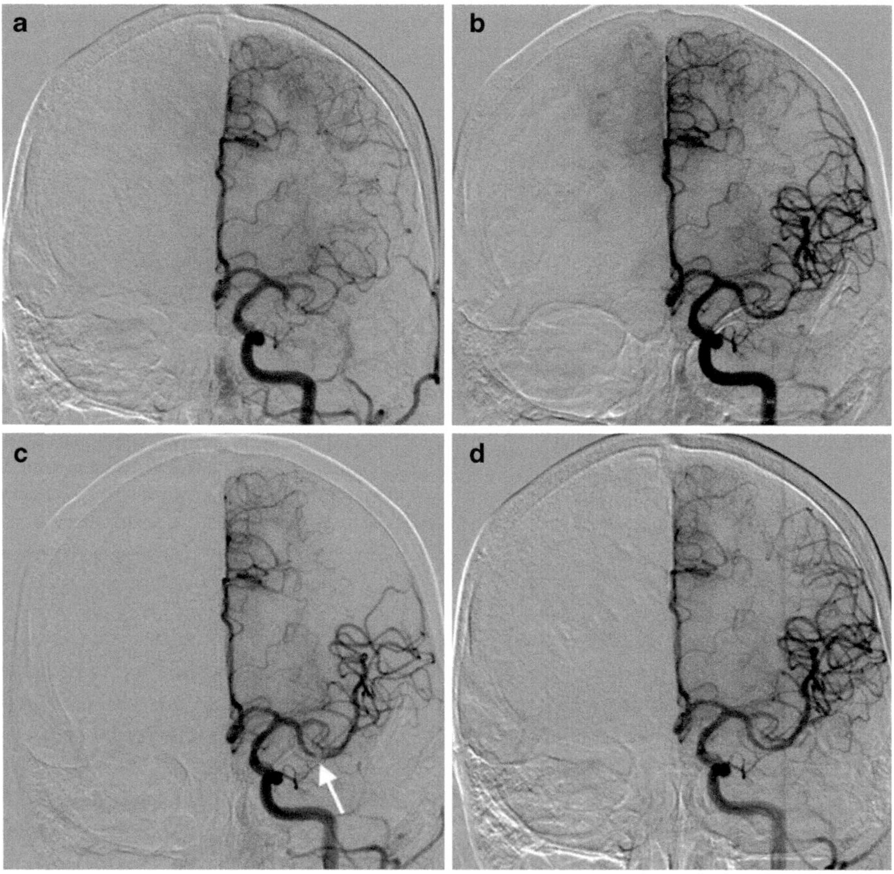

Fig. 21.2 (**a**) Left M1 middle cerebral artery occlusion with good collaterals. (**b**) After local direct aspiration, TICI 3 flow achieved. (**c**) Following reocclusion, several passes with stent-retrievers under local aspiration were attempted. However, reocclusion would occur quickly after reopening of the vessel. Subocclusive thrombus (white arrow) was seen as reocclusion occured. (**d**) Following administration of abciximab, dissolution of the thrombus was seen with TICI 3 flow achieved

This case illustrates that underlying endothelial injury can result in platelet activation, causing reocclusion. Neurointerventionalists should be prepared to administer glycoprotein IIb/IIIa inhibitors for this situation.

Case 3: A 58-year-old right-handed female with past medical history significant for prior right MCA stroke developed sudden-onset aphasia and right hand weakness that initially fluctuated in severity, returning to normal (initial NIHSS 0). She was not given tPA due to resolution of symptoms. Later, her exam continued to progress with expressive and ultimately global aphasia, accompanied by right upper extremity and right lower extremity drift (NIH 11.) CT head was only notable for encephalomalacia from old stroke. tPA was not given at this point as patient was out of the time window. CTA revealed ulcerative plaque and large thrombus, causing severe left ICA stenosis (>90%) (Fig. 21.3a). Hyperacute MRI revealed minimal punctate infarcts in the left MCA territory (Fig. 21.3b) and repeat MRA displayed left M3 opercular branch occlusion as well as poor signal in the left ICA, suggesting poor flow past the thrombus (Fig. 21.3c). Due to the large clinical deficit with minimal infarcts (clinical-diffusion mismatch), it was felt the carotid lesion was resulting in hypoperfusion with slow progressive infarction. After discussion with the

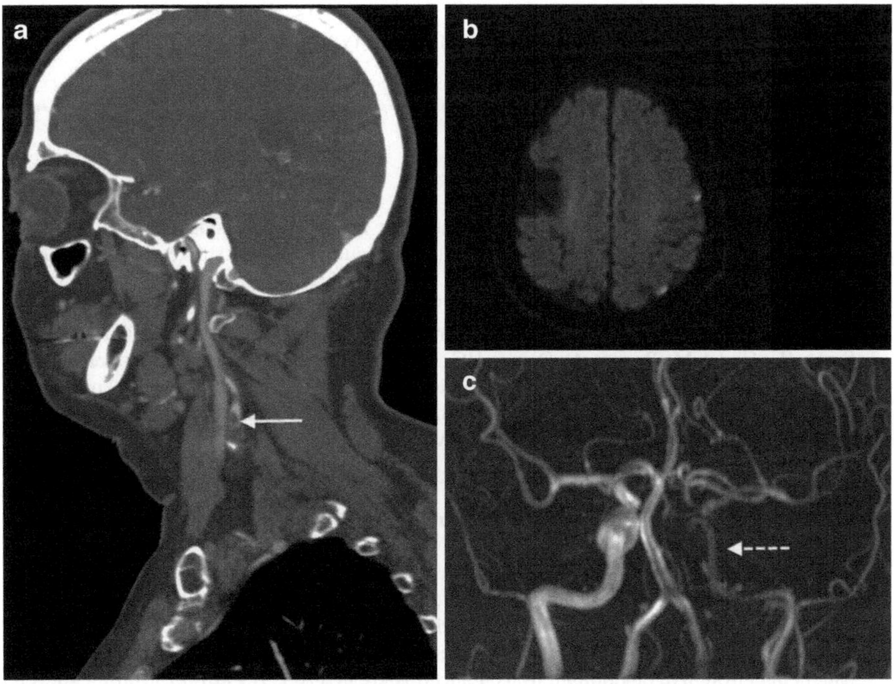

Fig. 21.3 (**a**) Large thrombus (solid white arrow) seen in the left ICA origin. (**b**) Hyperacute MRI revealed only small punctate infarcts despite large and worsening clinical deficit, suggesting clinical-diffusion mismatch. (**c**) Hyperacute MRA shows poor signal in the left ICA (dotted white arrow), suggesting poor flow around the thrombus

multidisciplinary team, it was decided to take the patient for emergent carotid endarterectomy with thrombectomy. Following clamping of the distal ICA, the CCA and ECA were clamped. An incision was made into the left carotid bulb, revealing a complex ulcerated plaque with thrombus. The endarterectomy was completed. By the following morning, the patient had greatly improved. Patient was ultimately discharged home with NIH 1 for mild aphasia.

This case illustrates the option of endarterectomy with thrombectomy for large proximal carotid thrombus. Though endovascular options could be also considered, in our experience, the likelihood of distal embolization with endovascular methods is high. If an endovascular approach is attempted, techniques to minimize embolization should be utilized, including balloon guide to arrest flow before crossing the thrombus and use of distal protection.

Conclusion

Mega clots are among the most challenging situations in neurointerventional practice. Understanding the underlying pathophysiological processes that lead to mega clot formation and employing strategies to deal with large thrombus burden can lead to success in dealing with these most devastating types of strokes.

References

1. Berkhemer OA, Fransen PS, Beumer D, van den Berg LA, Lingsma HF, Yoo AJ, et al. A randomized trial of intraarterial treatment for acute ischemic stroke. N Engl J Med. 2015;372(1):11–20.
2. Goyal M, Demchuk AM, Menon BK, Eesa M, Rempel JL, Thornton J, et al. Randomized assessment of rapid endovascular treatment of ischemic stroke. N Engl J Med. 2015;372(11):1019–30.
3. Saver JL, Goyal M, Bonafe A, Diener HC, Levy EI, Pereira VM, et al. Solitaire with the Intention for Thrombectomy as Primary Endovascular Treatment for Acute Ischemic Stroke (SWIFT PRIME) trial: protocol for a randomized, controlled, multicenter study comparing the Solitaire revascularization device with IV tPA with IV tPA alone in acute ischemic stroke. Int J Stroke. 2015;10(3):439–48.
4. Campbell BC, Mitchell PJ, Kleinig TJ, Dewey HM, Churilov L, Yassi N, et al. Endovascular therapy for ischemic stroke with perfusion-imaging selection. N Engl J Med. 2015;372(11):1009–18.
5. Jovin TG, Chamorro A, Cobo E, de Miquel MA, Molina CA, Rovira A, et al. Thrombectomy within 8 hours after symptom onset in ischemic stroke. N Engl J Med. 2015;372(24):2296–306.
6. Goyal M, Menon BK, van Zwam WH, Dippel DW, Mitchell PJ, Demchuk AM, et al. Endovascular thrombectomy after large-vessel ischaemic stroke: a meta-analysis of individual patient data from five randomised trials. Lancet. 2016;387(10029):1723–31.
7. Nogueira RG, Jadhav AP, Haussen DC, Bonafe A, Budzik RF, Bhuva P, et al. Thrombectomy 6 to 24 hours after stroke with a mismatch between deficit and infarct. N Engl J Med. 2018;378(1):11–21.

8. Albers GW, Marks MP, Kemp S, Christensen S, Tsai JP, Ortega-Gutierrez S, et al. Thrombectomy for stroke at 6 to 16 hours with selection by perfusion imaging. N Engl J Med. 2018;378(8):708–18.
9. Wolberg AS, Aleman MM, Leiderman K, Machlus KR. Procoagulant activity in hemostasis and thrombosis: Virchow's triad revisited. Anesth Analg. 2012;114(2):275–85.
10. Chung I, Lip GY. Virchow's triad revisited: blood constituents. Pathophysiol Haemost Thromb. 2003;33(5–6):449–54.
11. Nieswandt B, Pleines I, Bender M. Platelet adhesion and activation mechanisms in arterial thrombosis and ischaemic stroke. J Thromb Haemost. 2011;9(Suppl 1):92–104.
12. Chapin JC, Hajjar KA. Fibrinolysis and the control of blood coagulation. Blood Rev. 2015;29(1):17–24.
13. Arnold M, Nedeltchev K, Mattle HP, Loher TJ, Stepper F, Schroth G, et al. Intra-arterial thrombolysis in 24 consecutive patients with internal carotid artery T occlusions. J Neurol Neurosurg Psychiatry. 2003;74(6):739–42.
14. Yoo AJ, Andersson T. Thrombectomy in acute ischemic stroke: challenges to procedural success. J Stroke. 2017;19(2):121–30.
15. Levine SR. Hypercoagulable states and stroke: a selective review. CNS Spectr. 2005;10(7):567–78.
16. Nakashima MO, Rogers HJ. Hypercoagulable states: an algorithmic approach to laboratory testing and update on monitoring of direct oral anticoagulants. Blood Res. 2014;49(2):85–94.
17. Saqqur M, Uchino K, Demchuk AM, Molina CA, Garami Z, Calleja S, et al. Site of arterial occlusion identified by transcranial Doppler predicts the response to intravenous thrombolysis for stroke. Stroke. 2007;38(3):948–54.
18. John S, Burgess R, Cheng-Ching E, Wisco D, Taqui A, Bain M, et al. Last resort: case of clot translocation in intra-arterial stroke therapy. J Neurointerv Surg. 2014;6(10):e50.

Chapter 22
Challenges in Thrombectomy: Access Problems, Hard Clots, Relapsing Occlusions, and Embolization to New Territories

Tommy Andersson and Leonard Leong Litt Yeo

Introduction

Acute ischemic stroke (AIS) is still the number one cause of dependency in the world, but over the last few years, thrombectomy has become the first-line therapy for large vessel occlusion and changed the way acute stroke is managed [1–4]. The later versions of thrombectomy devices have been designed to improve the rates of recanalization. However, up to 20% of AIS patients treated with mechanical thrombectomy do not have successful recanalization and the rate of good functional outcomes is even less, remaining around 50% [5–10]. In addition, each failed thrombectomy attempt not only delay recanalization and have a progressing infarct size, with each additional pass, there are concerns for vessel injury, distal embolization from clot fragmentation, or embolization into unaffected territories [7, 9].

Disclosures This research received no specific grant from any funding agency in the public, commercial or not-for-profit sectors.
Tommy Andersson is a consultant for Ablynx, Amnis Therapeutics, Medtronic, Neuravi/J&J, Rapid Medical and Stryker.
Leonard Yeo has received substantial grant funding from the National Medical Research Council (NMRC), Singapore, substantial grant funding from ministry of health (MOH), Singapore, and a moderate grant funding from I²R, A-STAR, Singapore.

T. Andersson
Department of Clinical Neuroscience, Karolinska Institutet, Stockholm, Sweden

Department of Neuroradiology, Karolinska University Hospital, Stockholm, Sweden

Department of Medical Imaging, AZ Groeninge, Kortrijk, Belgium

L. L. L. Yeo (✉)
Department of Clinical Neuroscience, Karolinska Institutet, Stockholm, Sweden

Department of Neuroradiology, Karolinska University Hospital, Stockholm, Sweden

Divison of Neurology, National University Health System, Singapore and Yong Loo Lin School of Medicine, National University of Singapore, Singapore, Singapore

F. K. Hui et al. (eds.), *12 Strokes*, https://doi.org/10.1007/978-3-030-56857-3_22

It is important to understand the factors that prevent us from recanalizing the culprit vessel during acute stroke as restoring blood flow is one of the most powerful methods of improving outcomes in AIS. This can be accomplished by looking at all the elements, which make it difficult to open the vessel, from anatomical variations to the full spectrum of clot properties to try to find ways to more efficiently extract them [11]. In this study, we review the literature surrounding each of these factors and the potential solutions that have been tried in this new era.

Access Problems and Stroke Etiology

One of the commonly faced issues with failed thrombectomy is the problem of difficult vascular access. If the patient has problematic femoral arteries, an elongated unfolded aortic arch, or tortuous neck vessels, it can be challenging to reach the intracranial occlusion.

Variations of the aortic arch elongation can be classified according to the length measured vertically, of the beginning of the innominate artery to the top of the aortic arch [12]. The longer this is, the more difficult it can be to catheterize the cerebral vasculature. With higher grades, there is also a propensity for the guiding catheter to be less stable and collapse into the aortic arch during the procedure, requiring the operator to start over [13]. Other variations such as a bovine arch from the common origin of innominate artery and left CCA or the origin of the left CCA from the innominate artery can also exist and add to the complexity of the procedure [14]. After navigating the aorta, tortuosity of the carotid vessels can also be associated with failure of thrombectomy. This can be due to tortuous, looped, or kinked cervical vessels that prevent smooth navigation as well as take up a length of the catheter rendering them too short to reach the occlusion [15, 16].

In the intracranial circulation, the geometric anatomy of the middle cerebral artery can contribute to the inability of the stent to remove the clot; for example, a hair-pin loop can increase the friction of the clot and the vessel wall when it is being withdrawn, or a short vessel dilatation can trap the clot as it is being drawn past if the stent does not expand to accommodate the wider vessel [17, 18]. Similarly, an "S-configuration" vessel, withdrawal of a stentretriver may also pull on the vessel and cause avulsion injuries with bleeding of these small vessels (Fig. 22.1). Using an intermediate catheter will improve the vector of force and reduce the risk of avulsion injuries to the vessel or other complications such as inadvertent stent detachment (Fig. 22.2). In fact, this was the initial idea behind the creation of the distal access catheter (DAC) (Concentric Medical), rather than as a distal aspirate catheter or for the pinning technique.

This is why a pretreatment computed tomography angiogram (CTA) from the aortic arch to the intracranial vessel is a very useful tool for preplanning of the thrombectomy procedure. It can be used to predict anatomical difficulties, after which specific tools such as a Simmons types catheter or an alternative access site such as a radial, brachial, or carotid access can be prophylactically chosen

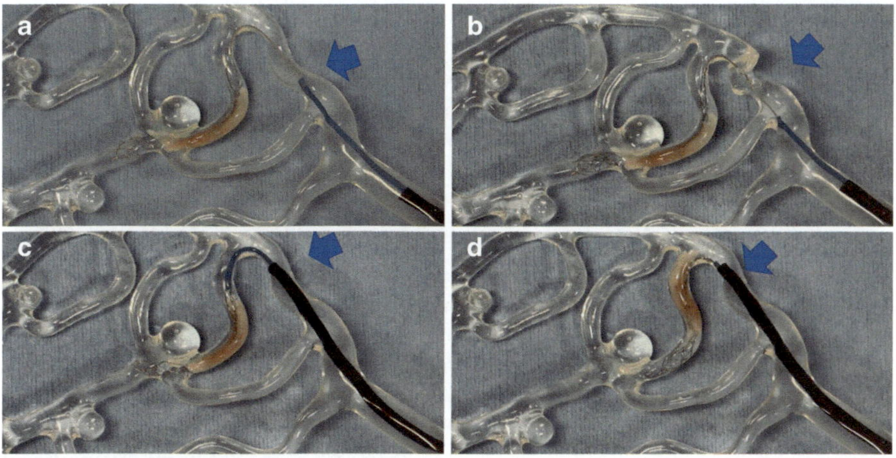

Fig. 22.1 (**a**) Stentretriver without using the intermediate catheter in a hair-pin turn of a flow model. (**b**) On withdrawal of the stentretriver, the friction causes traction and force to be applied perpendicular to the line of vessel with resultant severe deformation of the vessel without moving the clot. (**c**) Stentretriver with an intermediate catheter in a hair-pin turn of a flow model. (**d**) The change in the direction of force with an intermediate catheter allows for the clot to be removed without deformation of the vessel

[19–21]. Occlusions in certain vessel are sometimes much more easily reached with an alternative access site; a common example is a vertebral or basilar occlusion with an unfolded aorta, which can be better accessed via a radial approach. This will cut down on the length of the procedure, reduce complications, and diminish wastage by avoiding changing catheters or wires that are not suitable (Fig. 22.3).

Intracranial atherosclerotic stenosis is a possible etiology for refractory thrombectomy or immediate reocclusion post thrombectomy [22]. This problem is much more commonly seen in Asian populations compared to Caucasian populations, although hypertension, diabetes, and hyperlipidemia are well-known risk factors for intracranial atherosclerosis in any population [23–25]. Vascular luminal imaging such as a CT angiogram or a digital subtracted angiography can sometimes differentiate intracranial atherosclerotic occlusions from embolic occlusions and therefore the response to stentretriver thrombectomy [26]. In large vessel occlusion stroke due to underlying atherosclerotic lesions, there is a need to use other adjunct devices in addition to the stentretriver in most of the cases. Whereas in cardioembolic lesions, the stentretriver alone was successful in 83.3% of the patients. In the same study, the need for adjunct devices meant that atherosclerotic lesions had much longer procedure times, which can be up to 50 minutes longer on average [27]. Other rarer causes for failure of recanalization are underlying vessel wall pathologies such as vasculitis or early Moyamoya disease, which can render the thrombectomy devices ineffective [28, 29]. In such cases a high index of suspicion and early recognition is key to prevent futile procedures.

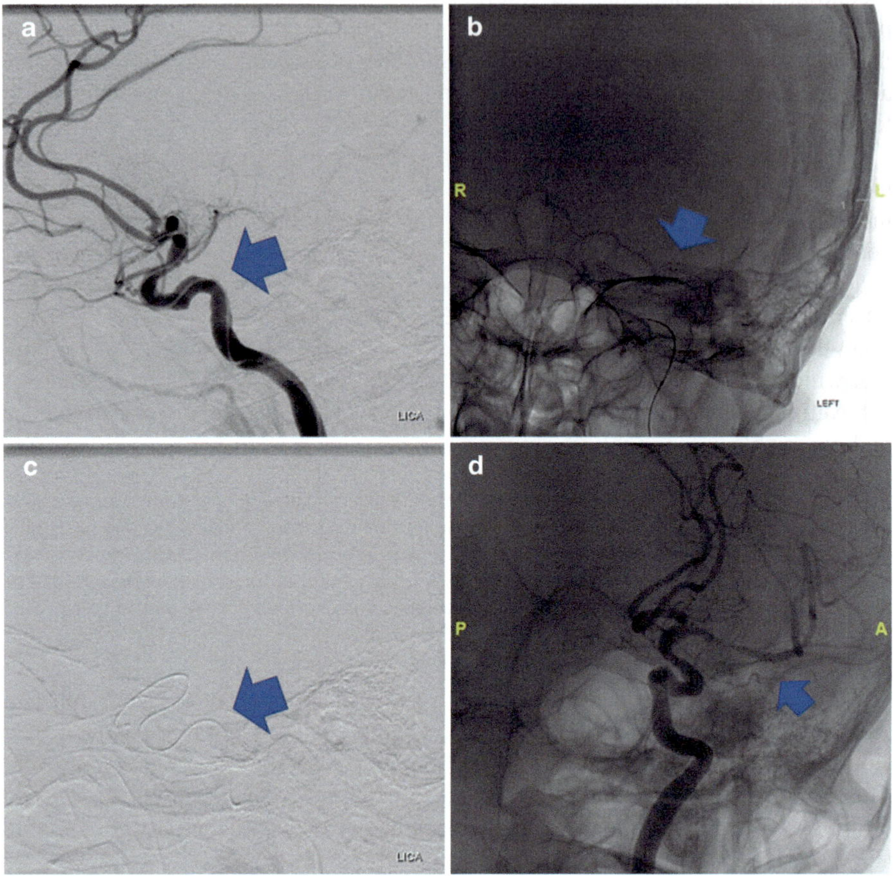

Fig. 22.2 (**a**, **b**) An angiogram showing an S-shaped tortuous vessel and the same winding path taken by the guidewire. (**c**, **d**) On stentretriver thrombectomy, the high friction between the stentretriver and the wall caused a complication of an inadvertent detachment of the stentretriver (arrow in **c** and **d**)

Finally, the anatomical location of the occlusion can determine the thrombus burden. For example, the volume of the thrombus is largest in the internal carotid artery occlusions and smaller in middle cerebral artery (MCA) occlusions [30]. Greater thrombus length would be expected to yield increased friction and adhesion given the larger surface area for thrombus-vessel interaction. However, the association between thrombus size and successful recanalization after endovascular treatment is inconsistent. A higher clot burden scores has shown an association with increased likelihood of recanalization [31–37], but worse outcomes were seen after aspiration thrombectomy of longer thrombi in the THERAPY trial, which excluded thrombus length shorter than 8 mm [38].

The size of the thrombectomy device should therefore be chosen to optimally accommodate the thrombus burden and avoid complications. For example, a smaller intermediate catheter can result in sides of the thrombus being sheared off when the

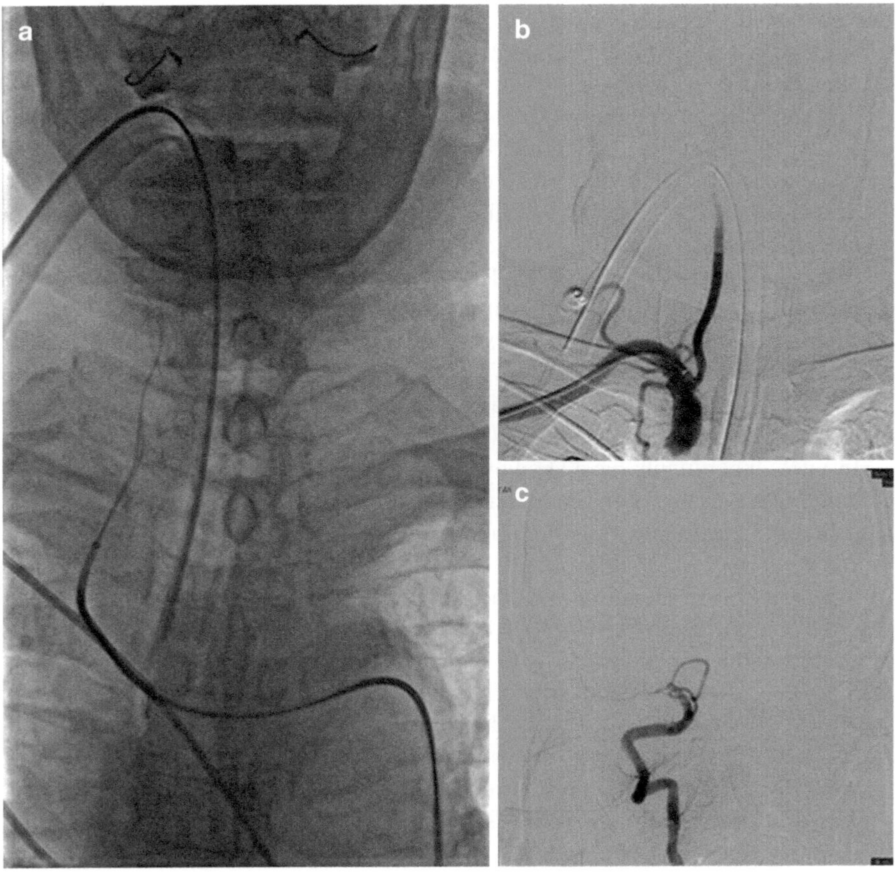

Fig. 22.3 (**a**) A widened unfolded aortic arch with difficulty advancing the guide catheter into the vertebral artery. (**b**, **c**) A radial access was chosen, which simplified the procedure

stentretriver is withdrawn into it. There is emerging evidence that the best thrombectomy technique may depend on the localization occlusion, whether it is an anterior circulation or posterior circulation occlusion, for example, or the shape of the vessel housing the proximal occlusion site [39, 40]. Some occlusions, which are refractory to one technique, may respond favorably to a different approach [39]. In the future, we may be able to tailor not only our device but also the technique used with respect to different clot locations and compositions.

Clot Properties

Thrombus composition is a key factor in determining its susceptibility to mechanical and pharmacological methods and thus the degree of successful recanalization. Unfortunately, the makeup of the clot is currently unknown prior to treatment and thus, all thrombi are approached in the same manner. Research to determine optimal thrombectomy methodology before the procedure is sorely lacking and is a crucial gap that needs to be addressed.

The composition of a thrombus is made up of many different substances largely dependent on its source, but primarily consists of three components: fibrin, red blood cells (RBCs), and white blood cells (WBCs) [41, 42].

The distribution of platelets and fibrin within a thrombus varies between an atherosclerotic vessel thrombus and a cardiac thrombus. In a thrombus, which originates from an atherosclerotic vessel, RBC tends to be massed near the center with a slim outer layer of fibrin-platelet complexes at the outer edges. Conversely, in cardiac thrombi, fibrin-platelet complexes are distributed throughout the thrombus with corresponding larger amounts of fibrin [43]. The proportion of fibrin relative to the red blood cells in a clot substantially alters its physical properties, which affects how it responds to thrombectomy [44, 45] (Fig. 22.4).

In vitro experiments have shown that fibrin-rich thrombi with <20% red cell content have a significantly higher coefficient of static friction [46]. The preliminary literature available on clot composition tends to suggest that the proportion of fibrin is especially relevant in determining successful clot retrieval, with hypodense, fibrin-rich thrombi demonstrating decreased revascularization rates regardless of the technique employed [44, 47]. A mature, clot high in fibrin is thus more firm and less deformable with higher frictional properties and on compression by the struts of a stent, the friction between the clot and the vessel wall increases. This renders subsequent device passes substantially less effective with each attempt [46, 48]. As it becomes more compact, it will have greater tendency to "roll" over the struts of the stentretriver as it is withdrawn or not get properly aspirated into a catheter. The result is the clot remaining in the same position during the thrombectomy attempt. Newer-generation stent retrievers with increased radial force or designed to scoop or capture the clot within its struts rather than penetrate the thrombus may be more effective in clots high in fibrin. In contrast, clots rich in red blood cells are soft but friable. They may be easier to remove but are prone to break off and cause distal embolization into the same or a previously unaffected territory.

The percentage of white blood cells (WBCs) in the thrombus is another characteristic that determines the ease of recanalization and, by association, the procedure time [49]. According to histological studies, the development of a thrombus begins with platelets at the site of vessel injury, attracting other platelets to form a platelet clump. WBCs invade the sides of the clump after which fibrin strands form and trap RBCs to form a solid thrombus [50, 51]. WBCs are therefore a marker of the age of the thrombus and in cardioembolic thrombi, a higher proportion of WBCs exist in the clot, which may be related to the increased length of time to mature in the heart chamber before embolizing. Moreover, WBCs have more time to invade the cardiogenic thrombus and this is associated with an increased degree of organization of the thrombus. This organization is closely associated with the stability of the clot and the friction to the vessel wall. More mature clots are therefore more difficult to remove [52].

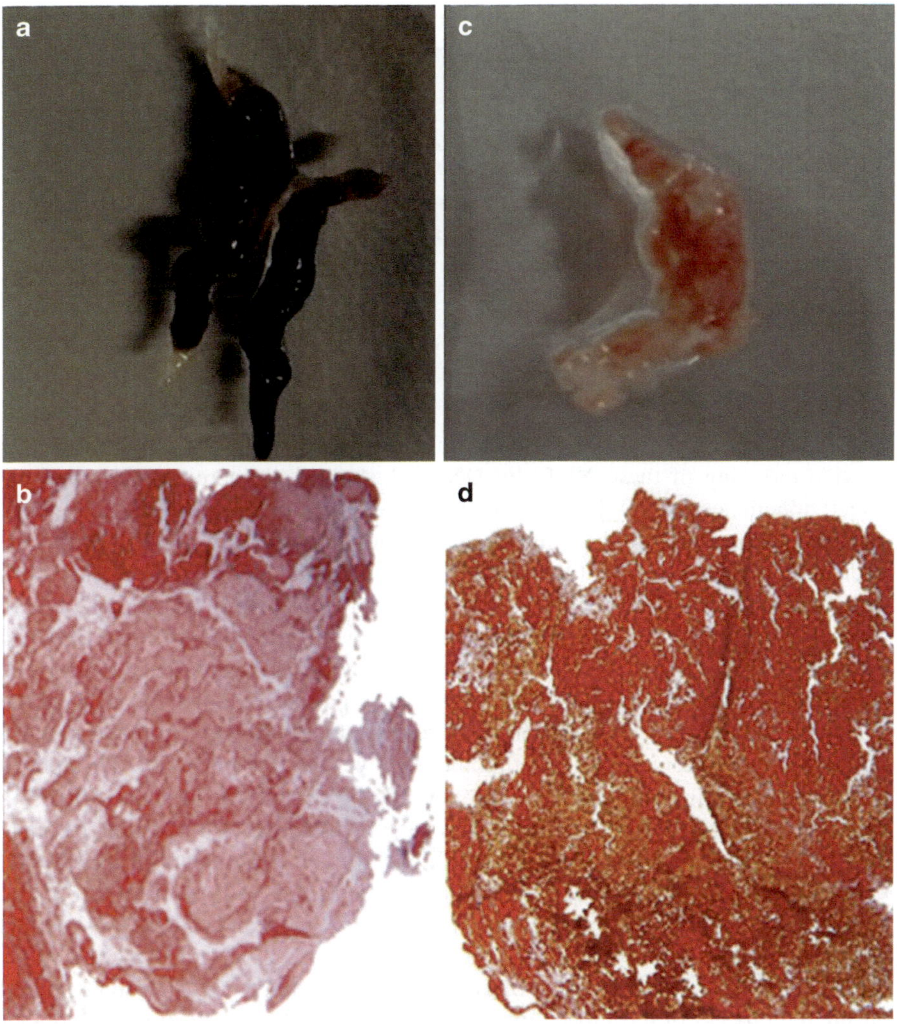

Fig. 22.4 (**a**) Clots comprised predominantly of red blood cells with the corresponding histology (**b**) and (**c**). Clots predominantly made of fibrin with corresponding histology (**d**)

While there are different types of WBCs, neutrophils in particular seem to be important in ischemic stroke. Neutrophils catalyze the thrombotic pathway by formation of neutrophil extracellular traps (NETs) [53]. These NETs are formed when neutrophils unleash decondensed DNA fibers into the extracellular matrix, which then act as supports for RBCs and platelets to bind to, and subsequently influence the coagulation cascade [54]. Studies recently showed that all thrombi contained NETs, but the neutrophil content in ischemic stroke thrombi was considerably higher, relative to coronary thrombi [54, 55]. A potential diagnostic use was put forth when an association between NETs and cardioembolic etiology was found

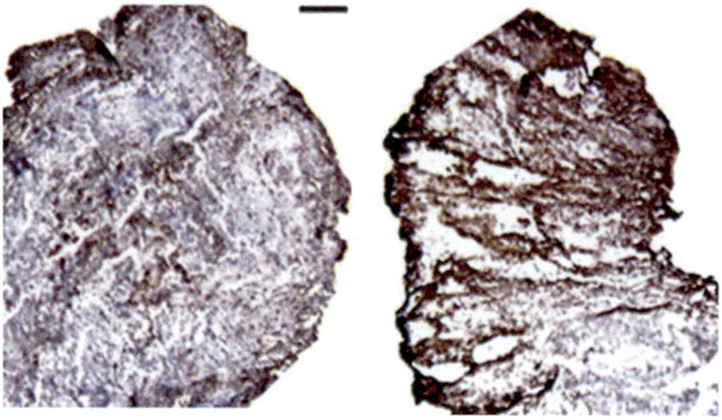

Fig. 22.5 Clots removed after a thrombectomy and stained for von Willebrand factor

[56]. The same study also had a potential therapeutic angle when it showed that ex vivo targeting of these NETs by DNase 1 showed an increased thrombolytic effect; nonetheless, this will have to be replicated in animal and human trials [56].

Clots contain many other substances besides fibrin, RBCS, and WBCs. One interesting study showed that the level of von Willebrand factor varied in clots. Von Willebrand factor is a large multimeric plasma glycoprotein that links platelets in conjunction with fibrin, which results in the clot becoming more organized and firmer (Figs. 22.4 and 22.5) [57, 58]. Another sign that can represent resistance to thrombolysis and mechanical thrombectomy is partial endothelialization at the edges of the thrombus. This is thought to represent early organization and maturation as the body attempts to grow endothelium over the thrombus [59]. Thrombi of nonthrombotic origin such as calcified or neoplastic content can be more difficult to remove [60, 61]. In a small series of cases with calcification of the plaque, multiple stent retriever attempts were unsuccessful, and adjunct treatment with intracranial balloon angioplasty was required. In one of the cases, a Solitaire FR became entrapped inside the dense calcification after its deployment and had to be resheathed with a microcatheter [44].

The distribution of the content of the clot and its architecture can also be altered during the process of thrombectomy. The longer the clot has to mature, the stickier it is and difficult to remove. This is amplified by the water-hammer effect of the systemic blood pressure that squeezes and compacts the thrombus, rendering it more recalcitrant to extraction. Failed thrombectomy attempts can also change the clot properties: for example, the clot can be compacted by the stentretriver and becomes more difficult to remove with each pass.

Imaging to Predict Thrombectomy Failure

As mentioned earlier, preprocedural imaging, whether CTA or magnetic resonance MR-angiography (MRA), is crucial for planning the thrombectomy. It can predetermine the best site for vascular access as well as anticipate any problems the operator is likely to face. Ideally, it can also determine which are the optimum tools and techniques to use, and prognosticate the chance of a successful recanalization or failed thrombectomy.

Historically, one of the earliest signs of an intracranial occlusion was the Hyperdense Middle Cerebral Artery Sign seen on a noncontrasted CT scan (Fig. 22.5). This correlated with a thrombus with a higher RBC content [44, 47, 62], although the proportion of fibrin, RBCs, and WBCs have all been shown to affect the thrombus density on a CT scan [44]. IV tPA has been shown to have be more effective with RBC-rich thrombi [63]. For endovascular thrombectomy, the literature available on CT thrombus density is conflicting especially with the older thrombectomy devices [32, 64, 65], although there is an association of stentrievers success with increased thrombus density [33]. RBC-rich thrombi can also be identified on MRI where the RBC in the thrombus induces a blooming artifact on GRE and SWI sequences. Longer and curved susceptibility vessel signs on MRI have been associated with reduced effectiveness of reperfusion therapies [66, 67].

Using thin-slice reconstruction, A non-contrasted CT can be used to estimate the thrombus length by minimizing partial volume averaging with adjacent lower density cerebrospinal fluid [68]. Another method of measuring the thrombus length is through the arterial filling defect on CT angiography. On a single phase CTA, the arterial filling defect is strongly dependent on the timing of imaging acquisition after the contrast and the presence of collaterals, which can allow the contrast to reach the distal end of the thrombus [69, 70]. In newer techniques such as the dynamic CT angiography or multiphasic CTA, this problem is less prominent as the delayed scans will allow the contrast time to reach the distal end of the thrombus [71]. As an alternative, the clot burden score is a semi-quantitative validated method of measuring clot burden on a single phase CTA, where points are subtracted for pre-specified vessel segments that are not opacified by contrast [72]. Longer and more proximally located thrombi are associated with worse clinical, imaging, and safety outcomes and are less successful recanalized by IV tPA [73, 74]. Longer thrombi have been shown to have better recanalization rates with aspiration thrombectomy when compared to IV tPA [74].

The perviousness of thrombus was determined by measuring the increase in Hounsfield unit (HU) on a CT scan before and after contrast administration. A study showed that a more pervious thrombus with an increase in HU $\geq$23 was associated with better recanalization, smaller infarct sizes and better functional outcome after IV tPA treatment [63, 71, 75]. A recent study done in vitro showed that fibrin-rich clots had a lower initial HU than RBC-rich clots but had a higher increase in HU after contrast was administered [76]. This imaging method can potentially be used to pre-determine clot characteristics and select devices more likely to capture such resistant clots, such as the later generation stentretrivers. This finding has yet to be replicated in vivo and will require clinical testing.

The angiographic pattern of occlusion can potentially help to determine the underlying pathology of the occlusion. A Korean group determined that an occlusion at the arterial bifurcation in an anterior circulation stroke (defined as a "branching type" occlusion) was more likely to be an embolic thrombus. Conversely an occlusion in the middle of the artery with clear distal visibility of all the branches

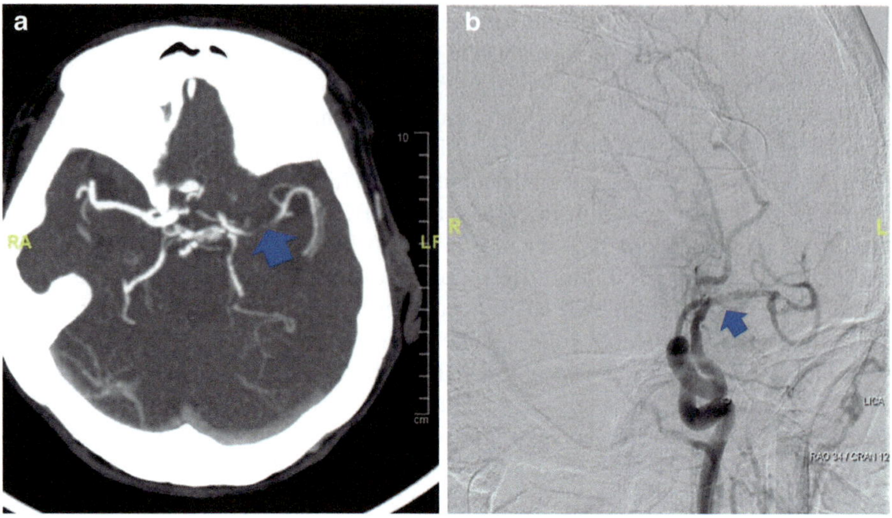

Fig. 22.6 (**a**) CT angiogram of an acute stroke with a gap indicating a "truncal" type occlusion of the MCA (arrow) with branches of the MCA bifurcation visible, rather than an "embolic" type where the branching portion would be unopacified. (**b**) The corresponding postthrombectomy angiogram showing an underlying atherosclerotic lesion (arrow)

was defined as a "truncal type" of occlusion (Fig. 22.6). This was associated with an underlying intracranial atherosclerotic cause of the occlusion. The authors noted that while truncal type occlusions were rarer, making up 12% of all angiographic occlusions, they were associated with a lower chance of stentriever's success. Branching type occlusions had an 80% chance of successful recanalization, compared to only 18.2% in truncal type occlusions. Truncal-type occlusion also had the propensity for immediate reocclusion after successful recanalization during stentriever-based endovascular procedures, which led to longer procedural times, more frequent adjunctive therapy use as well as poorer outcomes [77].

Good collaterals have been known to improve the chance of recanalization with IV tPA [78]. Good collateral circulation may also help in removing the thrombus in mechanical thrombectomy. It not only enhances thrombolytic penetration of the clot thereby softening it, but also breaks the water hammer effect of the systolic blood pressure and eliminating the pressure gradient across the clot. This enables easier withdrawal of the clot. A reflection of this was seen in the DAWN trial, which selected patients with good collaterals and had an 84% mTICI2b-3 rate [79].

Distal Emboli and Futile Revascularization

Secondary distal embolization to the same or previously unaffected territories is a feared complication during thrombectomy, which can result in poor outcomes even when the original thrombus is removed [80, 81]. There are various ways by which emboli can be generated during thrombectomy: Blood flow can break pieces off the clot. When the stentretriver is deployed, the struts can force pieces of the clot through the holes, thereby "cheese-grating" the clot using the mesh of the thrombectomy device. As the thrombus is withdrawn, the friction between the vessel wall and the thrombus may fragment it [81]. As the thrombus is withdrawn into a larger vessel from a smaller vessel, there can be a temporary loss of apposition between the stentretriver and the thrombus. Finally, the thrombus can be sheared off the sides of guide catheter if the lumen is too small as the thrombus is pulled into it.

Procedure-related embolic complications have been noted with various thrombectomy devices [82–85]. In the MR CLEAN study where a variety of different thrombectomy techniques were used, embolization to new territories was seen in 8.6% of the patients, which resulted in 5.6% developing new neurological deficits [1, 86]. For studies predominantly using stent retrievers, 5–22% had distal emboli with 0–7% of these into new vascular territories [4, 7, 87–90]. Older thrombectomy devices like the MERCI device or the initial iteration of the Penumbra system (Penumbra, Almeda, USA) fragmented the clot more and had worse outcomes compared to intra-arterial tPA thrombolysis, and therefore are no longer being used [86, 91–93].

Studies have shown that multiple distal emboli on the final angiographic runs are associated with worse functional outcomes [94]. However, in vitro bench studies have demonstrated that during a thrombectomy, the majority of clot fragments released are very small and not visible on standard digital subtracted angiography This means the actual incidence of distal emboli could be more than anticipated [91, 95]. These clots can block collateral flow to potentially salvageable tissue or even cause ischemia in a previously unaffected territory [87, 96–98]. The presence of these fragmented clots has been shown to be associated with worse clinical outcomes [96, 99].

Other causes of distal emboli are the use of conscious sedation, posterior circulation occlusions, and increased thrombus length. Patients who underwent thrombectomy with conscious sedation have more distal emboli than those under general anesthesia; this may be due to patient movement and its related technical difficulties [100]. Studies have shown that the use of balloon-guide catheter during a thrombectomy enables the operator to create a state of flow arrest, which reduces distal emboli and prevents emboli in new unaffected areas as well as interrupts the pressure gradient by breaking the forward force from the systemic blood pressure's water hammer effect and allows easier retrieval of the thrombus; this then translates into better functional outcomes [90, 101–103]. Posterior circulation occlusions are significantly associated with distal emboli likely due to the lack of flow arrest during such procedures [104]. Finally, the incidence of thromboembolic events into other vessels increases with the thrombus length. In in vitro experiments, the rate of thromboembolic events was 0% with 10-mm-long thrombi but increased to 7.4% with 20-mm thrombi and 14.8% with 40-mm thrombi [105].

A less obvious reason for futile revascularization is downstream injury caused by the reperfusion itself. Reperfusion into ischemic territory can activate the inflammatory pathway and produce a cascade of other factors, which may be detrimental to the brain. One such molecule is von Willebrand factor. We earlier described how it was associated with more organized clots, but it has also been linked to spontaneous thrombus formation in distal vessels. In the lab, blocking the function of von Willebrand factor in mice animal models was able to reduce damage due to stroke reperfusion [58, 106].

Solutions for Failed Thrombectomy

Patients who have an acute stroke but fail thrombectomy are prone to worse functional outcomes. Irrespective of the underlying cause, a rescue modality is necessary for such refractory cases. One such modality that has been used is intra-arterial infusion of glycoprotein IIb/IIIa inhibitor, which is commonly used as an adjunct in endovascular procedures to prevent thromboembolic complications and reocclusion of the vessel. Unfortunately, on its own, it appears relatively ineffective in acute stroke patients. In studies where mechanical thrombectomy had failed, a glycoprotein IIb/IIIa inhibitor achieved further successful recanalization in only 2.8–3.8% of cases [5, 107]. The decision to use glycoprotein IIb/IIIa inhibitors must also be tempered by the increased bleeding risk reported in studies using a combination of glycoprotein IIb/IIIa inhibitors and thrombolytics in stroke, as well as the poor results of the Abciximab in Emergency Treatment of Stroke Trial (AbESTT) [108–113].

Trifiban has been used as a strategy to treat recalcitrant cases where mechanical thrombectomy has failed [8]. When used intravenously in addition to mechanical thrombectomy or stenting, there was no improvement in the recanalization, but neither was there an increase in intracranial hemorrhage [114]. When it was used intra-arterially in conjunction with the next thrombectomy attempt, it appeared to prevent reocclusion after successful recanalization with no cases of symptomatic intracranial haemorrhage (ICH) [115]. This may be a viable strategy but needs to be validated in further clinical trials.

In the era before stent retrievers, recanalization of occluded intracranial arteries via stenting was initially used as an experimental treatment in AIS [112, 116–120], but this was quickly replaced by the newer superior thrombectomy devices and methods. Nonetheless, these early trials established that stenting in AIS with LVO could be a plausible method to restore the patency of vessels, which reocclude after thrombectomy.

Underlying intracranial atherosclerotic stenosis may render the occlusion refractory to recanalization with swift and immediate reocclusion once the stentretriver or aspiration device has been withdrawn. In such situations of recurrent occlusions, intracranial artery stent placement might be considered a feasible option. Initially, intracranial stenting was performed with off-label use of balloon-mounted cardiac stents [110, 111, 121, 122]. The problems with these stents are their rigidity, making navigation through the tortuous intracranial circulation difficult and prone to complications such as perforation [123, 124]. Levy et al. were the first to report the use of self-expandable stents in the setting of acute ischemic stroke [112]. The current iterations of intracranial self-expanding stents are made of nitinol and provide sufficient outward radial force at body temperatures to open up occluded vessels, yet are able to minimize the incidence of negative remodeling and in-stent restenosis that have been seen in the balloon mounted stents [112, 125].

Intracranial atherosclerotic stenosis is much more common in Asian patients and recently, a Korean series of patients have demonstrated a more favorable outcomes in the stented group than in the nonstented group of patients who failed thrombectomy (Fig. 22.7) [5]. Other case series reported good clinical outcomes with few complications using self-expanding stents such as the Enterprise self-expanding stent (Codman & Shurtleff, Raynham, Massachusetts), Neuroform (Stryker Neurovascular, Kalamazoo, Michigan), Solitaire FR and Wingspan stent (Stryker), or as a rescue treatment for failed thrombectomy patients [112, 116, 117, 126–128]. In a study, which compared permanent stenting with the Solitaire FR against other self-expanding stents, it managed to provide mTICI 2b–3 recanalization in 84.6% versus 78.6% of patient in whom mechanical thrombectomy had failed with a significantly shorter procedure time [129]. Another purported advantage of the Solitaire FR over other self-expandable stents is that it allows angiographic assessment of the patency of the vessel during its temporary placement before it is actually detached.

In another study, the author reported several patients where the Wingspan stenting was not able to navigate the tortuosity of cerebral vasculature. The author switched to the more navigable Enterprise stent, which was able to overcome this and be deployed at the occlusion site with good angiographic results. The author however mentioned that in this series, 50% of the patients required adjunctive angioplasty after deployment of the Enterprise stent, which the author attributed to the weaker radial force of the stent [119]. However is a series of patients from Sweden mostly using the Enterprise stent for rescue of failed thrombectomy, there was

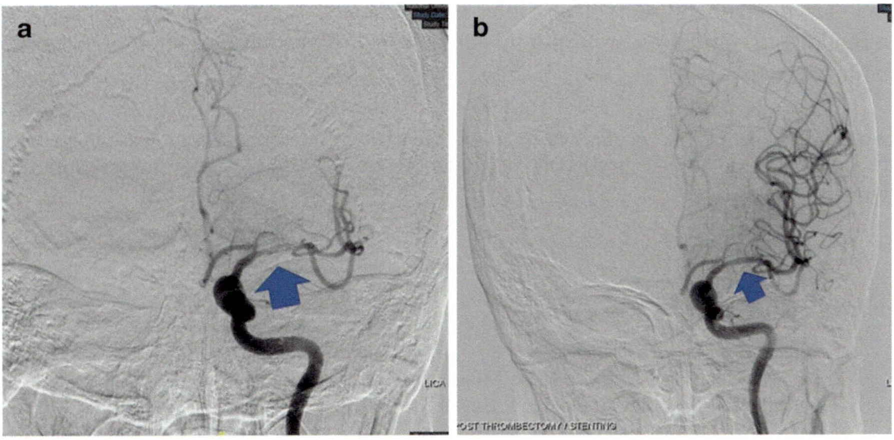

Fig. 22.7 (**a**) Post thrombectomy attempt, there is an underlying mid-MCA atherosclerotic stenosis seen on the final diagnostic angiogram, which keeps reoccluding after every pass. (**b**) Permanent stenting was performed under antiplatelet cover with TICI 3 recanalization

seldom a need for angioplasty after the stent was deployed. Over time the follow-up vessel imaging showed that the stent would gradually expand, and any stenosis tended to resolve itself [133]. For more distal occlusions, a series has shown that endovascular treatment with a Wingspan stent can be a safe potential solution for M2 occlusions [118]. However, it needs to be said that stenting in distal small intracranial arteries has a higher risk for vascular injury and subacute reocclusion or in-stent restenosis, this is exacerbated by the situation in an acute stroke where there is no opportunity to preload antiplatelet or test antiplatelet activity, and should be performed only when necessary and with some consideration of the risks [130, 131].

As with any other intracranial stents, dual antithrombotic therapy is recommended to prevent delayed thrombosis within the stent after rescue stenting for thrombectomy [132]. The optimum antiplatelet therapy after intracranial stenting is still controversial with no clear guidelines. There is nonetheless a higher potential risk of intracranial bleeding due to hemorrhagic conversion in the infarcted brain tissue and procedural complications [123]. A half-dose abciximab was safe and effective in a small series of patients from Sweden. In this series, three patients had abciximab used after treatment with IV tPA but did not lead to hemorrhage in these patients [133]. In another series of 42 patients, low-dose abciximab was associated with low risk of intracranial hemorrhage after permanent stenting for failed thrombectomy [134].

Conclusion

Acute stroke that is refractory to recanalization has poor outcomes with high dependency. There is an urgent need to develop techniques, medication, and devices that make it possible to more safely and efficiently remove these difficult clots. Ideally, this should be affordable with no need for extensive training so that it can be carried out in as many institutions as possible. The challenges highlighted here can serve as a roadmap to guide research into this area, which will translate into a high worldwide impact.

Acknowledgments We would like to thank Michael Gilvarry and David Vale at Neuravi/Cerenovus for use of their flow model images and Prof Simon De Meyer for the use of his clot histology images.

References

1. Jovin TG, Chamorro A, Cobo E, de Miquel MA, et al. Thrombectomy within 8 hours after symptom onset in ischemic stroke. N Engl J Med. 2015;372:2296–306.
2. Saver JL, Goyal M, Bonafe A, Diener HC, Levy EI, Pereira VM, et al. Stent-retriever thrombectomy after intravenous t-PA vs. t-PA alone in stroke. N Engl J Med. 2015;372:2285–95.
3. Goyal M, Demchuk AM, Menon BK, et al. Randomized assessment of rapid endovascular treatment of ischemic stroke. N Engl J Med. 2015;372:1019–30.

4. Berkhemer OA, Fransen PS, Beumer D, et al. A randomized trial of intraarterial treatment for acute ischemic stroke. N Engl J Med. 2015;372:11–20.
5. Baek JH, Kim BM, Kim DJ, Heo JH, Nam HS, Yoo J. Stenting as a rescue treatment after failure of mechanical thrombectomy for anterior circulation large artery occlusion. Stroke. 2016;47:2360–3.
6. Campbell BC, Mitchell PJ, Kleinig TJ, et al. Endovascular therapy for ischemic stroke with perfusion-imaging selection. N Engl J Med. 2015;372:1009–18.
7. Nogueira RG, Lutsep HL, Gupta R, et al. Trevo versus Merci retrievers for thrombectomy revascularisation of large vessel occlusions in acute ischaemic stroke (TREVO 2): a randomised trial. Lancet. 2012;380:1231–40.
8. Powers WJ, Derdeyn CP, Biller J, et al. 2015 American Heart Association/American Stroke Association focused update of the 2013 guidelines for the early management of patients with acute ischemic stroke regarding endovascular treatment: a guideline for healthcare professionals from the American Heart Association/American Stroke Association. Stroke. 2015;46:3020–35.
9. Saver JL, Jahan R, Levy EI, et al. Solitaire flow restoration device versus the Merci retriever in patients with acute ischaemic stroke (SWIFT): a randomised, parallel-group, non-inferiority trial. Lancet. 2012;380:1241–9.
10. Song D, Cho AH. Previous and recent evidence of endovascular therapy in acute ischemic stroke. Neurointervention. 2015;10:51–9.
11. Yoo AJ, Andersson T. Thrombectomy in acute ischemic stroke: challenges to procedural success. J Stroke. 2017;19(2):121–30.
12. Lam RC, Lin SC, DeRubertis B, Hynecek R, Kent KC, Faries PL. The impact of increasing age on anatomic factors affecting carotid angioplasty and stenting. J Vasc Surg. 2007;45:875–80.
13. Burzotta F, Nerla R, Pirozzolo G, et al. Clinical and procedural impact of aortic arch anatomic variants in carotid stenting procedures. Catheter Cardiovasc Interv. 2015;86:480–9.
14. Layton KF, Kallmes DF, Cloft HJ, Lindell EP, Cox VS. Bovine aortic arch variant in humans: clarification of a common misnomer. Am J Neuroradiol. 2006;27:1541–2.
15. Han HC. Twisted blood vessels: symptoms, etiology and biomechanical mechanisms. J Vasc Res. 2012;49:185–97.
16. Kaymaz Z, Nikoubashman O, Brockmann M, et al. Influence of carotid tortuosity on internal carotid artery access time in the treatment of acute ischemic stroke. Interv Neuroradiol. 2017;23:583–8. CrossRef Medline.
17. Schwaiger BJ, Gersing AS, Zimmer C, et al. The curved MCA: influence of vessel anatomy on recanalization results of mechanical thrombectomy after acute ischemic stroke. AJNR Am J Neuroradiol. 2015;36:971–6. CrossRef Medline.
18. Yamamoto S, Yamagami H, Todo K, et al. Correlation of middle cerebral artery tortuosity with successful recanalization using the Merci retrieval system with or without adjunctive treatments. Neurol Med Chir (Tokyo). 2014;54:113–9. CrossRef Medline.
19. Snelling BM, Sur S, Shah SS, et al. Transradial access: lessons learned from cardiology. J Neurointerv Surg. 2018;10:487–92. CrossRef Medline.
20. Mokin M, Snyder KV, Levy EI, et al. Direct carotid artery puncture access for endovascular treatment of acute ischemic stroke: technical aspects, advantages, and limitations. J Neurointerv Surg. 2015;7:108–13. CrossRef Medline.
21. Blanc R, Piotin M, Mounayer C, et al. Direct cervical arterial access for intracranial endovascular treatment. Neuroradiology. 2006;48:925–9. CrossRef Medline.
22. Bang OY. Intracranial atherosclerosis: current understanding and perspectives. J Stroke. 2014;16:27–35.
23. Holmstedt CA, Turan TN, Chimowitz MI. Atherosclerotic intracranial arterial stenosis: risk factors, diagnosis, and treatment. Lancet Neurol. 2013;12:1106–14.
24. Kim JS, Bonovich D. Research on intracranial atherosclerosis from the east and west: why are the results different? J Stroke. 2014;16:105–13.
25. Wong LK. Global burden of intracranial atherosclerosis. Int J Stroke. 2006;1:158–9.

26. Baek JH. Importance of truncal-type occlusion in stentriever-based thrombectomy for acute stroke. Neurology. 2016;87:1542–50.
27. Matias-Guiu JA, Serna-Candel C, Matias-Guiu J. Stroke etiology determines effectiveness of retrievable stents. J Neurointerv Surg. 2014;6:e11.
28. Jia B, Feng L, Liebeskind DS, et al. Mechanical thrombectomy and rescue therapy for intracranial large artery occlusion with underlying atherosclerosis. J Neurointerv Surg. 2018;10:746–50.
29. Lee JS, Hong JM, Lee KS, et al. Primary stent retrieval for acute intracranial large artery occlusion due to atherosclerotic disease. J Stroke. 2016;18:96–101. CrossRef Medline.
30. Kim EY, Yoo E, Choi HY, Lee JW, Heo JH. Thrombus volume comparison between patients with and without hyperattenuated artery sign on CT. AJNR Am J Neuroradiol. 2008;29:359–62.
31. Treurniet KM, Yoo AJ, Berkhemer OA, Lingsma HF, Boers AM, Fransen PS, et al. Clot burden score on baseline computerized tomographic angiography and intra-arterial treatment effect in acute ischemic stroke. Stroke. 2016;47:2972–8.
32. Spiotta AM, Vargas J, Hawk H, Turner R, Chaudry MI, Battenhouse H, et al. Hounsfield unit value and clot length in the acutely occluded vessel and time required to achieve thrombectomy, complications and outcome. J Neurointerv Surg. 2013;6:423–7.
33. Mokin M, Morr S, Natarajan SK, Lin N, Snyder KV, Hopkins LN, et al. Thrombus density predicts successful recanalization with Solitaire stent retriever thrombectomy in acute ischemic stroke. J Neurointerv Surg. 2014;7:104–7.
34. Jindal G, Miller T, Shivashankar R, Mitchell J, Stern BJ, Yarbrough K, et al. Relationship of thrombus length to number of stent retrievals, revascularization, and outcomes in acute ischemic stroke. J Vasc Interv Radiol. 2014;25:1549–57.
35. Soize S, Batista AL, Rodriguez RC, Trystram D, Tisserand M, Turc G, et al. Susceptibility vessel sign on T2* magnetic resonance imaging and recanalization results of mechanical thrombectomy with stent retrievers: a multicentre cohort study. Eur J Neurol. 2015;22:967–72.
36. Angermaier A, Michel P, Khaw AV, Kirsch M, Kessler C, Langner S. Intravenous thrombolysis and passes of thrombectomy as predictors for endovascular revascularization in ischemic stroke. J Stroke Cerebrovasc Dis. 2016;25:2488–95.
37. Mokin M, Levy EI, Siddiqui AH, Goyal M, Nogueira RG, Yavagal DR, et al. Association of clot burden score with radiographic and clinical outcomes following Solitaire stent retriever throm-bectomy: analysis of the SWIFT PRIME trial. J Neurointerv Surg. 2017;9:929–32.
38. Yoo AJ, Khatri P, Mocco J, Zaidat OO, Gupta R, Frei D, Lopes D, Shownkeen H, Berkhemer OA, Meyer D, Hak SS, Kuo SS, Buell H, Bose A, Sit SP, von Kummer R, THERAPY Trial Investigators. Impact of thrombus length on outcomes after intra-arterial aspiration thrombectomy in the THERAPY trial. Stroke. 2017;48(7):1895–900.
39. Gory B, Mazighi M, Blanc R, Endovascular Treatment in Ischemic Stroke (ETIS) Research Investigators, et al. Mechanical thrombectomy in basilar artery occlusion: influence of reperfusion on clinical outcome and impact of the first-line strategy (ADAPT vs stent retriever). J Neurosurg. 2018;12:1–10.
40. Consoli A, Rosi A, Coskun O, et al. Thrombectomy for M1-middle cerebral artery occlusion angiographic aspect of the arterial occlusion and recanalization: a preliminary observation. Stroke. 2018;49:1286–9. CrossRef Medline.
41. Marder VJ, Chute DJ, Starkman S, Abolian AM, Kidwell C, Liebeskind D, Ovbiagele B, Vinuela F, Duckwiler G, Jahan R, Vespa PM, Selco S, Rajajee V, Kim D, Sanossian N, Saver JL. Analysis of thrombi retrieved from cerebral arteries of patients with acute ischemic stroke. Stroke. 2006;37:2086–93.
42. Liebeskind DS, Sanossian N, Yong WH, Starkman S, Tsang MP, Moya AL, Zheng DD, Abolian AM, Kim D, Ali LK, Shah SH, Towfighi A, Ovbiagele B, Kidwell CS, Tateshima S, Jahan R, Duckwiler GR, Viñuela F, Salamon N, Villablanca JP, Vinters HV, Marder VJ, Saver JL. CT and MRI early vessel signs reflect clot composition in acute stroke. Stroke. 2011;42:1237–43.

43. Ahn SH, Hong R, Choo IS, Heo JH, Nam HS, Kang HG, et al. Histologic features of acute thrombi retrieved from stroke patients during mechanical reperfusion therapy. Int J Stroke. 2016;11:1036–44.
44. Liebeskind DS, et al. CT and MRI early vessel signs reflect clot composition in acute stroke. Stroke. 2011;42:1237–43.
45. Cline B, et al. O-027 Pathological analysis of extracted clots in embolectomy patients with acute ischaemic stroke. J Neurointerv Surg. 2013;5:A15–6.
46. Gunning GM, McArdle K, Mirza M, Duffy S, Gilvarry M, Brouwer PA. Clot friction variation with fibrin content; implications for resistance to thrombectomy. J Neurointerv Surg. 2018;10:34–8.
47. Brinjikji W, Duffy S, Burrows A, Hacke W, Liebeskind D, Majoie CE, et al. Correlation of imaging and histopathology of thrombi in acute ischemic stroke with etiology and outcome: a systematic review. J Neurointerv Surg. 2017;9:529–34.
48. Duffy S, Farrell M, McArdle K, Thornton J, Vale D, Rainsford E. Novel methodology to replicate clot analogs with diverse composition in acute ischemic stroke. J Neurointerv Surg. 2017;9:486–91.
49. Boeckh-Behrens T, Schubert M, Förschler A, Prothmann S, Kreiser K, Zimmer C, Riegger J, Bauer J, Neff F, Kehl V, Pelisek J, Schirmer L, Mehr M, Poppert H. The impact of histological clot composition in embolic stroke. Clin Neuroradiol. 2016;26(2):189–97.
50. French JE. The structure of natural and experimental thrombi. Ann R Coll Surg Engl. 1965;36:191–200.
51. Welch WH. The structure of white thrombi. Trans Path Soc Philadelphia. 1887;13:281.
52. Yuki I, Kan I, Vinters HV, Kim RH, Golshan A, Vinuela FA, Sayre JW, Murayama Y, Vinuela F. The impact of thromboemboli histology on the performance of a mechanical thrombectomy device. AJNR Am J Neuroradiol. 2012;33:643–8.
53. Martinod K, Wagner DD. Thrombosis: tangled up in NETs. Blood. 2014;123:2768–76.
54. Fuchs TA, Brill A, Duerschmied D, et al. Extracellular DNA traps promote thrombosis. Proc Natl Acad Sci U S A. 2010;107:15880–5.
55. Niesten JM, van der Schaaf IC, van Dam L, et al. Histopathologic composition of cerebral thrombi of acute stroke patients is correlated with stroke subtype and thrombus attenuation. PLoS One. 2014;9:e88882.
56. Laridan E, Denorme F, Desender L, François O, Andersson T, Deckmyn H, Vanhoorelbeke K, De Meyer SF. Neutrophil extracellular traps in ischemic stroke thrombi. Ann Neurol. 2017;82(2):223–32.
57. Denorme F, et al. ADAMTS13 destabilizes thrombi in a mouse model of thrombotic focal cerebral ischemia. J Thromb Haemost. 2015;13(Suppl 2):694–5.
58. De Meyer SF, et al. Von Willebrand factor: an emerging target in stroke therapy. Stroke. 2012;43:599–606.
59. Almekhlafi MA, Hu WY, Hill MD, Auer RN. Calcification and endothelialization of thrombi in acute stroke. Ann Neurol. 2008;64:344–8.
60. Dobrocky T, Piechowiak E, Cianfoni A, et al. Thrombectomy of calcified emboli in stroke: does histology of thrombi influence the effectiveness of thrombectomy? J Neurointerv Surg. 2018;10:345–50.
61. Judge C, Mello S, Bradley D, et al. A systematic review of the causes and management of ischaemic stroke caused by nontissue emboli. Stroke Res Treat. 2017;2017:7565702. CrossRef Medline.
62. Kirchhof K, Welzel T, Mecke C, Zoubaa S, Sartor K. Differentiation of white, mixed, and red thrombi: value of CT in estimation of the prognosis of thrombolysis phantom study. Radiology. 2003;228:126–30.
63. Santos EM, Dankbaar JW, Treurniet KM, Horsch AD, Roos YB, Kappelle LJ, et al. Permeable thrombi are associated with higher intravenous recombinant tissue-type plasminogen activator treatment success in patients with acute ischemic stroke. Stroke. 2016;47: 2058–65.

64. Moftakhar P, English JD, Cooke DL, et al. Density of thrombus on admission CT predicts revascularization efficacy in large vessel occlusion acute ischemic stroke. Stroke. 2013;44:243–5.
65. Froehler MT, Tateshima S, Duckwiler G, et al. The hyperdense vessel sign on CT predicts successful recanalization with the Merci device in acute ischemic stroke. J Neurointerv Surg. 2013;5:289–93.
66. Simons N, Mitchell P, Dowling R, Gonzales M, Yan B. Thrombus composition in acute ischemic stroke: a histopathological study of thrombus extracted by endovascular retrieval. J Neuroradiol. 2015;42:86–92.
67. Denorme F, Langhauser F, Desender L, et al. ADAMTS13-mediated thrombolysis of t-PA-resistant occlusions in ischemic stroke in mice. Blood. 2016;127:2337–45.
68. Riedel CH, Jensen U, Rohr A, et al. Assessment of thrombus in acute middle cerebral artery occlusion using thin-slice nonenhanced computed tomography reconstructions. Stroke. 2010;41:1659–64.
69. Mortimer AM, Little DH, Minhas KS, Walton ER, Renowden SA, Bradley MD. Thrombus length estimation in acute ischemic stroke: a potential role for delayed contrast enhanced CT. J Neurointerv Surg. 2014;6:244–8.
70. Kamalian S, Morais LT, Pomerantz SR, et al. Clot length distribution and predictors in anterior circulation stroke: implications for intra-arterial therapy. Stroke. 2013;44:3553–6.
71. Mishra SM, Dykeman J, Sajobi TT, et al. Early reperfusion rates with IV tPA are determined by CTA clot characteristics. AJNR Am J Neuroradiol. 2014;35:2265–72.
72. Tan IYL, Demchuk AM, Hopyan J, et al. CT angiography clot burden score and collateral score: correlation with clinical and radiologic outcomes in acute middle cerebral artery infarct. AJNR Am J Neuroradiol. 2009;30:525–31.
73. Seners P, Turc G, Maïer B, Mas J-L, Oppenheim C, Baron J-C. Incidence and predictors of early recanalization after intravenous thrombolysis: a systematic review and meta-analysis. Stroke. 2016;47:2409–12.
74. Mocco J, Zaidat OO, von Kummer R, et al. Aspiration thrombectomy after intravenous alteplase versus intravenous alteplase alone. Stroke. 2016;47:2331–8.
75. Santos EMM, Marquering HA, den Blanken MD, et al. Thrombus permeability is associated with improved functional outcome and recanalization in patients with ischemic stroke. Stroke. 2016;47:732–41.
76. Borggrefe J, et al. Differentiation of clot composition using conventional and dual-energy computed tomography. Clin Neuroradiol. 2018;28:515–22.
77. Khatri P, Abruzzo T, Yeatts SD, et al. Good clinical outcome after ischemic stroke with successful revascularization is time-dependent. Neurology. 2009;73:1066–72.
78. Yeo LLL, Paliwal P, Teoh HL, Seet RC, Chan BP, Ting E, Venketasubramanian N, Leow WK, Wakerley B, Kusama Y, Rathakrishnan R, Sharma VK. Assessment of intracranial collaterals on CT-Angiography in anterior circulation acute ischemic stroke. AJNR Am J Neuroradiol. 2015;36(2):289–94.
79. Nogueira RG, Jadhav AP, Haussen DC, et al. Thrombectomy 6 to 24 hours after stroke with a mismatch between deficit and infarct. N Engl J Med. 2018;378:11–21.
80. Chueh JY, Kühn AL, Puri AS, et al. Reduction in distal emboli with proximal flow control during mechanical thrombectomy: a quantitative in vitro study. Stroke. 2013;44:1396–401.
81. Mordasini P, Frabetti N, Gralla J, et al. In vivo evaluation of the first dedicated combined flow-restoration and mechanical thrombectomy device in a swine model of acute vessel occlusion. AJNR Am J Neuroradiol. 2011;32:294–300.
82. Turk AS, Frei D, Fiorella D, et al. ADAPT FAST study: a direct aspiration first pass technique for acute stroke thrombectomy. J Neurointerv Surg. 2014;6(4):260–4.
83. Tomsick TA, Khatri P, Jovin T, et al. Equipoise among recanalization strategies. Neurology. 2010;74:1069–76.
84. Mokin M, Kass-Hout T, Levy EI. Solitaire FR—a promising new device for acute ischemic stroke treatment. World Neurosurg. 2012;78:557–8.

85. Dorn F, Stehle S, Lockau H, et al. Endovascular treatment of acute intracerebral artery occlusions with the solitaire stent: single-centre experience with 108 recanalization procedures. Cerebrovasc Dis. 2012;34:70–7.
86. Furlan A, Higashida R, Wechsler L, et al. Intra-arterial prourokinase for acute ischemic stroke the PROACT II study: a randomized controlled trial prolyse in acute cerebral thromboembolism. JAMA. 1999;282:2003–11.
87. Akins PT, Amar AP, Pakbaz RS, et al. Complications of endovascular treatment for acute stroke in the SWIFT Trial with Solitaire and Merci devices. AJNR Am J Neuroradiol. 2014;35:524–8.
88. Gascou G, Lobotesis K, Machi P, et al. Stent retrievers in acute ischemic stroke: complications and failures during the perioperative period. AJNR Am J Neuroradiol. 2014;35:734–40.
89. Nguyen TN, Malisch T, Castonguay AC, et al. Balloon guide catheter improves revascularization and clinical outcomes with the Solitaire device: analysis of the North American Solitaire Acute Stroke Registry. Stroke. 2014;45:141–5.
90. Mazur MD, Kilburg C, Park MS, Taussky P. Patterns and clinical impact of angiographically visible distal emboli during thrombectomy with solitaire for acute ischemic stroke. Neurosurgery. 2016;78:242–50.
91. Penumbra Pivotal Stroke Trial Investigators. The penumbra pivotal stroke trial: safety and effectiveness of a new generation of mechanical devices for clot removal in intracranial large vessel occlusive disease. Stroke. 2009;40:2761–8.
92. Smith WS, Sung G, Saver J, et al. Mechanical thrombectomy for acute ischemic stroke: final results of the multi MERCI trial. Stroke. 2008;39:1205–12.
93. Ogawa A, Mori E, Minematsu K, et al. Randomized trial of intraarterial infusion of urokinase within 6 hours of middle cerebral artery stroke: the middle cerebral artery embolism local fibrinolytic intervention trial (MELT) Japan. Stroke. 2007;38:2633–9.
94. Gratz PP, Schroth G, Gralla J, et al. Whole-brain susceptibility-weighted thrombus imaging in stroke: fragmented thrombi predict worse outcome. AJNR Am J Neuroradiol. 2015;36:1277–82.
95. Chueh JY, Wakhloo AK, Gounis MJ. Effectiveness of mechanical endovascular thrombectomy in a model system of cerebrovascular occlusion. AJNR Am J Neuroradiol. 2012;33:1998–2003.
96. Kurre W, Vorlaender K, Aguilar-Perez M, Schmid E, Bazner H, Henkes H. Frequency and relevance of anterior cerebral artery embolism caused by mechanical thrombectomy of middle cerebral artery occlusion. AJNR Am J Neuroradiol. 2013;34:1606–11.
97. Soize S, Barbe C, Kadziolka K, et al. Predictive factors of outcome and hemorrhage after acute ischemic stroke treated by mechanical thrombectomy with a stent-retriever. Neuroradiology. 2013;55:977–87.
98. Todo A, Minaeian A, Sahni R, et al. Incidence and outcome of procedural distal emboli using the penumbra thrombectomy for acute stroke. J Neurointerv Surg. 2013;5:135–8.
99. Costalat V, Lobotesis K, Machi P, et al. Prognostic factors related to clinical outcome following thrombectomy in ischemic stroke (RECOST study). 50 patients prospective study. Eur J Radiol. 2012;81:4075–82.
100. Maegerlein C, Mönch S, Boeckh-Behrens T, et al. PROTECT: PRoximal balloon Occlusion TogEther with direCt Thrombus aspiration during stent retriever thrombectomy – evaluation of a double embolic protection approach in endovascular stroke treatment. J Neurointerv Surg. 2018;10:751–5.
101. Gralla J, Schroth G, Remonda L, et al. A dedicated animal model for mechanical thrombectomy in acute stroke. AJNR Am J Neuroradiol. 2006;27:1357–61.
102. Spiotta AM, Chaudry MI, Hui FK, Turner RD, Kellogg RT, Turk AS. Evolution of thrombectomy approaches and devices for acute stroke: a technical review. J Neurointerv Surg. 2015;7:2–7.
103. Brinjikji W, Starke RM, Murad MH, et al. Impact of balloon guide catheter on technical and clinical outcomes: a systematic review and meta-analysis. J Neurointerv Surg. 2018;10:335–9.

104. Yeo LL, et al. Posterior circulation occlusions may be associated with distal emboli during thrombectomy. Clin Neuroradiol. 2019;29(3):425–33. https://doi.org/10.1007/s00062-018-0679-z.
105. Gralla J, et al. Occlusion length is a crucial determinant of efficiency and complication rate in thrombectomy for acute ischemic stroke. AJNR Am J Neuroradiol. 2008;29:247–52.
106. De Meyer SF, et al. Binding of von Willebrand factor to collagen and glycoprotein Ibalpha, but not to glycoprotein IIb/IIIa, contributes to ischemic stroke in mice–brief report. Arterioscler Thromb Vasc Biol. 2010;30:1949–51.
107. Baracchini C, Farina F, Soso M, Viaro F, Favaretto S, Palmieri A, Kulyk C, Ballotta E, Nico L, Cester G, Causin F. Stentriever thrombectomy failure: a challenge in stroke management. World Neurosurg. 2017;103:57–64. https://doi.org/10.1016/j.wneu.2017.03.070.
108. Adams HP Jr, Effron MB, Torner J, Dávalos A, Frayne J, Teal P, Leclerc J, Oemar B, Padgett L, Barnathan ES, Hacke W, AbESTT-II Investigators. Emergency administration of abciximab for treatment of patients with acute ischemic stroke: results of an international phase III trial: Abciximab in Emergency Treatment of Stroke Trial (AbESTT-II). Stroke. 2008;39:87–99.
109. Eckert B, Koch C, Thomalla G, Kucinski T, Grzyska U, Roether J, Alfke K, Jansen O, Zeumer H. Aggressive therapy with intravenous abciximab and intra-arterial rtPA and additional PTA/stenting improves clinical outcome in acute vertebrobasilar occlusion: combined local fibrinolysis and intravenous abciximab in acute vertebrobasilar stroke treatment (FAST): results of a multicenter study. Stroke. 2005;36:1160–5.
110. Levy EI, Ecker RD, Horowitz MB, Gupta R, Hanel RA, Sauvageau E, Jovin TG, Guterman LR, Hopkins LN. Stent-assisted intracranial recanalization for acute stroke: early results. Neurosurgery. 2006;58:458–63.
111. Sauvageau E, Samuelson RM, Levy EI, Jeziorski AM, Mehta RA, Hopkins LN. Middle cerebral artery stenting for acute ischemic stroke after unsuccessful Merci retrieval. Neurosurgery. 2007;60:701–6.
112. Levy EI, Mehta R, Gupta R, Hanel RA, Chamczuk AJ, Fiorella D, Woo HH, Albuquerque FC, Jovin TG, Horowitz MB, Hopkins LN. Selfexpanding stents for recanalization of acute cerebrovascular occlusions. AJNR Am J Neuroradiol. 2007;28:816–22.
113. Kellert L, Hametner C, Rohde S, et al. Endovascular stroke therapy: tirofiban is associated with risk of fatal intracerebral hemorrhage and poor outcome. Stroke. 2013;44:1453–5.
114. Siebler M, Hennerici MG, Schneider D, von Reutern GM, Seitz RJ, Rother J, Witte OW, Hamann G, Junghans U, Villringer A, Fiebach JB. Safety of tirofiban in acute ischemic stroke: the SaTIS trial. Stroke. 2011;42:2388–92.
115. Kang DH, Kim YW, Hwang YH, Park SP, Kim YS, Baik SK. Instant reocclusion following mechanical thrombectomy of in situ thromboocclusion and the role of low-dose intra-arterial tirofiban. Cerebrovasc Dis. 2014;37(5):350–5.
116. Zaidat OO, Wolfe T, Hussain SI, et al. Interventional acute ischemic stroke therapy with intracranial self-expanding stent. Stroke. 2008;39:2392–5.
117. Brekenfeld C, Schroth G, Mattle HP, et al. Stent placement in acute cerebral artery occlusion: use of a self-expandable intracranial stent for acute stroke treatment. Stroke. 2009;40:847–52.
118. Sung SM, Lee TH, Lee SW, Cho HJ, Park KH, Jung DS. Emergent intracranial stenting for acute M2 occlusion of middle cerebral artery. Clin Neurol Neurosurg. 2014;119:110–5.
119. Dumont TM, Natarajan SK, Eller JL, et al. Primary stenting for acute ischemic stroke using the Enterprise vascular reconstruction device: early results. J Neurointerv Surg. 2014;6(5):363–72.
120. Kulcsár Z, Bonvin C, Lovblad KO, Gory B, Yilmaz H, Sztajzel R, Rufenacht D. Use of the enterprise™ intracranial stent for revascularization of large vessel occlusions in acute stroke. Clin Neuroradiol. 2010;20(1):54–60.
121. Ramee SR, Subramanian R, Felberg RA, McKinley KL, Jenkins JS, Collins TJ, Dawson RC, White CJ. Catheter-based treatment for patients with acute ischemic stroke ineligible for intravenous thrombolysis. Stroke. 2004;35:e109–11.
122. Gupta R, Vora NA, Horowitz MB, Tayal AH, Hammer MD, Uchino K, Levy EI, Wechsler LR, Jovin TG. Multimodal reperfusion therapy for acute ischemic stroke: factors predicting vessel recanalization. Stroke. 2006;37:986–90.

123. Qureshi AI, Siddiqui AM, Kim SH, Hanel RA, Xavier AR, Kirmani JF, Suri MF, Boulos AS, Hopkins LN. Re-occlusion of recanalized arteries during intra-arterial thrombolysis for acute ischemic stroke. AJNR Am J Neuroradiol. 2004;25:322–8.
124. Fiorella D, Albuquerque FC, Deshmukh VR, et al. In-stent stenosis as a delayed complication of Neuroform stent-supported coil embolization of an incidental carotid terminus aneurysm. AJNR Am J Neuroradiol. 2004;25:1764–7.
125. Henkes H, Miloslavski E, Lowens S, Reinartz J, Liebig T, Kühne D. Treatment of intracranial atherosclerotic stenoself-expandable stent with balloon dilatation and self-expanding stent deployment (WingSpan). Neuroradiology. 2005;47:222–8.
126. Levy EI, Siddiqui AH, Crumlish A, et al. First Food and Drug Administration- approved prospective trial of primary intracranial stenting for acute stroke: SARIS (stent-assisted recanalization in acute ischemic stroke). Stroke. 2009;40:3552–6.
127. Levy EI, Rahman M, Khalessi AA, et al. Midterm clinical and angiographic follow-up for the first Food and Drug Administration-approved prospective, single-arm trial of primary stenting for stroke: SARIS (Stent-Assisted Recanalization for Acute Ischemic Stroke). Neurosurgery. 2011;69:915–20.
128. Gonzalez LF, Jabbour P, Tjoumakaris S, et al. Temporary endovascular bypass: rescue technique during mechanical thrombolysis. Neurosurgery. 2012;70:245–52.
129. Woo HG, et al. Feasibility of permanent stenting with solitaire FR as a rescue treatment for the reperfusion of acute intracranial artery occlusion. AJNR Am J Neuroradiol. 2018;39:331–6.
130. Sugiura Y, Yamagami H, Sakai N, Yoshimura S, Committee of Recovery by Endovascular Salvage for Cerebral Ultra-acute Embolism (RESCUE)-Japan Study Group. Predictors of symptomatic intracranial hemorrhage after endovascular therapy in acute ischemic stroke with large vessel occlusion. J Stroke Cerebrovasc Dis. 2017;26(4):766–71.
131. Hussain MS, Lin R, Moskowitz S, Bain M, Gonugunta V, Rasmussen PA, et al. Symptomatic delayed reocclusion after initial successful revascularization in acute ischemic stroke. J Stroke Cerebrovasc Dis. 2010;19:36–9.
132. Bose A, Hartmann M, Henkes H, et al. A novel, self-expanding, nitinol stent in medically refractory intracranial atherosclerotic stenoses: the Wingspan study. Stroke. 2007;38:1531–7.
133. Cornelissen SA, et al. Intracranial stenting after failure of thrombectomy with the emboTrap® device. Clin Neuroradiol. 2019;29:677–83. https://doi.org/10.1007/s00062-018-0697-x.
134. Delgado Acosta F. Intracranial stents in the endovascular treatment of acute ischemic stroke. Radiologia. 2017;59:218–25.

Chapter 23
Challenges in Thrombectomy: Impossible Aortic Arches and Tortuous Vessels

Jaims Lim, Muhammad Waqas, Kunal Vakharia, and Adnan H. Siddiqui

Abbreviations

ADAPT A direct aspiration first-pass technique
AIS Acute ischemic stroke
BCA Brachiocephalic artery
CCA Common carotid artery
CT Computed tomography
DI Divergence index
ICA Internal carotid artery
MR Magnetic resonance
rtPA Recombinant tissue plasminogen activator
TI Tortuosity index

Introduction

The goal of endovascular treatment of acute ischemic stroke (AIS) is to achieve rapid, safe, and effective arterial recanalization of large intracranial vessel occlusions. The likelihood of recanalization with intravenous thrombolysis using

J. Lim · M. Waqas · K. Vakharia
Department of Neurosurgery, Jacobs School of Medicine and Biomedical Sciences, University at Buffalo, Buffalo, NY, USA

Department of Neurosurgery, Gates Vascular Institute at Kaleida Health, Buffalo, NY, USA

A. H. Siddiqui (✉)
Department of Neurosurgery, Gates Vascular Institute at Kaleida Health, Buffalo, NY, USA

Departments of Neurosurgery and Radiology, Jacobs School of Medicine and Biomedical Sciences, University at Buffalo, Buffalo, NY, USA

Jacobs Institute, Buffalo, NY, USA
e-mail: asiddiqui@ubns.com

F. K. Hui et al. (eds.), *12 Strokes*, https://doi.org/10.1007/978-3-030-56857-3_23

recombinant tissue plasminogen activator (rtPA) is about 46.2% [1]. Since 2014, the results of several randomized controlled trials have confirmed the benefit of mechanical thrombectomy for large-vessel occlusions in the anterior circulation, shaping current AIS management [2]. Techniques including a direct aspiration first-pass technique (ADAPT) and the use of stent retrievers has significantly increased the likelihood of recanalization with mechanical thrombectomy. However, the neurointerventionist must also be aware of the challenges in accessing, maintaining, and supporting catheters while negotiating difficult aortic arches and tortuous vasculature. In this chapter, we describe the different variations of the aortic arch anatomy and discuss strategies to overcome the tortuosity of the arch and associated vessels to gain rapid access to intracranial vasculature for mechanical thrombectomy.

Diagnosis

Ischemic stroke therapy relies heavily on imaging modalities to help determine viable brain tissue. Computed tomography (CT) perfusion imaging and magnetic resonance (MR) perfusion imaging are important diagnostic tools in establishing an understanding of cerebral vascular supply, reserve, and viable penumbra in cases of intracranial occlusive disease. CT perfusion imaging allows quick assessment of normal and ischemic cerebral territories based on cerebral blood volume and time-to-peak blood flow as well as providing 3-dimensional reconstructions of the cerebral and extracranial vasculature, including the aortic arch, which may indicate large-vessel cutoffs due to occlusion and indicate vessel tortuosity. When such occlusions are identified, neuroendovascular treatments are often pursued. MR perfusion can provide similar information but in the setting of AIS is reserved for cases in which CT perfusion imaging is not possible.

Preprocedure Imaging

CT angiography and magnetic resonance (MR) angiography are crucial in the assessment of aortic arch aberrancies and tortuosity of the vasculature when mechanical thrombectomy is a consideration for AIS treatment. They not only highlight the spatial organization of extracranial and intracranial vessels, but also they help the interventionists to assess the severity of the stenosis (occlusion), both of which become very important considerations when trying to obtain endovascular access through the aorta and the carotid and vertebral arteries.

Development of the Aortic Arch

The primitive aorta first begins to take shape on day 21 of gestation with the formation of the endocardial tube [3]. Two ventral and dorsal segments of the aorta bridge to form six pharyngeal arches that gradually appear and regress in cephalocaudal order. During development, the first and second arches regress by the fourth week of gestation to give rise to the maxillary and hyoid or stapedial arteries, respectively [3]. During the time of first and second pharyngeal arch regression, the fourth, fifth, and sixth arches also begin to form and grow [3]. The third pharyngeal arch ultimately regresses to form the common carotid artery (CCA) and proximal cervical portions of the internal carotid artery (ICA), and the fourth forms the final adult aortic arch [3]. The fifth pharyngeal arch completely regresses without forming any structures, while the sixth arch forms the ductus arteriosus and central pulmonary arteries [3].

Types of Aortic Arches

Congenital aortic arch variants are separated into three types: left-sided, right-sided, and double aortic arches. Each type is associated with specific branching patterns of the great vessels. Aortic sidedness is assigned and based on which bronchus, left or right, the aortic arch crosses over. The aortic arch forms with various regressions and remnant vessels in the fourth aortic arch, which bridges the primitive dorsal and ventral aorta. Different anomalies or variations of the aortic arch are shown in Figs. 23.1, 23.2, and 23.3.

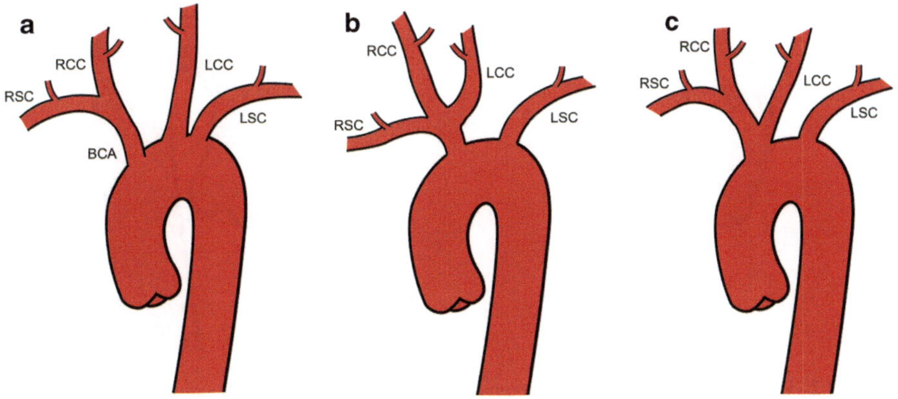

Fig. 23.1 (**a**) Common arch. (**b**) and (**c**) are two bovine arch anomalies. Abbreviations: BCA, brachiocephalic artery; LCC, left common carotid artery; LSC, left subclavian artery; RCC, right common carotid artery; RSC, right subclavian artery. (© University at Buffalo Neurosurgery)

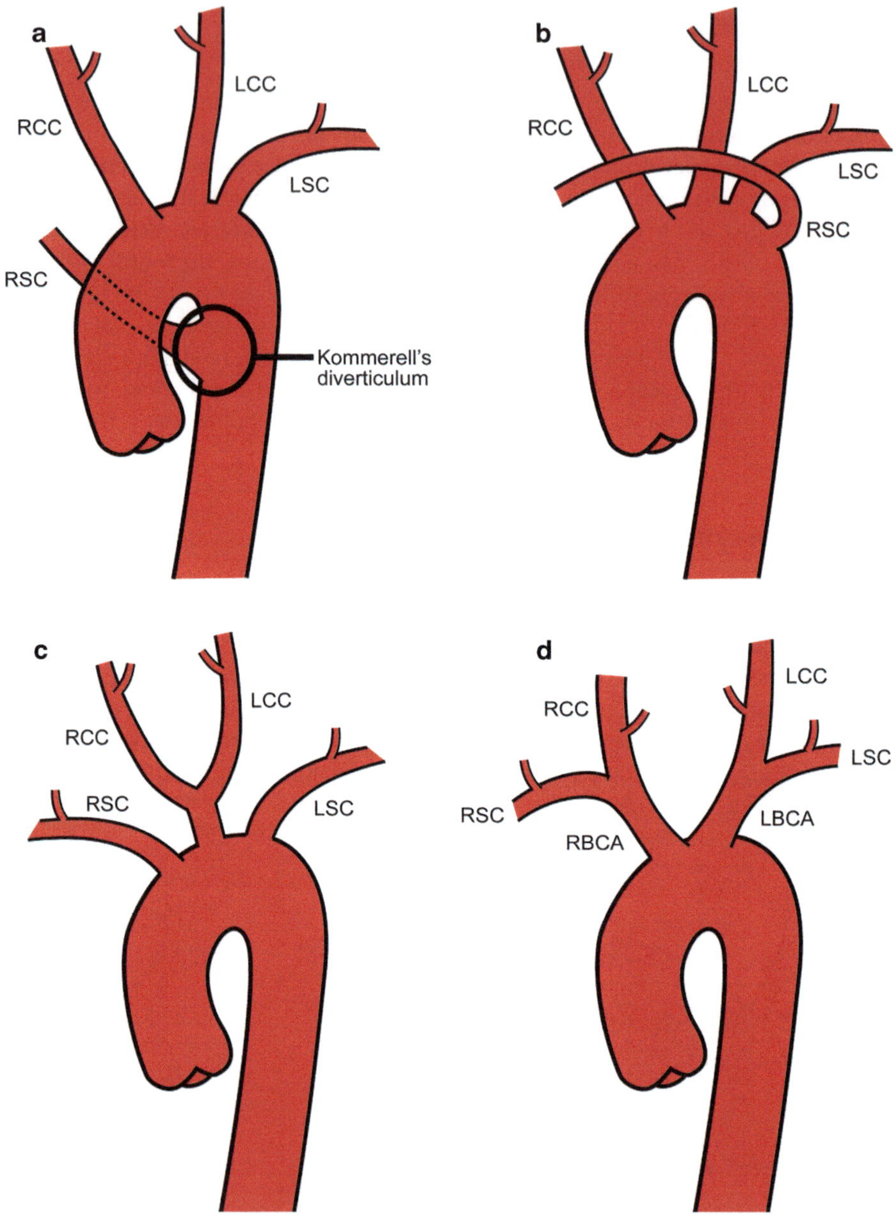

Fig. 23.2 Different variations in the anatomy of the left aortic arch. (**a**) Kommerell's diverticulum (circled) with an aberrant right subclavian artery. (**b**) Aberrant right subclavian artery. (**c**) Common origin of both common carotid arteries. (**d**) Bilateral brachiocephalic arteries. Abbreviations: LBCA, left brachiocephalic artery; LCC, left common carotid artery; LSC, left subclavian artery; RBCA, right brachiocephalic artery; RCC, right common carotid artery; RSC, right subclavian artery. (© University at Buffalo Neurosurgery)

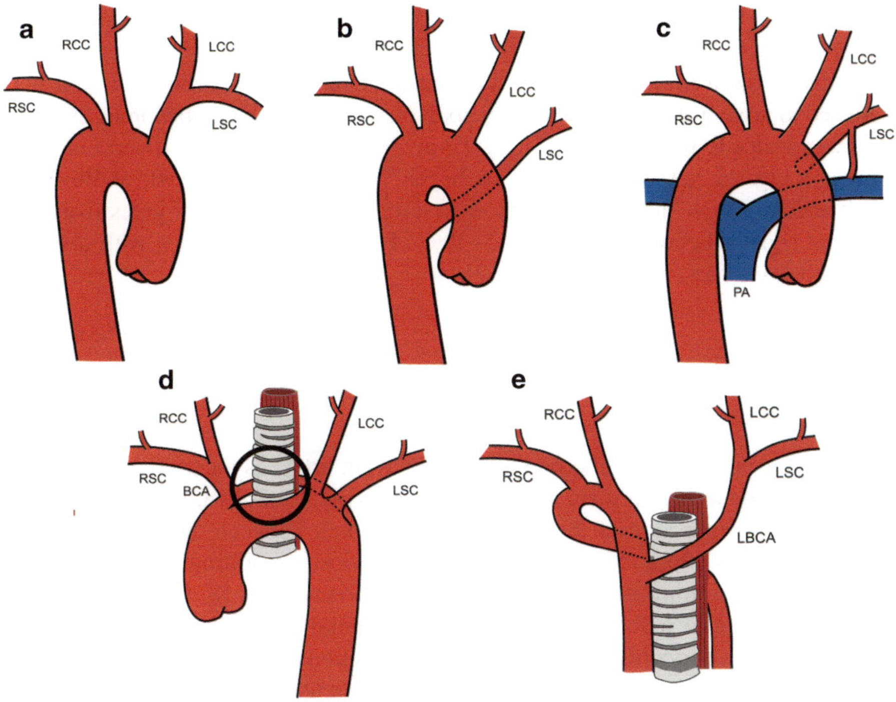

Fig. 23.3 (**a**) Right aortic arch with mirror image. (**b**) Aberrant left subclavian artery. (**c**) Isolated subclavian artery. (**d**) Double aortic arch with a vascular ring around the trachea and esophagus (*circled*). (**e**) Circumflex aortic arch. Abbreviations: BCA, brachiocephalic artery; LCC, left common carotid artery; LSC, Left subclavian artery; PA, pulmonary artery; RCC, right common carotid artery; RSC, right subclavian artery. (© University at Buffalo Neurosurgery)

The most common aortic arch is the left aortic arch (present in 70–80% of patients undergoing CT scanning for various reasons) (Fig. 23.1a), which results from the regression of the distal right fourth pharyngeal arch between the subclavian artery and the descending aorta, eliminating the right ductus arteriosus and right intersegmental artery. The remainder of the proximal fourth pharyngeal arch forms the proximal end of the right subclavian artery, and the left fourth pharyngeal arch forms the definitive aortic arch. The left subclavian artery originates entirely from the left seventh intersegmental artery with the left patent or ductus arteriosus bridging the proximal left pulmonary artery and the aorta just adjacent to the left subclavian artery [4].

Several variants of the left-sided aortic arches persist, with the most common being the left CCA arising directly from (in 9% of cases) or having a common origin with (in 13%) the right brachiocephalic artery, which is commonly referred to as the "bovine-type arch" (Fig. 23.1b, c) Another relatively common variant includes the left vertebral artery, which arises from the aortic arch proximal to the left subclavian artery (in 5–6% of cases) [5, 6].

Left Aortic Arch with Diverticulum of Kommerell

The diverticulum of Kommerell is a remnant of the dorsal aortic arch, and it is believed to arise from a persistent right sixth pharyngeal arch that becomes the right ductus arteriosus in most individuals (Fig. 23.2a). Kommerell's diverticulum is shown in Fig. 23.2a [7]. It is a retroesophageal outpouching that exists at the origin of an aberrant right subclavian artery with left aortic arches, and it gives rise to an aberrant right subclavian artery in 15–30% of all left aortic arches with aberrant right subclavian arteries (Fig. 23.2a) [7].

Left Aortic Arch with Aberrant Right Subclavian Artery

A left aortic arch with an aberrant right subclavian artery is a common congenital anomaly of the aortic arch (in 0.5–2% of cases) (Fig. 23.2b) [8, 9]. This anomaly occurs due to regression of the right pharyngeal arch between the right CCA and subclavian artery, eliminating the right ductus arteriosus, resulting in the distal right dorsal aorta becoming the proximal right subclavian artery [8, 9]. This anomaly sometimes may be associated with other congenital anomalies including aortic coarctation, patent ductus arteriosus, ventricular septal defect, and carotid or vertebral artery anomalies. Patients with this anomaly are usually asymptomatic but can at times have esophageal compression [8, 9]. Furthermore, patients with trisomy 21 (Down syndrome) have a high prevalence of this aberrancy (in 35%) [8, 9].

Right Aortic Arch with Aberrant Brachiocephalic Artery

This is a rare anomaly that results from regression of the fourth pharyngeal arch between the ascending aorta and the left CCA with a resultant persistent left dorsal aortic root and ductus arteriosus [7, 10]. Such a regression results in the development of the following aortic vessels, from right to left: the right CCA, right subclavian artery, and the left brachiocephalic artery; the aberrant brachiocephalic artery course left and posteriorly to the esophagus [7].

Right Aortic Arch with Mirror-Image Branching of the Arch Vessels

A right aortic arch with mirror-image branching of the arch is the second most common right aortic arch that results from interruption of the left pharyngeal arch during development, causing separation of the descending aorta and left subclavian artery [10]. Its incidence is 0.05–0.1% in normal population [11]. This creates a right aortic arch with three branches from left to right: a left brachiocephalic artery, a right CCA, and a right subclavian artery (Fig. 23.3a) [10]. This anomaly is commonly associated with a congenital heart disease in 98% of cases, usually Tetralogy of Fallot, truncus arteriosus, tricuspid atresia, and/or transposition of the great arteries with pulmonary valve stenosis [10].

Right Aortic Arch with Aberrant Left Subclavian Artery

Most common among right aortic arch variants is a right aortic arch with an aberrant left subclavian artery (Fig. 23.3b). The incidence in the general population is 0.025–0.5%. This is often an isolated anomaly that results from regression of the left arch between the left CCA and subclavian artery [7, 10]. This results in the proximal portion of the left arch to develop into the left CCA, while the distal portion of the left arch persists as an enlargement, interchangeably known as the diverticulum of Kommerell (as mentioned above) [7, 10]. From this diverticulum, the left subclavian artery arises at the borders of the right arch and descending aorta [7, 10].

Right Aortic Arch with Isolation of the Left Subclavian Artery

The rarest of the right aortic arch aberrancies is a right aortic arch with an isolated left subclavian artery, which results from interruption and regression of the left arch at two levels between the left CCA and left subclavian artery and distal attachment of the left ductus arteriosus [7, 12]. The proximal portion of the left arch forms the left CCA as the first branch of the right aortic arch followed by the right CCA and right subclavian artery (Fig. 23.3c) [7, 12]. This results in the left subclavian artery branching off the left pulmonary artery through the left ductus arteriosus [7, 12].

Double Aortic Arch

A double aortic arch results from the right and left pharyngeal arches failing to connect. This results in each arch giving rise to separate pairs of carotid and subclavian arteries [3]. Typically, only one ductus arteriosus persists from the sixth pharyngeal arch in a double aortic arch. Clinically, this anomaly is the most common cause of a symptomatic vascular ring due to completely encircling the trachea and esophagus (Fig. 23.3d) [3]. The ascending aorta divides and reunites, forming a circle around the esophagus and trachea. Infants with this congenital vascular anatomy present with wheezing, stridor, and dysphagia often worsened with tachypnea [3]. A double aortic arch is rarely associated with congenital heart disease, unlike a right aortic arch with mirror-imaging, which is usually associated with Tetralogy of Fallot [3].

Circumflex Aortic Arch

A circumflex aortic arch is also known as a right aortic arch with a left descending aorta and left ductus arteriosus. Rather than crossing the subclavian artery, the aortic arch crosses over the midline posteriorly to the esophagus above the carina (Fig. 23.3e). This deviant anatomy is due to one of two regressions during development [3, 10]. First is the regression of the left dorsal aorta between the left carotid and left subclavian arteries, which results in the formation of a circumflex aorta with an aberrant left subclavian artery. Second, there can be regression of the left fourth pharyngeal arch between the left subclavian artery and the left ductus arteriosus.

There are two possible branching patterns with a circumflex aorta depending on whether the left subclavian artery is aberrant [10]. With no aberrant left subclavian artery, the first vessel ascending from the arch is the left brachiocephalic followed by the right carotid artery and the right subclavian artery, respectively. In the presence of an aberrant left subclavian artery, the first ascending vessel is the left carotid artery, followed by the right carotid artery, right subclavian artery, and lastly, the aberrant left subclavian artery [13].

Origin of Carotid and Vertebral Arteries

The ICAs form and materialize approximately 24 days into gestation with fusing of the fourth branchial arch arteries and the distal segments of the two dorsal aortas. The ventral segment of the second branchial (pharyngeal) arch detaches from the dorsal aorta at the base of the ICA artery and becomes the ventral pharyngeal artery. The ICAs then combine with ventral pharyngeal arteries at the proximal origins of both arteries to form the CCA. The ventral pharyngeal artery becomes the external carotid artery.

Occipital lobe and brainstem growth further stimulates the posterior division beginning with development of the basilar artery followed by vertebral artery development. The hind and posterior brain is supplied by two parallel arteries that are supplied by numerous carotid-vertebrobasilar anastomoses and connecting arteries including the trigeminal artery, otic artery, hypoglossal artery, and proatlantal artery. These anastomosing connecting arteries disappear, resulting in the creation of a single basilar artery, except for the proatlantal artery. The proatlantal artery later disappears after the transverse anastomoses form between the cervical intersegmental arteries down to the sixth pair of intersegmental arteries, which ultimately become the origin of the vertebral arteries from the subclavian arteries [14, 15].

Endovascular Access

Cerebral endovascular procedures are conducted with the patient under general anesthesia or conscious sedation. It is imperative that the patient does not move during the procedure to ensure an accurate road map for assessment of the anatomy and origin of the vessels, particularly the distal branches. There are several options for vascular access, including femoral, radial, brachial, and direct carotid access. The femoral artery is the most common entry location for endovascular carotid and cerebral access [16]. Scenarios in which transfemoral access become difficult are iliac or femoral artery stenosis, coexisting abdominal aortic aneurysms, severe aortic atherosclerosis, elongated or calcified aortic arches, and congenitally anomalous aortic arches [17]. When such aforementioned obstacles are identified, other endovascular access points are sought, including radial, brachial, and direct carotid access. These approaches can be selectively utilized to gain successful endovascular access to the carotid and cerebral system in the setting of tortuous vessels and aortic arch anatomy.

Radial Access

Radial artery access to the carotid and distal cerebral vasculature has been shown to be technically feasible and a successful method of cerebrovascular access that could bypass tortuous aortic arch anatomy and vessels such as a tortuous right carotid artery or bovine left carotid artery [17, 18]. Technical considerations of this approach include the acute angle at the origin of the CCA once the catheter is at the left or right subclavian artery. Folmar et al. proposed a 2-step strategy that entails the use of a diagnostic catheter (S1 catheter; Cook Medical, Bloomington, Indiana) over an extra support guidewire into the external carotid artery [17]. A standard guidewire is then positioned through the S1 catheter into the external carotid artery for catheter exchange and deployment of a Shuttle sheath (Cook Medical) into the distal ICA system.

Radial artery access has great utility in patients with right ICA or bovine left carotid artery disease [19]. However, radial access can be difficult in patients with tortuous or occluded subclavian arteries, congenitally anomalous radioulnar loops or hypoplasia, or severe vasospasm with adequate collateral flow. Complications associated with radial access include radial artery vasospasm and occlusion, and thromboembolic events including stroke [20].

Brachial Access

Brachial artery access has been effective in cases where transfemoral access is unsuccessful due to tortuous aortas and severe peripheral vascular disease. Brachial access is also more preferable to transradial access due to the large arterial diameter of the brachial artery (vs. the radial artery) as well as the shortened distance for access to the aortic arch and carotid vasculature. After initial catheter access through the brachial artery, the guide catheter is advanced proximally into the subclavian artery into the aortic cusp followed by careful guidance into either CCA. The retrograde-engagement method is commonly used in which the proximal guide catheter is curved and supported by the right coronary cusp of the aortic valve, which allows distal access with the proximal guiding catheter into the carotid vessels [21].

Investigators in several studies have utilized transbrachial access for carotid access and endovascular treatment with complication rates ranging from 0% to 5% [18, 20, 22, 23]. Complications associated with brachial access include median nerve palsy, brachial artery occlusion, and pseudoaneurysm of the brachial artery [22, 24].

Direct Carotid Access

Direct percutaneous puncture and transcervical access to the carotid artery is another method of cerebral endovascular access that bypasses tortuous vessels and aortic arch anatomy. This technique has been successfully utilized in conjunction with mechanical thrombectomy in the setting of AIS, and it can be conducted in several ways.

Carotid access can be obtained using a simple percutaneous approach, as done with a femoral or transbrachial approach, or an open surgical cut-down approach to the carotid artery proposed around the idea of decreasing the risk of soft tissue hematoma formation [25, 26]. Surgical cut-down access takes more time than percutaneous access and delays the time to recanalization of an occluded vessel in the setting of AIS. Furthermore, direct surgical access places patients with AIS who have received intravenous thrombolysis at high risk for bleeding complications [27].

Transcervical access has been successfully used in intracranial endovascular treatments and has been considered safe with no significant increased risk of complications but has been associated with various complications including carotid artery dissections, cervical hematomas, puncture-related vasospasm, and small aneurysm formation at the puncture site [28–31]. Potential explanations for such complications include the unavailability of a dedicated vascular closure device for direct cervical carotid artery access. Although vascular closure systems such as the StarClose SE (Abbott Vascular, Chicago, Illinois) are available, the additional muscle and soft tissue layers in the cervical region make the closure challenging [15]. Direct carotid access is a viable method for cerebral access after femoral or transbrachial access has failed in the setting of tortuous vessel and aortic arch anatomy.

Case Illustration

A case of direct carotid access for mechanical thrombectomy in a patient with severe CCA tortuosity is illustrated in Fig. 23.4. The patient in this case is an 84-year-old woman who presented with the sudden onset of left hemiparesis. Her National Institutes of Health Stroke Scale score at presentation was 16. A CT angiogram showed a right middle cerebral artery occlusion. Mechanical thrombectomy was planned. Right femoral access was obtained (Fig. 23.4a). Right brachiocephalic and CCA injections showed extreme tortuosity of the CCA (Fig. 23.4b, c).

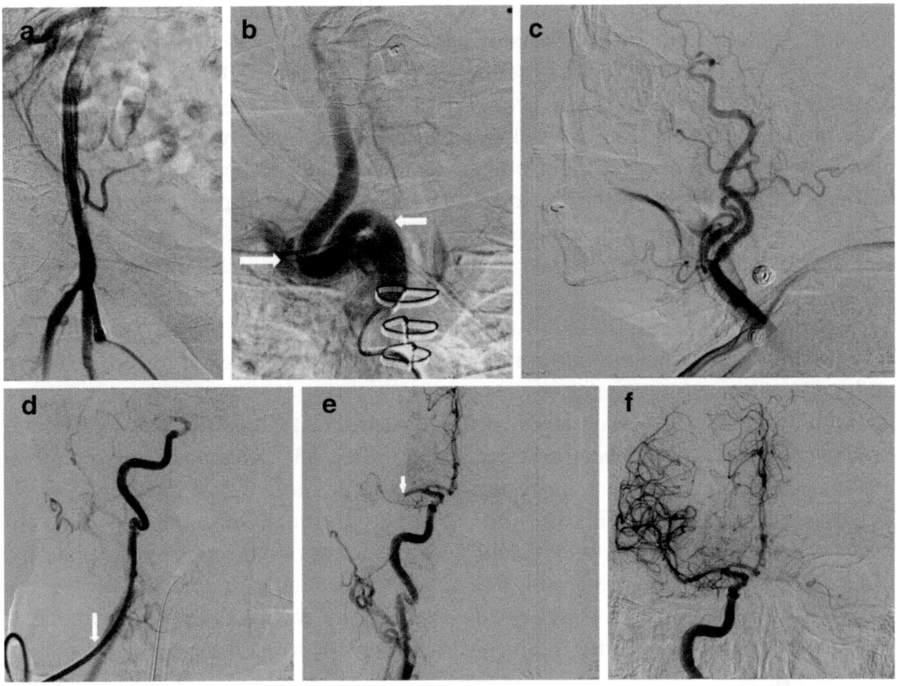

Fig. 23.4 Case illustration. (**a**) Right femoral artery access. (**b**) Right brachiocephalic artery and (**c**) common carotid artery injections show the extreme tortuosity of the common carotid artery (*arrows in* **b**). After attempts with multiple Select catheters (Penumbra Inc., Alameda, California) failed to achieve further access, a decision was made to utilize a direct carotid access approach. (**d**) 8-French sheath placed in the common carotid artery (*arrow*). (**e**) An M1 cutoff was identified (*arrow*). The clot was successfully removed with a direct aspiration first-pass technique (ADAPT) using the Sofia PLUS system (MicroVention, Aliso Viejo, California). (**f**) Postthrombectomy angiographic run shows thrombolysis in cerebral infarction (TICI) grade 3 revascularization

Catheterization with multiple Select catheters (Penumbra Inc. Alameda, CA) was tried, but further access could not be achieved. A decision was made to pursue direct carotid access. An 8-French sheath was placed in the CCA (Fig. 23.4d). An M1 cutoff (occlusion) was identified (Fig. 23.4e). A Sofia PLUS system (MicroVention) was used, and the clot was successfully removed with a direct aspiration first-pass technique (ADAPT). Complete revascularization was achieved (thrombolysis in cerebral infarction [TICI] grade 3) (Fig. 23.4f). The patient improved after the procedure to a modified Rankin scale score of 1 at 90 days.

Access in Types I, II, and III Aortic Arches

Another classification of aortic arches is based on the distance of the brachiocephalic artery origin from the top of the aortic arch and pertains to endovascular access. The Type I aortic arch gives rise to vessels from the outer curvature of the top of the arch in the same horizontal plane, and the vertical distance from the origin of the right brachiocephalic artery to the top of the arch is less than 1 CCA diameter (Fig. 23.5a). Types II and III are acquired variations of the arch. In a Type II aortic arch, the arch vessels arise between parallel planes defined by the outer and inner curves of the arch, and the right brachiocephalic artery is between 1 and 2 CCA diameters from the top of the aortic arch (Fig. 23.5b). In a Type III aortic arch, the arch vessel origins are from the proximal arch or at the top of the ascending aorta, and the vertical distance from the origin of the right brachiocephalic artery and the top of the aortic arch is greater than 2 left CCA diameters (Fig. 23.5c). Before attempting any approach for endovascular access, a CT angiogram can very helpful in assessing the aforementioned aortic arch types and the angles of tortuosity of the arch and the ascending greater vessels.

Arch anomalies are associated with increased technical difficulties and higher procedural risk of complications and failure [32, 33]. There are no definitive evidence-based techniques or materials proven to be more efficacious for Types II and III aortic arch access. However, the use of an 8-French Simmons-2 guide catheter has been shown to effectively achieve distal access in tortuous aortic anatomy. Femoral access is obtained, and the diagnostic catheter is exchanged for the Simmons-2 guide catheter, which is advanced up the aorta. This unique catheter is easy to form into the needed shape, which allows it to gain access across sharp angles [34].

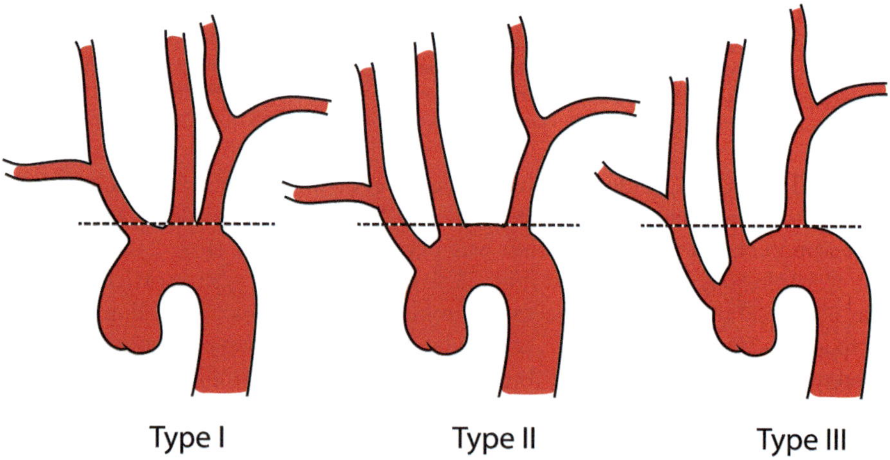

Fig. 23.5 Classification of aortic arches based on the distance of the brachiocephalic artery origin from the top of the aortic arch among aortas with typical anatomy: (**a**) Type I arch. Note that the origin of the brachiocephalic artery and top of the aortic arch are on the same plane. (**b**) Type II arch. The distance between the brachiocephalic artery origin and the top of the aortic arch is within 1–2 diameters of the common carotid artery. (**c**) A Type III arch is more than 2 diameters of the common carotid artery arch. (© University at Buffalo Neurosurgery)

Access in Bovine Arches

Endovascular access into a bovine arch can be technically challenging with traditional femoral access due to the right brachiocephalic trunk and left CCA sharing a common vessel origin off the aortic arch. The double tight turn between the aortic arch and the right subclavian artery is challenging in addition to access to the distal right subclavian artery and the left CCA.

It is recommended that a CT angiogram is obtained prior to endovascular access to better access vessel angles and tortuosities. The transfemoral approach is attempted if the angle between the right brachiocephalic artery and left CCA is <50°. If unsuccessful or the angle is found to be wide, transradial or transbrachial access should be attempted. There is documented success of carotid access and stenting in patients with bovine arches with either radial or brachial access [35]. Brachial access may be preferable due to the aforementioned transradial complications. If all three access approaches fail, transcervical access can be obtained through the CCA, either with the simple percutaneous or open-surgical approaches [36].

Access to Tortuous Proximal and Distal Carotid Arteries

There are documented reports in which carotid artery stenting procedures were aborted due to proximal and distal carotid artery tortuosity [37–41], but there has been a lack of tools and visual assessments that could aid in access and endovascular decision making. First explained by Dougherty and Varro, the tortuosity index (TI) of the carotid vasculature is utilized to measure and predict carotid stenting technical failure [42]. The TI in carotid stenting planning is a quantitative measurement of carotid artery tortuosity and is defined as the sum of all angles diverging from the ideal straight axis of a vessel from one end to the other. Carotid vessel tortuosity can be further specified by proximal and distal TI. The proximal TI is defined as the TI measured from the aortic arch to stenotic ICA area. The distal TI is defined as the TI from the distal stenotic ICA area) to distal location of filter deployment [43]. Although the TI has not been used in assessing technical failure rates in AIS and large-vessel occlusion thrombectomies, this index has the potential to be utilized as a quantitative predictor for successful access in tortuous proximal and distal carotid arteries in such cases.

Tower of Power

Difficult and tortuous aortic arches and vessels are responsible for 4–6% of failed endovascular cases. In response, various techniques have been described. The most standard is the exchange of a diagnostic catheter over a stiff exchange wire [44].

However, this method commonly fails with Type III aortic arches due to the higher vessel tortuosity that causes guide catheter and wire pushback, thereby preventing distal cervical vasculature access. A newer technique, referred to as the "Tower of Power," has had great success for navigation through difficult vessels [45]. This technique entails consecutively passing three smaller-diameter microguidewires together in parallel to secure and support wire access. The three smaller wires create a stable construct in which a distal wire allows passage of a diagnostic catheter or guide catheter. The three wires collectively act as one larger wire, termed the "Tower of Power;" the kickback force seen with a single larger wire is also resolved. This system has been shown to be beneficial because of the support it provides for the use of different types of different catheters (depending upon the requirement of a specific procedure) [45, 46].

Access to the Vertebral Artery and Posterior Circulation

Guidance and access to tortuosities of the vertebral artery and posterior circulation are not well described in the current literature. In 1 case report and technical note, the use of ultrasound-guided direct percutaneous puncture of the vertebral artery was described in the treatment of a basilar artery occlusion [47]. A regular micropuncture access needle was successfully placed into the vertebral artery, and a micropuncture sheath was successfully inserted to allow stiff wire exchange and distal access to the occlusion. Other reports of posterior circulation access include the use of direct percutaneous punctures (without ultrasound guidance) and open surgical approaches [24, 48]. Complications associated with direct access to the posterior circulation include pseudoaneurysm formation at the puncture site, injury to the caudal loop of the posterior inferior cerebellar artery, vasospasm secondary to arterial disruption, and cervical hematomas [49–51].

Access in Vessels with Proximal Stenosis

When femoral access cannot to be obtained due to proximal stenosis secondary to iliac artery stenosis or abdominal aortic atherosclerosis, other routes of access including transradial, transbrachial, and direct transcervical are options, as mentioned in previous sections [27, 52]. These routes can be used to bypass the stenotic area or arch anomaly [24, 27]. The endovascular interventionist should be wary of each patient's unique vascular anatomy and medical history when resorting to other options. Supplementary CT angiography, MR angiography, CT, and MR imaging will further aid in such decision making.

Conclusion

The goal of endovascular treatment is to achieve rapid and safe revascularization of brain tissue at risk for irreversible ischemic injury. Aortic arch anomalies can pose a difficult challenge to rapid access to the site of arterial occlusion. Therefore, it is important to study the anatomy of the aortic arch and its branches. A CT angiogram before endovascular intervention is valuable. Distal access in a type III arch is particularly difficult due to the higher pushback force of the guide catheter and wire. This can be overcome by using the "Tower of Power" technique, which utilizes three small wires acting together to provide greater stability against pushback force. Direct carotid access should be considered whenever timely access to the site of arterial occlusion through a conventional route is not possible.

References

1. Rha JH, Saver JL. The impact of recanalization on ischemic stroke outcome: a meta-analysis. Stroke. 2007;38:967–73.
2. Mokin M, Rojas H, Levy EI. Randomized trials of endovascular therapy for stroke – impact on stroke care. Nat Rev Neurol. 2016;12:86–94.
3. Kau T, Sinzig M, Gasser J, Lesnik G, Rabitsch E, Celedin S, Eicher W, Illiasch H, Hausegger KA. Aortic development and anomalies. Semin Intervent Radiol. 2007;24:141–52.
4. Jakanani GC, Adair W. Frequency of variations in aortic arch anatomy depicted on multidetector CT. Clin Radiol. 2010;65:481–7.
5. Matula C, Trattnig S, Tschabitscher M, Day JD, Koos WT. The course of the prevertebral segment of the vertebral artery: anatomy and clinical significance. Surg Neurol. 1997;48:125–31.
6. Turkvatan A, Buyukbayraktar FG, Olcer T, Cumhur T. Congenital anomalies of the aortic arch: evaluation with the use of multidetector computed tomography. Korean J Radiol. 2009;10:176–84.
7. Shuford WH, Sybers RG, Edwards FK. The three types of right aortic arch. Am J Roentgenol Radium Therapy, Nucl Med. 1970;109:67–74.
8. Polguj M, Chrzanowski L, Kasprzak JD, Stefanczyk L, Topol M, Majos A. The aberrant right subclavian artery (arteria lusoria): the morphological and clinical aspects of one of the most important variations – a systematic study of 141 reports. ScientificWorldJournal. 2014;2014:292734.
9. Tsai IC, Tzeng WS, Lee T, Jan SL, Fu YC, Chen MC, Lin PC, Liao WC, Chen CC. Vertebral and carotid artery anomalies in patients with aberrant right subclavian arteries. Pediatr Radiol. 2007;37:1007–12.
10. Hanneman K, Newman B, Chan F. Congenital variants and anomalies of the aortic arch. Radiographics. 2017;37:32–51.
11. Ebner L, Huber A, Christe A. Right aortic arch and Kommerell's diverticulum associated with acute aortic dissection and pericardial tamponade. Acta Radiol Short Rep. 2013;2:2047981613476283.
12. Rad EM. Goldenhar syndrome with right circumflex aortic arch, severe coarctation and vascular ring in a twin pregnancy. Ann Pediatr Cardiol. 2014;7:217–20.
13. Yadav JS, Wholey MH, Kuntz RE, Fayad P, Katzen BT, Mishkel GJ, Bajwa TK, Whitlow P, Strickman NE, Jaff MR, Popma JJ, Snead DB, Cutlip DE, Firth BG, Ouriel K, Stenting,

Angioplasty with Protection in Patients at High Risk for Endarterectomy Investigators. Protected carotid-artery stenting versus endarterectomy in high-risk patients. N Engl J Med. 2004;351:1493–501.
14. Luh GY, Dean BL, Tomsick TA, Wallace RC. The persistent fetal carotid-vertebrobasilar anastomoses. AJR Am J Roentgenol. 1999;172:1427–32.
15. Choi HM, Hobson RW, Goldstein J, Chakhtoura E, Lal BK, Haser PB, Cuadra SA, Padberg FT, Jamil Z. Technical challenges in a program of carotid artery stenting. J Vasc Surg. 2004;40:746–51; discussion 751.
16. Noble S, Roffi M. Overcoming the challenges of the transfemoral approach in transcatheter aortic valve implantation. Interv Cardiol. 2013;8:131–4.
17. Folmar J, Sachar R, Mann T. Transradial approach for carotid artery stenting: a feasibility study. Catheter Cardiovasc Interv. 2007;69:355–61.
18. Wu CJ, Hung WC, Chen SM, Yang CH, Chen CJ, Cheng CI, Chen YH, Yip HK. Feasibility and safety of transradial artery approach for selective cerebral angiography. Catheter Cardiovasc Interv. 2005;66:21–6.
19. Etxegoien N, Rhyne D, Kedev S, Sachar R, Mann T. The transradial approach for carotid artery stenting. Catheter Cardiovasc Interv. 2012;80:1081–7.
20. Wu CJ, Cheng CI, Hung WC, Fang CY, Yang CH, Chen CJ, Chen YH, Hang CL, Hsieh YK, Chen SM, Yip HK. Feasibility and safety of transbrachial approach for patients with severe carotid artery stenosis undergoing stenting. Catheter Cardiovasc Interv. 2006;67:967–71.
21. Hayashi K, Kitagawa N, Morikawa M, Kawakubo J, Hiu T, Tsutsumi K, Nagata I. Carotid artery stenting using the transbrachial approach: technical case report. No Shinkei Geka. 2008;36:233–7.
22. Nanto M, Tsuura M, Takayama M, Hirayama K, Okada H, Naka D, Kamei I. Carotid artery stenting via a transbrachial artery: techniques and problems. No Shinkei Geka. 2007;35:155–60.
23. Tietke MW, Ulmer S, Riedel C, Jansen O. Carotid artery stenting via transbrachial approach. Rofo. 2008;180:988–93.
24. Dorfer C, Standhardt H, Gruber A, Ferraz-Leite H, Knosp E, Bavinzski G. Direct percutaneous puncture approach versus surgical cutdown technique for intracranial neuroendovascular procedures: technical aspects. World Neurosurg. 2012;77:192–200.
25. Sfyroeras GS, Moulakakis KG, Markatis F, Antonopoulos CN, Antoniou GA, Kakisis JD, Brountzos EN, Liapis CD. Results of carotid artery stenting with transcervical access. J Vasc Surg. 2013;58:1402–7.
26. Mokin M, Snyder KV, Levy EI, Hopkins LN, Siddiqui AH. Direct carotid artery puncture access for endovascular treatment of acute ischemic stroke: technical aspects, advantages, and limitations. J Neurointerv Surg. 2015;7:108–13.
27. Blanc R, Piotin M, Mounayer C, Spelle L, Moret J. Direct cervical arterial access for intracranial endovascular treatment. Neuroradiology. 2006;48:925–9.
28. Guimaraens L, Theron J, Casasco A, Cuellar H. Carotid artery stenting by direct percutaneous puncture. J Vasc Surg. 2011;54:249–51.
29. Perez-Arjona EA, DelProsto Z, Fessler RD. Direct percutaneous carotid artery stenting with distal protection: technical case report. Neurol Res. 2004;26:338–41.
30. Nii K, Kazekawa K, Onizuka M, Aikawa H, Tsutsumi M, Tomokiyo M, Iko M, Kodama T, Matsubara S, Go Y, Tanaka A. Direct carotid puncture for the endovascular treatment of anterior circulation aneurysms. AJNR Am J Neuroradiol. 2006;27:1502–4.
31. Saleem T, Baril DT. Vascular access closure devices. In: StatPearls. Treasure Island: StatPearls Publishing LLC; 2018.
32. Lin SC, Trocciola SM, Rhee J, Dayal R, Chaer R, Morrissey NJ, Mureebe L, McKinsey JF, Kent KC, Faries PL. Analysis of anatomic factors and age in patients undergoing carotid angioplasty and stenting. Ann Vasc Surg. 2005;19:798–804.
33. Chang FC, Tummala RP, Jahromi BS, Samuelson RM, Siddiqui AH, Levy EI, Hopkins LN. Use of the 8 French Simmons-2 guide catheter for carotid artery stent placement in patients with difficult aortic arch anatomy. J Neurosurg. 2009;110:437–41.

34. Shaw JA, Gravereaux EC, Eisenhauer AC. Carotid stenting in the bovine arch. Catheter Cardiovasc Interv. 2003;60:566–9.
35. Montorsi P, Galli S, Ravagnani P, Ghulam Ali S, Trabattoni D, Fabbiocchi F, Lualdi A, Ballerini G, Andreini D, Pontone G, Annoni A, Bartorelli AL. Carotid stenting through the right brachial approach for left internal carotid artery stenosis and bovine aortic arch configuration. Eur Radiol. 2009;19:2009–15.
36. Brismar J. Persistent hypoglossal artery, diagnostic criteria. Report of a case. Acta Radiol Diagn (Stockh). 1976;17:160–6.
37. Chong PL, Salhiyyah K, Dodd PD. The role of carotid endarterectomy in the endovascular era. Eur J Vasc Endovasc Surg. 2005;29:597–600.
38. Halabi M, Gruberg L, Pitchersky S, Kouperberg E, Nikolsky E, Hoffman A, Beyar R. Carotid artery stenting in surgical high-risk patients. Catheter Cardiovasc Interv. 2006;67:513–8.
39. Henry M, Amor M, Klonaris C, Henry I, Masson I, Chati Z, Leborgne E, Hugel M. Angioplasty and stenting of the extracranial carotid arteries. Tex Heart Inst J. 2000;27:150–8.
40. Sztriha LK, Voros E, Sas K, Szentgyorgyi R, Pocsik A, Barzo P, Szikra P, Makai A, Szolics A, Elek P, Rudas L, Vecsei L. Favorable early outcome of carotid artery stenting without protection devices. Stroke. 2004;35:2862–6.
41. Dougherty G, Varro J. A quantitative index for the measurement of the tortuosity of blood vessels. Med Eng Phys. 2000;22:567–74.
42. Faggioli G, Ferri M, Gargiulo M, Freyrie A, Fratesi F, Manzoli L, Stella A. Measurement and impact of proximal and distal tortuosity in carotid stenting procedures. J Vasc Surg. 2007;46:1119–24.
43. Vitek JJ, Roubin GS, Al-Mubarek N, New G, Iyer SS. Carotid artery stenting: technical considerations. AJNR Am J Neuroradiol. 2000;21:1736–43.
44. Rangel-Castilla L, Shakir HJ, Siddiqui AH. Initial experience with a multiple parallel guidewire support system for complex tortuous aortic arch navigation and great vessel catheterization: technical note. Neurosurg Focus. 2017;42:E14.
45. Harrigan MR, Deveikis JP. Extracranial cerebrovascular occlusive disease. In: Handbook of cerebrovascular disease and neurointerventional technique. New York: Springer; 2018. p. 957–1014.
46. Lozano JD, Massari F, Howk MC, de Macedo Rodrigues K, Brooks C, Perras M, Rex DE, Wakhloo AK, Kuhn AL, Puri AS. Utilization of a new intracranial support catheter as an intermediate aspiration catheter in the treatment of acute ischemic stroke: technical report on initial experience. Cureus. 2016;8:e617.
47. Sasaki K, Yoshida M, Mino M, Tashiro R. Coil embolization of vertebral artery aneurysm using direct percutaneous puncture of vertebral artery: a technical report. No Shinkei Geka. 2018;46:599–605.
48. Haider AS, Osumah T, Thakur R, Vayalumkal S, Shail MS, Khan U, Sumdani H, Hise J, Layton KF. Percutaneous vertebral artery access for embolization of cerebrovascular dsease: illustrative case and operative technique. Cureus. 2017;9:e1621.
49. Vergouwen MD, Algra A, Pfefferkorn T, Weimar C, Rueckert CM, Thijs V, Kappelle LJ, Schonewille WJ, Basilar Artery International Cooperation Study Study Group. Time is brain(stem) in basilar artery occlusion. Stroke. 2012;43:3003–6.
50. Brinjikji W, Cloft H, Kallmes DF. Anatomy of the posterior inferior cerebellar artery: relevance for C1-C2 puncture procedures. Clin Anat. 2009;22:319–23.
51. Al-Mubarak N, Vitek JJ, Iyer SS, New G, Roubin GS. Carotid stenting with distal-balloon protection via the transbrachial approach. J Endovasc Ther. 2001;8:571–5.
52. Levy EI, Kim SH, Bendok BR, Qureshi AI, Guterman LR, Hopkins LN. Transradial stenting of the cervical internal carotid artery: technical case report. Neurosurgery. 2003;53:448–51; discussion 451–442.

Index

F. K. Hui et al. (eds.), *12 Strokes*, https://doi.org/10.1007/978-3-030-56857-3

GPSR Compliance

The European Union's (EU) General Product Safety Regulation (GPSR) is a set of rules that requires consumer products to be safe and our obligations to ensure this.

If you have any concerns about our products, you can contact us on ProductSafety@springernature.com

In case Publisher is established outside the EU, the EU authorized representative is:

Springer Nature Customer Service Center GmbH
Europaplatz 3
69115 Heidelberg, Germany

Batch number: 10726135

Printed by Printforce, the Netherlands